Clinical Psychiatry

For E and S

BY THE SAME AUTHOR

Lecture Notes on Psychiatry
Blackwell Scientific Publications, 1974

Drug Dependence
Faber & Faber, 1969

Addicts: Drugs and Alcohol re-examined
Pitman, 1973

JAMES H. WILLIS

MB, FRCP(Edin), FRCPsych, DPM

Consultant Psychiatrist
King's College Hospital London
Guy's Hospital London and
Bexley Hospital Kent

Clinical Psychiatry

BLACKWELL
SCIENTIFIC PUBLICATIONS
OXFORD LONDON EDINBURGH MELBOURNE

© 1976 Blackwell Scientific Publications
Osney Mead, Oxford OX2 0EL
85 Marylebone High Street, London W1M 3DE
9 Forrest Road, Edinburgh EH1 2QH
P.O. Box 9, North Balwyn, Victoria, Australia

ISBN 0 632 00761 3
First published 1976

Distributed in the U.S.A. by J. B. Lippincott Co.,
Philadelphia; and in Canada by
J. B. Lippincott Co. of Canada Ltd, Toronto

Set in Monotype Garamond

Printed in Great Britain by Western Printing Services Ltd,
Bristol and bound by Kemp Hall Bindery, Oxford

Contents

Preface   vii

1   Introduction   1

2   History of psychiatry   5

3   Concept of psychiatric illness   19

4   Language of psychiatry   27

5   Psychiatric history and examination   53

6   Causes of psychiatric disorder   77

7   Organic cerebral syndromes   111

8   Affective disorders   161

9   The neuroses   189

10   Schizophrenia   223

11   Normal and abnormal personalities, and psychopathy   269

12   Alcoholism and drug addiction   285

13 Mental subnormality   313

14 Disorders of childhood and adolescence   327

15 The psychiatrist in the general hospital   335

16 Psychiatric disorders in old age   355

17 Psychosexual disorders   367

18 Management of psychiatric disorders   373

19 Rare syndromes—classifiable and unclassifiable   415

20 Psychiatry and the law   421

      References—contents   435

      References   436

      Index   463

Preface

I have attempted to write a book that gives a reasonably wide coverage of clinical psychiatry in a concise and at times provocative form. The book deals mainly with the clinical aspects of adult psychiatry and I have only referred briefly to topics such as disorders of childhood and adolescence, mental handicap and psychosexual disorders since these are all subjects in their own right with their own extensive literature.

The manuscripts were typed by Audrey White, Vera Barber, Jill Donovan and Doreen Harlow to whom I am extremely grateful.

I should also like to thank Messrs. Roche Ltd for their permission to use the material on Drug Dependence and Alcoholism which originally appeared in *An Encyclopaedia of Psychiatry for General Practitioners*. Also I should like to thank the Oxford University Press for permission to reproduce tables which appeared in *Psychiatric Illness in General Practice* by Shepherd, Cooper and Brown.

Finally I would like to thank the publishers for their patience and encouragement.

London, 1975   *James Willis*

I

Introduction

Psychiatry is in a muddled state. It has not proved to be a cure-all despite its record of steady achievement in terms of the humane handling of problems and symptoms that trouble and disturb people. Twenty years ago it seemed that psychiatry was an established medical specialty in which a 'medical model' of disordered human experience and behaviour was totally acceptable as a way of diagnosing and treating 'mental illness'. This was backed up by the discovery of effective psychotropic drugs which could alter weird behaviour, block hallucinosis and restore calm, *i.e.* the *neuroleptic drugs.* These were followed by *antidepressant* drugs and by the vast range of tranquillisers used to wipe out the symptoms of anxiety.

At the same time the mental hospital changed its image and became less of an 'institution' and more like a 'real hospital'. This encouraged the general acceptance of a medical model of psychiatric disorder *i.e.* 'it's just the same as pneumonia/cancer/diabetes' and led to a more tolerant and accepting view of people who behaved oddly, heard voices, couldn't think clearly or seemed inexplicably sad. So the idea spread that these abnormalities were illnesses. Unhappily the results of the new treatments were not as good as had been expected, also the results of research into biochemical causes of 'mental illness' were conflicting and hard to interpret. But after all research is time consuming, difficult, often tedious and frequently unproductive; psychiatry is no worse off in this respect than most other disciplines.

The next problem was raised by the dissatisfaction with orthodox psychiatry voiced by those who have come to regard it as a process of social degradation—even political persecution.

At this stage someone has to say 'enough'. Doctors, on the whole do not seek out or advertise for patients. And *psychiatry* like it or not is a medical specialty that has developed over the years as a practical way of management, counselling, advice and *treatment* of troubled, ill, deluded, lost, unhappy people who go to doctors and ask for help. It begins and ends in that doctor–patient relationship. The basic medical training of the psychiatrist encourages him to use a medical framework of diagnosis, treatment and prognosis and to study the natural history of psychiatric disorder.

In some cases a medical model is the most useful *e.g.* in organic psychoses, in others it is less useful, and the patient is seen as someone with a problem in living which is the outcome of a variety of psychosocial influences. Doctors and medical students still find it hard to accept and understand psychiatry—a subject that often comes up late in their training, usually competing for more tangible topics or near the time of final examinations. Until comparatively recently a medical student's only encounters with psychiatric patients and their problems were limited to a course of lectures and a series of visits to mental hospitals where chronic psychotic patients were paraded like circus performers and invited to talk to the visitors.

The announcement by a patient that he was the Emperor of all the Russias would bring forth a mixed response in which embarrassment and laughter competed with a general feeling of unease that this seemed to have little to do with medicine since medicine is about the recognition of diseases that seem remote from the plight of a patient who may have spent 20 or more years in a mental hospital. But times and ideas change, and the contemporary medical student is unlikely to witness such degradations.

An introduction to clinical psychiatry at out-patient clinics and in general hospital units is now a more likely first encounter with psychiatric patients, to hear them talk about themselves and to learn something of their problems and illnesses. However, even this is not adequate.

The student rarely has enough time to get to grips with the subject and also may be put off by the apparent lack of a sound body of psychiatric knowledge since much of medical education is based on science and applied science and includes a vast range of fascinating information that can satisfy the intellectual curiosity of any intelligent student. The whole of the student's training is geared to a scientific view of disease processes and their interaction with 'the patient'. Admittedly in more recent times many medical schools have tried to emphasise the role of social and emotional factors in illness and to stress the importance of 'whole person' medicine *i.e.* viewing the patient and his illness in the light of physical aetiology and his personal and total social problems. But this is as yet hardly more than a top dressing on a formal education that relies on the natural sciences as basic guide lines. This means that in general the newly qualified doctor has had a good quality training in scientific and clinical methods all aimed at the recognition of disease processes which cause malfunction in one or other bodily system. The doctor tends to construe illness as a concept in mechanical terms, to value tangible and measurable indices of illness, to mistrust intuition and to be wary of emotions, feelings and 'odd behaviour', mainly because they do not readily lend themselves to any system of measurement. In fact if they were honest many doctors would say that they only have any dealings with psychiatric patients and their problems because they have to and not from choice.

This is unfortunate since people tend to consult doctors if they feel 'depressed' or 'anxious' or 'mixed up' and doctors know this but tend to feel uncertain and helpless when the patient comes to them. The reasons for this, as we shall see, are partly related to the history of science and partly to the history of medicine and psychiatry.

Psychiatry is on the one hand regarded as a medical specialty where doctors trained in the subject are able to identify and treat psychiatric disorders, yet at the same time there exists the uncomfortable suspicion that terms like 'psychiatric illness' are labels and little more, and also that psychiatry may have overstepped the limits of available knowledge; that psychiatrists have made excessive claims for their subject and that perhaps doctors ought to stick to physical illnesses and leave 'psychiatric patients' to someone else.

The *concept of psychiatric illness*—of disorders of the mind and the emotions—is an old one and also it is one that has practical value and meaning. Certain altered forms of behaviour, experience and feelings may, as we shall see, reasonably be regarded as *syndromes of disorder* which can be *treated*, but this only remains reasonable so long as the concept of psychiatric syndromes is not permitted to become ossified into a rigid system that codifies human behaviour into 'sick' and 'normal', always regarding the sick person as someone who has an illness that needs treatment. To adopt this view of psychiatry is self-defeating since the notion of 'treatment' may become unjustifiably expanded. It is more honest to regard psychiatry as a discipline that is concerned with the recognition of and management of abnormal states of mind that may reasonably be regarded as illnesses. This is always with the proviso that psychiatry is not the only way of dealing with such people and their problems, that the only reason that psychiatry *is* regarded as one of the main methods is largely a historical accident and that not everyone who comes to see a psychiatrist is *ill*. Illness and abnormality, in psychiatric terms, are words that should have a fairly limited meaning which may be summarised thus:

Illness implies a state of change—the personality *changes*, the person's behaviour *changes*, his feelings *change* etc. This is as true of psychiatric disorders as of physical disorders, it is merely that a different time scale operates.

Abnormality is a term that is used entirely in a statistical sense—the *normal* represents the commonly accepted ranges of behaviour, feeling, perception and intellectual function, *i.e. the mean*. The *abnormal* lies outside the mean of common acceptance and expectation. Thus a 'psychiatric abnormality' needs always to be qualified in the light of the expectation of the particular culture.

So the doctor who is starting to study psychiatry usually has very good reason to feel muddled and perplexed; often this is caused by the simple experience of working amidst colleagues who use psychiatric jargon in ordinary conversation as well as in professional discussion and expect the newcomer to pick it up as he goes along. And despite the energetic efforts in postgraduate education this is still very much the case. It may seem odd to discuss the needs of the medical student and of the postgraduate all in one breath but their needs are not so different for both start from total ignorance. The student has to pick up what knowledge he can in the time available and the doctor has to immerse himself in a new subject which people seem reluctant to explain to him in a simple way, some even go so far as to object to the idea of simple explanations. It is the author's belief that if a topic cannot be explained simply it probably isn't worth explaining anyway and it is in the hope of assisting those students who would like at least to have a chance of simple explanations that this book has been written since the privilege of teaching nurses, medical students, social workers and doctors has confirmed his belief that simple explanations are welcomed because they help the student to take the next step in learning about the subject in depth. But if they are fobbed off with instructions to look up obscure papers they are put off. Knowledge is not a Holy Grail, it is something that is meant to be shared.

2

History of psychiatry

Psychiatry and History—an embarrassing conjunction

The study of primitive cultures suggests that man's early notions of illness were largely influenced by beliefs in the supernatural. Illness was thought to be the result of divine interference through the spirits of dead ancestors or as punishment for misdeeds. Magic became the preferred form of treatment—often used to avert calamity either with rituals or by the use of talismans and amulets worn to ward off the malignant effects of unseen powers.

Accounts of this usually refer to the importance of the *shaman*, a medicine man who was the forerunner of the spiritualist medium. The shaman was an intermediary through whom spirits spoke in seances usually preceded by drinking and dancing. Here the ill person could ask for relief, confess sin or release pent-up feeling. The crisis of the seance occurred with the liberation of the 'unhealthy spirit' from the sufferer—with no doubt considerable relief all round—and a degree of relief about which perhaps we need not feel unduly superior. This should lead to a free admission that our present knowledge of the nature of mental illness and its treatment is insubstantial, no matter how we try to dress it up in often rather ill-fitting scientific clothing.

With man's emergence from primitive ways to more structured societies influenced by philosophy, organised religion and the beginnings of science, the concepts of illness became more surely established and eventually based on theories related to available scientific knowledge. But this took a long time. 'Scientific Medicine' is 100 years old and 'Scientific Psychiatry' is a good deal younger.

The history of psychiatry may be reviewed in six periods:
1 Ancient Greece and Ancient Rome
2 The Middle Ages
3 The Renaissance
4 The 17th and 18th Centuries
5 The 19th Century
6 The 20th Century

Ancient Greece and Ancient Rome

Greece and Rome gave the world art, science, philosophy, poetry, prose, laws, administration and the foundations of medicine. Science in Ancient Greece was bounded only by the relative insufficiency of the methods of measurement available at the time. Whichever way we look at it the Greeks left for all time an aura of inspired genius which becomes more impressive the more closely we examine it. But the Greek genius for inspired thinking was modified, even codified by the equally impressive if somewhat dispiriting Roman genius for putting things in their right place and justifying the activity in formal, even platitudinous, statements. The Greeks were original and clever, the Romans methodical and bureau-cratic and each left its mark on Western civilisation in terms of art and knowledge and also in terms of survival capability. It is hardly surprising then that we look for the beginnings of psychiatry in both these cultures—skillfully, it is hoped, sidestepping the fact that the very term psychiatry is a Greek derived word meaning the healing of the spirit.

In Greece popular ideas of mental illness were influenced by beliefs in goddesses such as Mania. People saw madness as the end product of divine wrath—to be alleviated by appropriate observances. Thus the mad-man was regarded as sacred and his infirmity something to be healed by purification ceremonies. This was the cultural view of madness. The literary view remained unstated until the concept of the soul was pro-claimed by Heraclitus who regarded dreams as therapeutic—a view that awaited 2000 years until rediscovery. The Greek literary concepts of psychosis incorporated souls and dreams in a surprisingly vague way until Socrates looked at human behaviour and experience in a provocative way relating virtue to intellectual ability. However it was Plato who took the bold step, reiterated ever since, of describing types of madness.

Plato's four types of madness were the erotic, the prophetic, the ritual and the poetic. Poetic madness was thought to arise from possession by the Muses, no doubt today it would be labelled as 'overvalued inspiration' or such; ritual madness was thought to be a result of excessive exposure to Corybantic Rites. Aristotle viewed human behaviour in a rational way and stressed the importance of the release of feeling in catharsis. However Hippocrates had started the medical association with psychiatry by regarding mental illness as the outcome of the interaction between four factors (humours), *blood, black bile, yellow bile* and *phlegm*, and suggested a theory of personality based on this interaction. He descriped epilepsy but rejected its *sacred* quality. He also gave clear accounts of depression and delusional states. Later Greek writers, particularly the stoic philosophers emphasised the positive qualities of imperturbability—stating an ideal of 'ataraxia', *i.e.* a state of calm acceptance of life.

Ancient Rome

The Romans were pragmatic, clear headed and unimaginative as compared to the Greeks but left behind them a number of important basic observations on human behaviour. Cicero for instance suggested that there might be an underlying reservoir of drive and emotion—animus and proposed the use of the term 'libido' as a store of unconscious energy. He also suggested that a confluence of 'perturbatio' (conflicting feeling) could lead to morbi (illnesses). This remains a challenging idea for 20th Century man, near enough verified we may suppose by Pavlov's drowning dogs or Freud's simmering ladies. But the day-to-day aspects of psychiatry concerned the Romans who were the first to recognise that the mentally ill needed the protection of the law and that their responsibility for criminal acts might be diminished by drunkenness and mental illness.

The Corpus Juri Civilis was a practical expression of this, it was a set of laws that classified mental states that caused diminished responsibility and empowered judges to define the extent of responsibility. Roman influences on treatment lagged until Soranus (1st–2nd Century AD) advocated a commonsense attitude to mentally disturbed patients. Later Roman physicians speculated about the possibility that the brain might be the organ of the mind. The most sophisticated of the late Romans was St. Augustine, not merely because of his relentless self-scrutiny, but because he antedated later contributions to the understanding of human behaviour by his sensible detachment and threw out ideas for others to think about. He was, by any standards, perceptive on such lively topics as education, being a child and the hidden joys of swimming. Nowadays many are untouched by his observations on the central importance of the will, but it is intriguing to speculate about those programmes of psycho-therapeutic and social rehabilitation that employ the concept of will without acknowledging its possible existence, *i.e.* by implying that patients need to employ their own degree of choice and responsibility for their actions.

The Middle Ages

To many the Middle Ages seem to have been a paradigm of scholarship gone slightly crazy—epitomised by a timorous confidence in the more rigid and unattractive aspects of theology and organised religion. This is fair comment but at the same time we cannot dismiss the beau ideal of the time which was of contemplative ascetic monasticism as the high point of intellectual life. Thus the contemplative life became highly valued and produced an interesting psychiatric side effect namely 'accedie', a complex of pessimistic indecisive gloom centring on loss of hope, doubt, mental inertia and inability to comprehend the incomprehensible that was first described in the Middle Ages as a mental state peculiar to young monks. Though the term is no longer used the condition has intriguing similarities to existential dread—the fear of non-being.

The main effect of the religious theories of the Middle Ages was disastrous since its end point was the explanation of abnormal behaviour in terms of demonic possession and witchcraft, these ideas persisted well into the 13th and 14th Centuries. The demonic theories found their ulti-mate expression in the *Malleus Maleficarum* (1487) written by the monks Sprenger and Kramer. This was the witch spotters' *vade mecum*, a catalogue of descriptions of the eccentric behaviour of people whom many would now regard as ill, and an unintended mine of sexual pathology. Its hideous accounts of tortures inflicted on 'witches' remains a sinister foretaste of the more subtle persecution of the socially deviant or politically unacceptable that is the present day equivalent.

However the Middle Ages were not all darkness. They were en-lightened for instance by the writings of the scholastic philosopher St. Thomas Aquinas (1225–1274), a man who was ahead of his time; an intellectual giant whose observations on human behaviour and personality structure were original and perceptive.

He related all psychological events to physical precipitants regarding the soul as an inviolable prime mover which was by definition exempt from illness since its perfection was incompatible with disease. Hence, he deduced, mental disturbance could arise either from physical causes or from inappropriate reasoning. In his view psychic structure was three tiered: the physiological; *the anima vegetiva* (approximately equivalent to the autonomic nervous system), the perceptual; perception, sense-data collection, memory and fantasy covered by the *anima sensitiva* and finally the ability to solve problems and learn from experience; the *anima intellectiva*.

This separation of three types of psychological function which acknowledged that their ultimate expression needed integration was a big step ahead which had to await Hughlings Jackson for a contemporary restatement.

The Renaissance

The Renaissance was not just the result of artistic and scientific ferment but also a prolonged sequel to the diminished influences of feudalism and fragmented religious orthodoxy.

Since action and reaction are equal and opposite it is not surprising that witchcraft and demonology received a fillip before they went; their influence increased even when humanism and science were emerging as powerful.

At the end of it all, superstition, torturing the sick and all the grisly paraphernalia of sadism had to go on for some time before people began to suspect that perhaps eccentrics, the solitary, the weird might be deserving of compassion and concern rather than torture. But it did take some time.

Actually the cheerful Christian torturers might well have looked to Islam for guidance since the prophet Muhammed had stated that the insane were loved by God. This had led to the establishment of asylums, which were, by any standards enlightened and humane. Also the mentally ill were treated in general hospitals attached to medical schools so that by the 10th Century AD visitors to Adrianapolis could marvel at the cheery atmosphere in which the mentally ill were treated and had been treated for over 400 years. Meanwhile Europe acquired its first mental hospital in 1409 in Valencia in Spain with the hospital founded by Fr. Gilabert Joffre. Fr. Joffre's influence spread through Spain and France to Mexico City.

The 17th and 18th Centuries

In England the most important medical influence came from Thomas Sydenham (1624–1689) who emphasised the importance of history taking and examination as major contributions to the concept of the natural history of disease.

Thus he took medicine away from being an erratic exercise in taxonomy and made it into a craft where illness could be regarded as a developing system, a dynamic interaction between host and agent. Sydenham also wrote about the usefulness of the clinical method as applied to the study of emotional and mental disorder. In psychiatry nowadays we take this for granted but Sydenham stated the idea clearly and forcefully, not only as a practical clinical exercise but also as something that could have applications in research.

Until Sydenham physicians had gradually forgotten Hippocrates' ideas about diagnosis and prognosis and had become bogged down in recognition of disease without trying to understand it as a process. And sadly, despite Sydenham's observations, for the next two centuries, doctors went on 'disease spotting'—leading in psychiatry to an almost obsessive concern with classification, as a sort of human stamp collecting, often with a total disregard for the expectation that psychiatric disorders could change in any way.

Sydenham had been ahead of his time in his observations on hysteria—he pointed out that hysteria was found not only in women but also in children and in men—he commented also on the pleomorphism of hysteria. In the 16th and 17th Century literary comments on mental disorder were no doubt still lagging behind the classic self-description and analysis of depressive states set out by Richard Burton in his *Anatomy of Melancholia*. Literary descriptions of psychiatric disorders often give the doctor a *trompe l'oeil* illustration of illness. The creative genius of an inspired writer can set out in a few lines a synthesis of human psychopathology which baffles the scientist with its untestable accuracy. This should neither deter the scientist nor make the writer over confident. Psychiatry is still reeling from the excesses of inspired guessers compounded by the natural timidity of the honest scientist. But the insights of literature and science are not mutually exclusive.

The writer can make shrewd observations on behaviour without being constrained by the requirements of scientific method, in the same way that the scientist must rely on method and distrust his intuition. By the end of the 18th Century in England medical involvement in mental illness was well established, more or less by accident. This started in 1601 when the Poor Law Act put the poor and mentally ill into the care of local authorities as opposed to the monasteries who cared for them before the Reformation.

The consequence was as might be expected—vagrants and mentally ill were unwelcome in communities fearing the cost of caring for them, and were driven out. They became a growing social problem and thus forced themselves on to doctors as needing care. Hospitals became diverse in their patterns of care; it was not all pure custodialism and neglect by any means. By the late 18th and early 19th Centuries open wards were taken for granted and the value of occupation and family contact were recognised. But, overall the 17th and 18th Centuries were bad times for the psychotic—hospital stay was usually compulsory, often prolonged and above all marked by violence, restraint, ill-treatment and neglect.

The 19th Century

The scientific developments in medicine of the late 19th Century turned medical attention to the possibility of finding causes for mental illness. If bodily illness could be shown to be caused by infection, metabolic disturbance, etc. then it was reasoned mental illness could be caused in similar ways. There is good sense in this; after all general paresis, long thought to be a 'mental' illness, was found to be caused by *Treponema* and was soon found to be treatable, thus reducing the mental hospital population more or less at a stroke and encouraging the idea of physical aetiology in mental illness. The dominant influence in psychiatric treatment in the early 19th Century had been the *moral treatment of the insane i.e.* treating madmen like human beings, using commonsense and humanity as guide lines. But in the scientific revolution of the latter half of the 19th Century this influence was lost; humanity was overtaken by the pathological laboratory—patients became the dehumanised objects of paternalistic custodial care. The patient was ill; he had no responsibility by definition and was denied the option of developing self-reliance and independence.

However the better influences of the 19th Century were really impressive—the rights of the individual and a practical concern for his welfare had been stated by philosophers such as John Stuart Mill. So it is not surprising to find that hospitals such as the Retreat were reported by Samuel Tuke (1812) in his classic work *Description of the Retreat,* a straightforward account of the humane treatment of mentally ill people.

In 1839 John Connolly (1794–1866), superintendent of Hanwell Asylum, published a straightforward account of his method of coping with supposedly aggressive patients in *Treatment of the Insane without Mechanical Restraint*. Connolly emphasised the importance of permitting patients in a mental hospital the luxury of leading a decent and civilised existence where independence and self-reliance could be encouraged rather than ruled out as beyond the capabilities of the 'lunatic'. Connolly suggested that it should be possible to preserve the patient's links with reality, to provide him with sensible and absorbing occupation and above all deal with the patient in a tolerant and humane fashion. This is what the 'moral treatment of the insane' was all about, but unhappily this humanity disappeared when scientific medicine seemed to offer so much.

But this dehumanising process was accelerated by other changes. The overcrowded industrial towns of the latter half of the 19th Century produced a society that had no place for, nor patience with, the chronic sick particularly those who were mentally disturbed. Such patients could not survive in an industrial state whose materialistic ethic equated capitalist expansion with a vigorous self-reliant religiosity and a level of public compassion that led to the poor, the vagrant, and the mentally ill to be no one's concern beyond the pinchpenny charity of pietistic Local Authorities as described by novelists such as Dickens. All the lessons of the 'moral treatment of the insane' were lost and compounded by scientific doctors who thought physiology would explain human behaviour and who speculated about such trivia as the stigmata of degeneracy *i.e.* poor people are morally unsound, less gifted and *worse* than their middle and upper class benefactors.

The inhumanity of the time was total except for the stirrings of non-conformists—a disturbing reminder that the middle classes contain the seeds of social revolution. But for the mentally ill society created a series of clean and well run warehouses where the sexes were segregated except for formal religious observance and dull pleasure and where even in the 1930s in England a former superintendent could recall his early days when there were separate hospital shops for men and women.

Large hospitals became the accepted mode of containing the mentally ill and the socially disadvantaged, even a cursory glance at case notes of the day supports this. The photographs, the accounts of the patient's history are a constant repetition of well meaning custodialism applied to the ill and the not-so-ill—and all carried out with the best of intentions in a society where the poor were categorised into the deserving and the non-deserving—an intriguing philosophical exercise which still astounds many but is still used by many.

However these large mental hospitals *did* attract thinking doctors. In England Daniel Hack Tuke's *Manual of Psychological Medicine* and *Dictionary of Medical Psychology* were based on his clinical experience and still survive as bonuses to be removed from library shelves by anyone with a taste for history and a simple prose style.

In Germany however, psychiatry had become established as a subject that could be taught and studied by university professors, something that had to be delayed until the 1960s for discovery by the universities in England. The great German academic psychiatrist of the 19th Century was Emil Kraepelin (1855–1926). Kraepelin broke through the quagmire of 19th Century psychiatry, where diagnosis had become uninspired taxonomy, by using his clinical observations to make good prognostic sense out of diagnosis and achieved his tour de maitre (obvious *now* but not *then*) by differentiating between dementia praecox (schizophrenia) and manic depressive psychosis. He left a diagnostic scheme about which many express doubt but which most psychiatrists still use even though they may raise objections. Before Kraepelin diagnosis was a lucky dip; Kraepelin made psychiatric diagnosis into a more certain and scientific activity.

The 20th Century

Although many regard the 20th Century as a breakthrough for psychiatry where doctors rediscovered the possibility that events, conflict and suppressed feeling might lead to emotional disorders the plain fact is that the *first* and most influential psychiatric *discovery* of the century linked artificially induced fever to the treatment of general paresis. This gave to history the first and to date last psychiatrist to become a Nobel Prize winner and later the only psychiatrist to gaze upon an unsuspecting public from the fairly unlikely setting of a postage stamp. Nowadays psychiatrists on television are two a penny but rarer than Penny Blacks, and many would add, nowhere as pretty. The 19th Century led to the emergence of 'psychological medicine' *i.e.* psychiatry well within a strictly medical model. The scientific climate of the age, and the evolutionary theory of Darwin favoured the idea that the brain and mind were the end products of an evolutionary process. Hughlings Jackson proposed a theory of *central nervous activity* which emphasised its integrated function but also related its integrative nature to an evolutionary theory of brain function in which the acquisition of higher functions was linked to an evolutionary time scale. Hughlings Jackson postulated a theory of brain activity which stated this in understandable clinical terms. In his schema of brain activity damage would be revealed by the loss of newly acquired functions and by the appearance of 'older' reflex responses. This was a fundamental statement which helps to explain not only the ways in which the human brain shows signs of damage but also is clearly related to man's place in the evolutionary hierachy. His highest order activities are related quite simply to the size and complexity of his brain and account for the diversity of his capabilities in language, intelligence, learning and memory.

The psychodynamic movement in psychiatry was greatly influenced by the theories of neurologists such as Hughlings Jackson who postulated an integrative theory of central nervous activity and also by earlier neurologists whose clinical experience of hysterical disorders led them to speculate about *levels* of central nervous activity. It now seems fairly certain that hysterical disorders were more common 100 years ago than now. This is probably because the medical attitudes of the time encouraged symptoms that implied a 'physical' rather than a 'psychological' aetiology. Neurologists and psychiatrists became absorbed in the study of hysteria and the beginnings of a psychodynamic concept of hysteria started in neurological clinics. Charcot (1825–1893) was a neurologist who was intrigued by the possible relationship between hypnotism and hysteria. He discounted the relevance of 'psychological' factors in hysteria and was a bitter rival of Bernheim (1840–1919) who thought, correctly, that many of the signs of hysteria described by Charcot were artefacts implanted in the patient by Charcot's powers of suggestion.

However one of the most significant influences in advancing a psychological theory of hysteria was provided by Pierre Janet (1859–1946) who had studied under Charcot. Janet viewed neurotic disorders as being related to deficiencies in 'psychic tension'. This was thought to be a reservoir of energy which preserved the integrity of consciousness—it was an energy source which could be depleted at various levels—moderate depletion would cause hysteria and severe depletion would cause 'psychasthenia'. Janet introduced the idea of *dissociation of consciousness* in which consciousness became split in a way that led discrete elements of consciousness to become autonomous and manifest in syndromes where a person lost a function but was unaware of the nature of the functional loss *e.g.* in hysterical fugue, hysterical paralysis (see hysteria).

The best known exponent of psychodynamic theory was Sigmund Freud (1856–1939). Freud's early interest in neurology led him to study under Charcot in Paris and then to return to Vienna to work with Breuer who was the first physician to suggest that hysterical symptoms might be related to childhood experience. This was a novel idea at the time. Some idea of just how novel it was may be gained from the fact that in those days much of what would now be regarded as normal history taking just did not occur, in fact certain areas of human life were regarded as being unfit for discussion amongst respectable people. This was true of sexual life where the cultural atmosphere of the 19th Century established a curious double standard of values as exemplified by the child prostitutes, brothels, etc. of Victorian London in contrast to polite society where sexual matters were taboo and people put cloth covers around piano legs!

Breuer and Freud were intrigued to find that some of their patients recalled early childhood experiences in which they described sexual advances from close relatives. These clinical observations led Freud to speculate about the relevance of the unconscious in the causation of psychiatric disorders. Thereafter psychiatry was influenced by an increasing concern for the importance of the unconscious in shaping mental life.

Freud's theories will be referred to in more detail later; the important point to make at this stage is that they seemed to offer better understanding of psychiatric disorders at a time when clinical psychiatry seemed to many to be a sterile exercise. Freud's ideas on treatment, his theory of psychoanalysis, offered hope at a time when doctors who took up psychiatry were regarded as second rate men who could not get ahead in medicine. This simple statement is really a criticism of the sort of people who go into medicine rather than of psychiatry.

It would be hard for anyone to estimate the real extent of Freud's influence in psychiatry. He illuminated murky areas and cut across much of the stuffy self-righteousness of the worst aspects of descriptive psychiatry. Psychiatry had lost the philosophical impetus of earlier days and clinical work had become rather like stamp collecting except that patients were stuck in warehouses, not revered as rare specimens, but treated in an atmosphere of arid contemptuous superiority. So that when Freud offered seemingly zany theories of the aetiology of psychosis these were seized on by enthusiastic doctors and by many whose appetite for change was too easily relieved by the strange diet later served up by the psychodynamic movement.

Freudian theories seemed to clarify mainly because they were insightful and novel but they lost out later because Freud's followers became too antiscientific and the whole psychoanalytic school became dogmatic. If the revealed truth was not believed then clearly the non-believer was a heretic and a sick heretic whose only hope of cure lay in further psycho-analysis. This reduced the credibility of psychoanalytic theory.

Since the early 20th Century psychiatry has been influenced by biology and sociology and by scientific method. The last is probably the most important influence. Medicine and psychiatry stand or fall by the use of scientific method. There is an attractive quality about the detailed study of the individual but facts about behaviour and experience are gained from the study of large numbers—a practice which does *not* dehumanise psychiatry but which ultimately renders it more human by teaching psychiatrists a proper respect for human similarities and human differences.

Physical treatment in psychiatry revived interest at a time when the early promise of psychoanalytic theory and treatment had fallen. Out of the blue, or so it seemed, there arrived the strange finding that electric shocks across the head could relieve depression, reduce the mortality of puerperal psychosis and bring schizophrenics temporarily into contact with reality. The apparent success of electroconvulsive therapy reinforced the medical model of psychiatry, as did the use of insulin coma treatment in schizophrenia. But in fact the most important medical influence on psychiatry has been the development of the *psychotropic drugs* starting in 1952 with the discovery that chlorpromazine could alter behaviour, calm agitation and block hallucinosis without altering consciousness. This made it easier for nurses and doctors to relate with patients whom they could now reach without bludgeoning them into stupor. Since that time and the discovery of antidepressant drugs and tranquillisers it has become easier to study the epidemiology and the manifestations of psychiatric disorders since it is no longer necessary to spend so much time acting as the patient's custodian. It has led ironically to a move away from a medical model of psychiatric disorder and a tendency to look more closely at social factors and social models of psychiatric disorder.

We are left with the inconvenient fact that we use a medical model of psychiatric illness, we use physical treatments but at the same time we have serious doubts about their ultimate value. However, as doctors we have to do the best we can for people who consult us as patients. To be effective the best we can do is to try and summarise the patient's mental state in the light of history and our examination—to state a diagnosis, offer a prognosis and offer treatment. It is as simple and a difficult as that—and this is what this book is about.

3

Concept of psychiatric illness

WHAT IS PSYCHIATRIC ILLNESS?

It will be realised that there is considerable disagreement about *the notion of psychiatric illness*—how justified are we in labelling certain forms of aberrant behaviour as illness? Is 'psychiatric illness' a term that is convenient to the spirit of the present times to explain away something that is badly understood—and if this is the case what are the consequences? This topic cannot be shirked; it is no longer good enough (if it ever was) to proclaim that certain people who behave oddly are 'mad' *i.e.* ill and need treatment and leave it at that.

Siegler and Osmond (1966) reviewed 'models of madness' systematically; referring particularly to psychosis but their observations have a general application to psychiatry.

They propose six models: **Medical; Moral; Psychoanalytic; Family interaction; Conspiratorial;** and **Social.** In each case a model is defined and it is shown how 'madness', its aetiology, treatment, prognosis, etc. can be explained in terms of a model based on a specific philosophical, scientific or social system of ideas. This is a valuable demonstration of the various ways in which inexplicable behaviour may be construed. The six models may be condensed into three, purely for the purposes of illustration: **Medical/analytic** model; **Family/social** model; and **Political/conspiratorial** model.

The medical/psychoanalytic model

In this the aberrant or abnormal behaviour is defined as *sick*, *i.e.* as a type of illness, and on the whole this is more the case for 'organic psychiatry' than for psychoanalysis—the differences lie in the theory of illness in either instance.

The 'organic' school of psychiatry sees the diagnosis and classification as a task of fundamental importance, and is sceptical about aetiology which is viewed in eclectic terms. Genetics, brain damage and biochemical disturbance are held to be the most measurable aetiologies whilst social and dynamic factors are regarded as being relevant but unlikely to be primary causes, even though *multifactorial aetiology* is thought to be the most acceptable notion. *Treatment* is mainly medical with emphasis on physical methods and the role of doctors and nurses in a therapeutic team. The psychoanalytic model may be seen as an outgrowth of the medical model since despite its allegiance to psychodynamic theory the behaviour abnormality is regarded at least as a form of illness. Causes are looked for in faulty personality development early in childhood and *treatment* is based on the relationship between therapist and patient, resolution of conflict and the interpretation of fantasy and symbolic behaviour but though many psychoanalysts might disclaim a medical model they behave as if they believe in one, using hospital admission, medication etc. in times of crisis.

The family/social model

In this model the patient is not regarded as a sick individual but as a member of a group whose disturbed communication network has resulted in one member of the group behaving in a way that needs help or correction; the 'illness' is faulty behaviour, *e.g.* as in the 'double bind' theory of schizophrenia where the 'patient' is a victim of bewildering and conflicting messages that leave him no option except to behave in a 'psychotic' way.

Treatment involves the whole group committing itself to a procedure— *family therapy* in which the attempt is made to unravel the tangled communication net and try to sort out the complicated roles and relationships of family members, aiming ultimately not so much at 'cure' but at finding an optimal level of function of all members of the family group. Thus taking the 'heat' off the 'sick member' and enabling him to come to terms with himself and the family and vice versa. This has found its most logical expression in the school of family psychiatry as expounded in the pioneer works of Howell (1960).

The social model of psychiatry extends beyond the family however and into the whole area that encompasses the effects of social forces on the individual; *social psychiatry* where the individual illness is viewed in terms of its aetiology caused by social forces and also in the diverse ways in which social and environmental forces may be mobilised in the rehabilitation of the psychotic patient and also where the effects of the patient's supposedly therapeutic environment, *e.g.* a hospital, are examined to determine how this environment may have reinforced his role as a sick person and in many instances made it worse.

The political/conspiratorial model

This is an extension of the social model in which the psychotic or the social deviant is viewed as the unwitting victim of the times and of the existing political/social system. The basic premise of this school is that 'psychiatric diagnosis' is a social judgement and that indices of supposed abnormality have nothing to do with individual pathology and everything to do with the requirements of a society which defines abnormality in an arbitrary way enabling family and colleagues etc. to deny the 'patient' liberty if he does not conform to their expectations of how he should behave. Behaviour norms are determined by political/social requirements and roles, *e.g.* a docile working class, an industrious bourgeoisie, a patrician aristocracy etc. Thus when a person is said to be 'abnormal' he is *ipso facto* less than responsible and can lose his rights and liberty whether in hospital or prison. The process of being in hospital dehumanises him and confirms society's expectations and predictions. He becomes 'worse' by becoming more dependent. The writings of Goffman (1954), Szasz (1959) and R. D. Laing (1970) have described these processes in arresting fashion and have caused doubt, dismay and anger amongst many psychiatrists.

Now to some extent all psychiatric disorders can be described in terms of these models. Some are obviously medical, *e.g.* organic cerebral syndromes, others such as the neuroses are indeterminate and can neither be seen as organic illnesses nor as the result of sociopolitical persecution. However the 'eccentric', the 'hippie', the student protester who is labelled as a 'psychopath' because of extreme political views must wonder at least whether their diagnostic labels serve some need for a society that cannot tolerate them.

None of these models is entirely satisfactory. The *medical model* is most commonly used since it is practical, is humane and is directed towards the individual. Sensibly used the *medical model* still has much to offer as long as it is used in a spirit of *clinical simplicity* and *intellectual honesty* with no aura of implied medical superiority over other disciplines.

PSYCHIATRIC DIAGNOSIS—CERTAIN OR UNCERTAIN

A central problem in psychiatry is the importance of diagnosis. Is the diagnosis of psychiatric illness a reasonable exercise or is it a total failure based on ill-comprehended philosophical theory backed up by faulty logic? This is no idle question but a real one which questions the usefulness of psychiatry as a scientific discipline since as we have seen in the summary of the history of psychiatry man has for centuries looked for practical explanations of persistently odd or abnormal behaviour. At present in Western society there is general acceptance of the notion that abnormal behaviour *can* signify illness, though not inevitably so, but we are entitled to question what we mean by psychiatric illness and see how useful classification may be.

A useful start is to examine the concept of physical disease—something that we take for granted. Physical illness is classified and codified reasonably accurately in a way that can be used in planning health care. The proper diagnosis of physical illness is itself only an accurate exercise since aetiology has become more clearly understood. Diagnosis is not a pure exercise in taxonomy, if this were the case 'fractured neck of femur' would be a term that would imply aetiology, *i.e.* traumatic or pathological. Similarly the term 'pneumonia' is general and tells us nothing of causes until we know the site, infecting organism etc. On the other hand there remain large areas of physical diagnosis that are purely anatomical and imply a process without specifying aetiology, *e.g.* carcinoma of the bronchus, multiple sclerosis etc. Disease as a concept is based on the idea of altered function whether by cell destruction, metabolic disorder, new growth and so on.

The problem in psychiatry is to decide whether alterations in behaviour, feeling, thinking and perception can reasonably be called illnesses. Obviously they are when the alteration in function is due to brain damage, *i.e.* organic cerebral syndromes. But in the case of the majority of psychiatric disorders no such organic damage or malfunction has to date been identified. So how *did* the theory of psychiatric illness start? Most would say that psychiatric illnesses are biological events characterised by specific symptoms and signs, and this is about as near as we can get, that is syndromes that can be recognised but not explained.

Classification of psychiatric disorder

The classification of psychiatric illness started in earnest in the late 19th Century, influenced by German psychiatrists such as Emil Kraepelin and Karl Jaspers, who emphasised the careful *phenomenological* study of mental illness.

Some however discard the whole idea of psychiatric diagnosis saying that anyone's disorder is peculiar to him, and cannot be compared to anyone else's. The dispute is basically a philosophical one started by Aristotle who defined the concept of genus and species—for centuries since people have argued whether general terms have any existence beyond words, and this argument persists wherever the question of psychiatric diagnosis is disputed. However doctors are pragmatic men and are concerned with ill people as summarised by Mayer-Gross, Slater and Roth (1969) '. . . when it leaves the study of the sick patient psychiatry ceases to be psychiatry.'

A classification of psychiatric disorders is needed first of all to estimate prevalence rates, and to assess the results of treatment, as pointed out by Florence Nightingale to the doctors of her day that informed medical care could only be sensibly organised if directed at an identifiable sick population. Classification may be arbitrary or systematic. Arbitrary classification is useless, systematic classification uses scientific method to bring order to chaos. Brill (1967) commenting on the history of psychiatric classification has related it to the evolution of thought over the past 4500 years. Modern psychiatric classification really started in the 18th Century with Pinel who described melancholia, mania without delirium, dementia and idiocy.

But as already mentioned classification became more detailed in the 19th Century influenced by Griesinger, Alzheimer, Wernicke, Korsakov and Boenhoffer and finally arriving at Emil Kraepelin's system which, like it or not, is the basis of our present broad classification into:

1 Schizophrenia
2 Affective disorders
3 Organic syndromes
4 Mental subnormality (mental retardation)
5 The neuroses
6 Personality disorders

And this remains the basis of conventional psychiatric classification though in the USA many influential psychiatrists such as Karl Menninger have eschewed such a diagnostic scheme in favour of a relatively simple division into psychotic and neurotic behaviour. The current state of diagnostic practice in England and Wales has been commented on by Kendell (1973) who examined two samples of 1000 first admissions to mental hospitals in the years 1968 and 1971 in the expectation that this might reveal some change in diagnostic practice that could have been influenced by recent changes in international classification of psychiatric disorders. In fact no significant changes were found—in the author's words 'English psychiatrists tend to use a small number of simple diagnostic terms like depression and schizophrenia, which reflect a distrust of elaborate diagnostic distinctions, new or old, a distrust of aetiological assumptions, and a lack of interest in formal nomenclatures.'

However psychiatrists such as Thomas Szasz (1957, 1960, 1970) have criticised the whole question of psychiatric nosology in simple, logical and uncompromising terms, which have infuriated the psychiatric establishment by their very simplicity. Szasz' position is quite clear and starts with the whole concept of psychiatric illness which implies a medical model, something which he finds unacceptable and inconsistent. In his view medical concern with 'psychiatric disorder' should begin and end with *organic cerebral disorders* since the term psychiatry is ambiguous, *i.e.* is it a part of medicine or is it the study of human relationships? Szasz is fiercely critical of the ways in which psychiatry has stepped outside the boundaries of absolute knowledge.

Psychiatric diagnosis

The essential problem of psychiatric diagnosis has been perfectly stated by Sir Aubrey Lewis (1972) in his introduction to the New York/London diagnostic study in two quotes:

'The wit of man has rarely been more exercised than in the attempt to classify the morbid phenomena covered by the term *insanity*' (Hack Tuke).

and

'The best rule, however, for everybody to observe when attempting to form a judgement on any particular case of insanity, is to take care and preserve his own faculties clear, and as free from the mysticism of speculate philosophy as from the trammels of nosology' (Burrows, 1828).

Two pieces of sound advice that any psychiatrist ignores at his peril!

The US/UK diagnostic survey (Cooper *et al*, 1972) is based on psychiatric and demographic data from two comparable hospitals, Brooklyn State in New York and Netherne in the South of London. In each place 250 admissions were examined (excluding those under 20 and over 59). The diagnostic differences were striking with twice as many schizophrenics and six times as many alcoholics in the New York series and five times as many psychotic depressives and twelve times as many manics in the London sample. Even allowing for cultural differences the study confirmed that the diagnostic differences were related to differing diagnostic practices. In New York schizophrenia is a much broader concept than in London and includes patients that in England would be diagnosed with depression, neurosis and personality disorder. This is in line with the author's personal experience in a New York State Mental hospital where patients presented at case conferences as 'difficult to treat' schizophrenics turned out to be people who responded well to antidepressants and/or ECT.

There has been much comment and speculation about the reliability and validity of psychiatric diagnoses (Beck, 1962; Copeland *et al*, 1971; Gauron & Dickinson, 1966; Kendell *et al*, 1968; Kreitman *et al*, 1961). However, Kendell (1973) has pointed out that there has been little interest taken in the *practical* aspects of diagnosis as a decision-making process. Kendell showed videotapes of 5-minute interviews with 28 patients to audiences of *experienced* psychiatrists and also used audiotapes and written transcripts for other experienced psychiatrists. He found that the raters final diagnoses were the same as the *hospital* diagnosis in 48% to 50% of cases at 2 minutes of the interview and 60% to 64% after 5 minutes. Also inter-rater agreement was over 75% under all three rating conditions. Kendell concluded that diagnoses made by adequately trained psychiatrists 'are more reliable than the literature would indicate' and that 'an

B

accurate diagnosis can be made within the first few minutes of an interview'. However, the author pointed out that the first interview is not concerned merely with diagnosis alone but with many other matters that concern the patient's past, present and future.

The dispute is by no means settled—at the moment it is practical to try and treat patients' complaints and try and assort them into syndromes, so long as one does not assign to a syndrome an existence of its own. So for the moment, until we get something better, most psychiatrists are prepared to make do with Kraepelin's nosology.

4

Language of psychiatry

The language of psychiatry contains as much jargon as any specialised subject whether it is ceramics or stamp collecting, the only difference being that psychiatric language is extensive and has frequently become part of everyday speech, so that terms like 'neurotic', 'psychotic', 'paranoid' and 'deluded' are used quite freely by large sections of the population. Yet at the same time there is often a general impression especially among doctors that psychiatrists use a highly specialised language which serves only to dress up simple truth in obscurity and that the language is only partially understood by psychiatrists themselves. It is true that professional jargon often is used in the first way and it is also true that professionals often use jargon that they barely understand but this is not confined to psychiatrists; it runs right through medicine. Some words, especially those that sound good or are colourful continue to be used and imply nothing, *e.g.* 'water hammer pulse'—how many doctors know what a water hammer is? or 'hardbake spleen'—how many know what hard bake means? Others include meteorism, titubation, hypertelorism and angina—all of which have lost their meaning.

However, in psychiatry the meaning of the words used is even more important since mostly the psychiatrist relies on words to arrive at a diagnosis and treat the patient. The science of psychiatric disorder is called psychopathology. This section attempts to set out the meanings and applications of some of the more important terms used in describing psychiatric abnormalities, but before going any further it is necessary to mention one or two of the most widely used terms since they recur

27

throughout psychiatry and they need brief definition before more elaborate discussion.

Anxiety   This is a feeling of fear or apprehension usually accompanied by autonomic disturbance. Anxiety may be felt by healthy subjects in the face of stress such as examinations etc., but is described as morbid anxiety when it pervades the mental life of an individual.

Depression   This is pathological mood disturbance resembling sadness or grief. Depression is described as *reactive* or neurotic when it can be related to an apparent causal agent, and *endogenous* when it appears out of the blue. The mood change is accompanied by characteristic disturbance of sleep, energy and thinking.

Dementia   This is progressive, irreversible intellectual impairment caused by organic brain disease.

Delirium   This is an organic mental state in which altered consciousness is combined with psychomotor overactivity, hallucinosis and disorientation.

Depersonalisation   This is a subjective feeling of altered reality of the self.

Derealisation   This is a subjective feeling of altered reality of the environment.

Delusion   This is a false belief which is inappropriate to an individual's sociocultural background and which is held in the face of logical argument. True delusions commonly have a paranoid colouring and are held with extraordinary conviction. Delusion is thus a primary and fundamental experience in which incorrect judgements are made. The experience of delusion proper precedes its expression in words and hence, when stated, is incomprehensible and beyond argument.

Delusional ideas   Delusional ideas differ from true or primary delusions in that instead of arising out of the blue they occur against a background of disturbed mood and are entirely explicable in that context.

Flight of ideas   This is accelerated thinking, characteristically seen in hypomanic and manic illness. The association between ideas are casual, and are determined by puns and rhymes. However, links are detectable and the flight can be followed.

Hallucinations   This is a perception occurring in the absence of an outside stimulus (*e.g.* hearing a voice outside one). They occur in organic and other psychoses.

Hypochondriasis   This is preoccupation with fancied illness. Hypochondriacal features are common in depression and may be found in schizophrenia. It seems likely that hypochondriasis does not exist on its own but is usually a manifestation of some underlying psychiatric condition.

Illusion   This is a perceptual error or misinterpretation. These commonly occur in organic mental states, particularly delirium.

Ideas of reference   The patient who has ideas of reference experiences events and perceives objects in his environment as having a special significance for himself.

Neurosis and psychosis   Although widely used the terms lack precise definition and give rise to disagreement. A working definition would be that neurotic illnesses are states in which anxiety, mild mood change and preservation of contact with reality are the rule. The neurotic patient is only too aware of his illness, and never loses contact with reality. In psychotic states, the patient loses contact with reality, there is a tendency towards the more bizarre manifestations of psychiatric disturbance as a common finding. Mood change when present is likely to be profound. Thus it appears that we base our definitions of neurosis and psychosis on severity of symptoms rather than anything else.

Obsessional phenomena (obsessive compulsive phenomena)   These are contents of consciousness of an unpleasant and recurrent sort which the patient experiences but which he resists. These contents may include words, ideas, phrases and acts.

Paranoid   This is a widely known psychiatric term and about as widely misused. It derives from the Greek *para nous i.e.* beyond reason. It has been used for years to describe 'classic' signs of psychosis particularly those that encompass delusions of grandeur or those of a fantastic sort.

Recent use of the term has tended to assign to it the meaning of 'persecutory', thus paranoid delusions become delusions of persecution and suspicion, oversensitive people are regarded as 'paranoid'. This is no doubt related to the fact that ideas of persecution are commonplace in psychosis so that by a process of condensation paranoid=psychotic=persecuted. But this is an incorrect way of using the term which is better applied to psychoses.

Passivity feeling   This is a feeling of bodily influence or control by outside agents.

Schizophrenia   This is a syndrome, occurring mainly in young people, in which are found characteristic disturbances of thinking, perception, emotion and behaviour. The illness tends to lead to disintegration of the personality.

Schizophrenic thought disorder   This is a characteristic type of disturbance of thinking, found only in schizophrenia, in which there is a basic disturbance of the process of conceptual thinking.

We may now examine some of these and other conditions in more detail in an attempt to use them sensibly and fairly.

Affect

The terms affect and emotion tend to be used interchangeably to describe a person's mood state although some restrict the word affect to imply the feeling associated with a particular emotion, *e.g.* the *feeling* of anger, of love, of despair etc. Therefore it is easy to see why it is usually difficult to describe a patient's affective state since one cannot *know* how he feels. On the other hand it is possible to find out and describe changes in affect, *i.e.* is the mood sustained or is it changeable? Also it is possible to find out whether or not the person's mood is responsive to the surroundings and other people, *e.g.* if sad can he be cheered up, if excited can he be calmed by being with quiet people? Again it is possible to observe whether a person's affective state is constant or changeable (labile) or whether it is appropriate or inappropriate to his circumstances or whether the emotional display is narrow, restricted or 'flattened'. In psychiatry affective symptoms are accorded considerable importance and rightly so since they are common.

Mood disturbance is something that patients notice and complain about particularly depressive mood disturbance; although some depressed patients may be so full of self-blame that they see their own sadness and lethargy as laziness. But generally people are aware of their feelings and describe them fairly accurately. The most common symptom of affective disorder is undoubtedly depression, a word which is used in a number of ways (Storey 1968): firstly to describe a normal emotional reaction, secondly a symptom, and thirdly a syndrome or for that matter an illness. Confusion arises because of the different ways in which the word *is* used.

For instance in common usage people often say that they feel 'depressed'—this usually means they have had a short lived bout of low spirits, part of the normal range of feeling. On the other hand a bereaved person may be described as 'depressed' when in fact he is showing a normal emotional reaction to loss. The term *depression* should really be restricted by clinicians at any rate to include disorders where there is a sustained mood change, akin to sadness or grief, which exceeds in extent and duration the customary variations and which is accompanied by other symptoms of physiological disturbance such as weight loss, sleeplessness, lack of energy etc. and other psychological symptoms such as anxiety, self-blame, feelings of guilt, hypochondriasis etc.

Depressed mood may be significant on its own or may precede disorders such as schizophrenia. So that the statement 'I feel depressed' or 'I am depressed' may mean a lot or may mean very little. The affective state may be *labile* as previously mentioned, *i.e.* changing quickly from one extreme to another. This may be a personality characteristic or it may occur in organic cerebral disease and in schizophrenia.

Euphoria is a mood of pleasant well being—normal, *e.g.* when following good news etc. or following the use of alchohol or drugs. Swings of mood can *also* be normal though they *may* be pathological in *cyclothymic personality* and *are* pathological in some manic depressive psychoses. *Elation* is a more serious and extreme elevation of mood found in mania and heavy intoxication with amphetamines.

There are also states of ineffable bliss and cosmic union, *i.e. ecstasy.* States of ecstasy are rare—the psychiatrist is not concerned with the ecstasy of saintliness but with the pathological ecstasies of schizophrenia and temporal lobe epilepsy. Other important affective symptoms include the feeling of having lost feeling, apathy and intense shades of feeling. All of these may occur in affective disorders and in schizophrenia.

Incongruity of affect is the term usually applied to the inappropriate emotional responses of the schizophrenic whose emotional reactions frequently extend beyond the inappropriate into total incongruity (laughing at bad news) or more usually in chronic schizophrenia a dulling of emotional response one way or the other usually called 'flattening of affect'.

Finally it needs to be said that despite the cultural influences of middle and upper class English upbringing, feelings are generally neither divorced from experience nor thought. People do not and cannot escape from their feelings no matter how hard they try.

Anxiety

Anxiety is an emotion, a psychophysiological phenomenon that is so widespread that many find it hard to distinguish between normal and morbid anxiety; a distinction which has to be made if the term is to be used sensibly.

Normal anxiety is experienced by everyone in situations of unaccustomed stress, *e.g.* examinations, interviews etc. but it goes further than that. Everyday indecision under pressure, irritability and discontent are often part of normal anxiety hardly to be regarded as morbid since these feelings are common and are relatively harmless. But morbid anxiety is different altogether, in extent and duration; the morbidly anxious person suffers more intensely and for longer, also his anxiety may be triggered off by trivia.

The feeling of anxiety is like fear or apprehension, it is unpleasant, directed towards the future and is often accompanied by physical symptoms of adrenergic overactivity (tachycardia, dry mouth, diarrhoea etc.). Attacks may be episodic ('panics') or the anxiety may colour affective disorders and *less commonly*, be found in organic mental states and schizophrenia.

Levitt (1968) has pointed out that a useful distinction may be made between 'trait anxiety' and 'state anxiety'. The former is a general tendency to be anxious, while the latter is to do with the experience of being acutely anxious. So that the remark 'I suppose I'm anxious' may have many meanings, *e.g.* 'I feel tense; I feel tense sometimes; I'm afraid; Sometimes I get fearful; Some things really tense me up; I feel uncertain; and I'm a worrier' etc. Therefore the clinician needs to evaluate 'anxiety' symptoms and complaints of 'anxiety' very carefully.

Delusion

Since ancient times delusion has been regarded as the classic sign of madness. In the past it was held that someone who was deluded was mad and that mad people had delusions as a matter of course. But it is not as simple as that—a clear understanding of the concept of delusion is basic to psychiatry and goes beyond the mere definition of a delusion and leaving it at that. The delusion is an abnormality which has important social and cultural aspects. Where anyone is described as deluded, implicit in the description there should always be sensible recognition of the culture bound relations of the term.

The usual definition of a delusion is that it is a belief which is demonstrably false, which is held with absolute conviction, which is not appropriate to the person's sociocultural background and which is not understandable as a result of a primary disturbance of mood.

To have a true appreciation of the psychopathological significance of delusion we need to step outside the psychiatrist's consulting room. A convenient starting point is the *awareness of reality*. This is based first on the realisation of existence and secondly on the signals of reality—the perceptions that are picked up, integrated and analysed by the central nervous system. The certainty of reality, taken for granted, most of the time, is probably based on the sensory perception/integration system which enables us to make predictions about the 'concreteness' of reality. This is most simply illustrated by the fact that a man in clear consciousness can appreciate his own reality and the reality of his environment and shares this with others.

If we accept *some* agreement about reality we may consider next the processes of thinking and forming judgements. No one can *define* thinking but we do know that thought contents are in part influenced by the input to the brain. Simple experiments in total sensory deprivation not only cause perceptual disturbance but also considerable difficulty in thinking and concentrating. In delusion there is probably a basic flaw in the mode of thinking and making judgements so that a person develops an incorrect belief, held with certainty and immune to rational argument. The term delusion should therefore be restricted to ideas that fulfill these fairly strict criteria (*i.e.* incorrect, unshakeable, inappropriate and unrelated to mood change).

However the concept of delusion *is* subject to basic criticism. For instance it might be thought that the term could be used to categorise contentious beliefs in general—if this is true then the concept is useless since anyone else's opinions could be called delusions. This criticism cannot be sidestepped, the concept of delusion is challenged by those who reject any medical model of psychiatric disorder and regard delusions as labels used by psychiatrists to label understandable eccentricity. But a delusion is more than this: it is an error in judgement based on the personality change that is the central feature of psychosis. The term delusion is not applied to difference of opinion nor for that matter a shared belief, *e.g.* religious beliefs are not to be dismissed as delusions even though some think them erroneous. The crucial point about delusions is that they are peculiar to the individual, they are never part of a shared system of belief even though their content is influenced by the prevailing culture, *e.g.* a person may believe that his mind is controlled by television. For someone in this state this highly individual experience in no way binds him to other deluded people. These and other qualities of the delusion have been commented on by writers such as Jaspers (1962) who stressed the alien quality of delusions which 'remain largely incomprehensible, unreal and beyond our understanding.'

Deluded people are often aware of an ineffable change in the environment and themselves—the 'something is going on' phenomenon. The meaning and significance of reality assume a different value. This definite, immediate certainty of altered reality is thought to be the basis of the experience of being deluded.

Jaspers (1962) considered the importance of three other aspects of the delusional experience referred to by him and the German School as

1 Delusional perception
2 Delusional reference
3 Delusional awareness

Delusional perception: 'Direct experiences of meaning whilst perception itself remains normal and unchanged.' In other words the event, object etc. is perceived clearly but assumes an abnormal significance, *e.g.* 'I saw a dog and knew that it was no ordinary dog. It meant I was the Saviour.'

Delusional reference: Here the person perceives his environment clearly but judges it to have special significance and meaning realted directly to himself.

Delusional awareness: This is a state in which a person develops singular knowledge and awareness of far reaching events of cosmic significance; of special revelations made only to him.

In practice many object to these distinctions as being unduly pedantic. This is less than fair. When we describe abnormalities in the mental state we need to be accurate so that the patient can be fairly assessed and protected from being casually described as deluded. Whether or not we accept the usefulness of Jasper's observations there is no doubt of the importance of distinguishing between true delusions and delusional ideas.

Delusional ideas are ideas based on some other psychological change such as a primary mood disturbance. The best example being in severe depression where the pessimistic mood of the patient colours his entire outlook so that he comes to believe that he is damned and doomed to rot in Hell, *i.e.* these are explicable and understandable delusions as opposed to true delusions which are always inexplicable alien experiences with which we cannot empathise.

Clinical recognition of delusions

Delusions are properly recognised only when they fulfil the criteria already described always bearing in mind the importance of the cultural milieu; a patient in London who says he is bewitched is likely to be deluded. In Southern Italy or Tribal Africa the diagnosis is less certain since the culture favours a belief in witchcraft. Another important aspect of delusion is the extent to which the person gets involved in the ideas. Deluded people do not lose their ideas in face of persuasion, torture and persecution. Delusions can be classified according to content.

Paranoid delusions are *para nous* (Greek), *i.e.* beyond reason. The term paranoid has been used in various ways, and has been reviewed by Lewis (1970) who noted that it should be applied to fantastic and grandiose delusions.

Persecutory delusions are common and this has led to 'paranoid' being used in the sense of persecutory. The problem here is that the meaning of the word has become condensed, but we need not be unduly perturbed over this, the meaning of words *does* change with usage. Sir Aubrey Lewis (1970) epitomised the use of the word paranoid by suggesting that it should be used only for the formal description of delusions and syndromes characterised by 'persecution, grandeur, litigation, jealousy, love, envy, hate, honour or the supernatural'. Without labouring the point the essence of the paranoid deluded experience is that the person becomes convinced of special significance, of being singled out whether by persecution, grandeur etc.

Kraupl Taylor (1966) listed six types of paranoid delusions:

1 Persecutory
2 Jealousy and envy
3 Erotic
4 Grandiose
5 Reference
6 Litigious

Persecutory delusions   Ideas of persecution are common in psychosis. The *psychotic depressive* comes to believe that he is scrutinised by unseen agencies who are punishing him for his misdeeds. In *organic psychosis* a persecutory flavouring is common. The delirious patient sees the nurses as dangerous people and is sure that bedside consultations are really whispered conspiracies. But these *persecutory delusional ideas* are not only explicable but are also loosely held and transient, disappearing as the primary disorder improves or is treated. On the other hand the *true delusions of schizophrenia* are not only held with conviction but may be carefully concealed. They may be revealed only after convoluted exchanges between patient and doctor or sometimes proclaimed insistently and noisily in a torrent of angry words. The depressive may glimpse at hope, the delirious patient may have moments of clarity but the paranoid schizophrenic *knows* that he is surrounded by an intricate web of conspiracy.

Jealousy and envy   Here the person becomes convinced of the jealous attention of others eager to supplant him, take his job, denigrate him and reduce his status and influence. It is interesting to speculate as to whether such delusions are becoming more common in a competitive and materialistic society.

Erotic   The delusion of being admired, courted and secretly loved is an ancient one and one that tends too often to invite derisive dismissal. Of all delusions the erotic type seem frequently to be projections of unfulfilled desire. The patient is in reality pathetic and wretched, often quirkish and unloved.

Grandiose   Delusions of grandeur are not hard to recognise. The person who announces that he is a monarch, the Saviour etc., is making such an absurd statement that any layman will agree that he must be ill. They occur in schizophrenia and are common in mania in consequence of the elevated mood.

Delusions of reference These are common in schizophrenia where trifling and insignificant events are given special and referent meaning for the patient who feels he is singled out in a sinister way. Newspaper headlines are not what they seem but refer to the patient, the television ceases to entertain and becomes a vehicle that refers to him etc.

Litigious delusions The querulous litigant who goes on suing, changes his lawyers and relentlessly involves himself with legal processes etc. is a character well known to lawyers. Some such people are abnormal and eccentric personalities but *litigious delusions* can and do occur, but are rare nowadays.

The most important clinical point is that the *diagnosis of delusion should never be made lightly* and only after careful examination of the patients mental state and in the light of the fullest available history.

Depersonalisation and derealisation

These terms are taken together since the two symptoms often occur to-gether. In both cases the symptom is one in which the person experiences an altered sense of reality. When the symptom refers to the self it is called depersonalisation and when referred to the environment it is called derealisation.

The subjective change in awareness of reality may be quite marginal in the sense that the person feels only very slightly unreal or the surround-ings seem only slightly so. But whatever the extent may be the experience is one that most people find very unpleasant and hard to bear possibly because the barrier between feeling real and not real may be tantalisingly fuzzy.

Depersonalisation tends to be a persistent, unpleasant and baffling symptom which usually makes the sufferer more and more preoccupied with his sufferings and talk about them persistently, often because he feels unable fully to communicate to others just exactly what it is he does feel. In normal life depersonalisation is commonly experienced by people when tired, in childhood or when under the influence of alcohol and drugs such as cannabis, mescaline or lysergic acid. The psychiatric significance of depersonalisation as a symptom is probably most easily appreciated by saying that this is a symptom that can be found in a number of psychiatric disorders. In the early stages of schizophrenia, for instance people may often experience feelings of unreality—the diagnosis of schizophrenia will naturally depend on the discovery of further schizophrenic sympto-matology—thinking disturbance, delusions and so on.

Depressed patients may also experience feelings of unreality and when they do many consider that this indicates the need for urgent treatment since the depressive may seek escape from this very unpleasant symptom by suicide.

In temporal lobe epilepsy episodic depersonalisation is common and part of the spectrum of disturbed perception that can occur in this condition.

Patients with obsessional disorders may develop not only deper-sonalisation but also elaboration of the symptom in an obsessional way so that they find themselves endlessly ruminating about their awareness of their altered reality in a repetitive unhappy way.

One variety of *adverse reaction to hallucinogenic drugs*, particularly lysergic acid is characterised by persistent depersonalisation and anxiety. It is common in more common toxic states such as alcoholic hangovers and has been reported as a troublesome symptom during and after steroid psychoses. It has also been reported by people with high therapeutic doses of salicylates and is probably reinforced by the tinnitus. In fact an altered sense of reality is very commonly experienced with any mind altering drug whether sedative, stimulant or hallucinogenic, the more carefully it is enquired after in these cases, the more striking is its pre-viously unsuspected existence probably since it is more or less taken for granted by the person who experiences it.

Again in ordinary life, shifts in daily routine, expected or unexpected often produce in people definite feelings of unreality: return from a holi-day, or hospital, the first day in a new job being common examples. However psychiatric opinion is divided between those who regard de-personalisation which can be a primary syndrome in its own right and those who see depersonalisation always as a symptom of an underlying psychiatric disorder. This was the view of Ackner (1954) who thought that depersonalisation was always a manifestation of some psychiatric state such as depression, hysteria or schizophrenia. This was in contrast to the views previously put forward by Shorvon *et al* (1946) who had pro-posed a specific primary syndrome of depersonalisation.

Roth (1960) reported on 135 cases of a syndrome of phobic anxiety and depersonalisation. The symptomatology of the syndrome was analysed, thus 74% of the patients had headache and insomnia, 60% mild obses-sional symptoms, 53% a depressive colouring and 45% hypochondriacal self-scrutiny. He observed too that the syndrome was positively associated with an insecure type of personality characterised by immaturity, undue depenedency, anxiety prone and obsessionality.

Sedman *et al* (1963) noted a definite association between depersonalisation, depressed mood and insecure personality and in an investigation of the association of depersonalisation in obsessional personalities and again noted that depersonalisation was most common in cases where depression coexisted with an underlying insecure personality structure. Davison (1964) reported on seven patients in whom depersonalisation occurred as an almost isolated symptom and that such cases could be fairly regarded as 'depersonalisation syndrome'.

Hallucinations

Hallucinations are perceptions which occur in the absence of any external stimulus. It is wrong to suppose that hallucinations are peculiar to the mentally ill, certain types are part of normal experience (Jaspers, 1962; Kraupl Taylor, 1966). Dreams are 'normal' hallucinations, as are the visual after-image seen after looking at a lamp. Less common normal hallucinations occur in childhood where the child is able to see and describe in great detail something remembered; 'eidetic imagery'. Though relatively common in childhood it fades with age though it is found in some artists. Other normal hallucinations are commonly experienced whilst falling asleep (hypnagogic) or waking up (hypnopompic).

Hallucinations may occur in any sensory modality—sight, hearing, touch (haptic), taste and smell. It is important always to note all details of hallucinosis, not merely its occurrence. Thus the modality is obviously important and also the relation of the hallucination to the person experiencing it. Is it perceived as outside the body or within it? Also it is important to assess the associated affect and to what extent the hallucination is thought to be real.

Hallucinations do not usually occupy the whole content of perception —this is an important point often overlooked—they appear alongside or interspersed with normal perceptions. Also true hallucinations tend to be regarded as real; a point stressed by Jaspers who emphasised a difference between true hallucinations and pseudo-hallucinations. The latter carry a lesser conviction of reality, and are found in hysteria and in organic psychoses. A good example of a pseudo-hallucination was the following description.

'Well its the black cloud you see. I mean there's this black cloud. Its been there for some time, for some months I think. It's quite black, oval in shape with white bits. No I don't see it quite outside me and I know its not real—I suppose I sort of see it in my mind's eye. I suppose I think its my soul—I don't know—but the black cloud is there.'

Hallucinosis as a clinical phenomenon is therefore not quite as clear a sign as some may suppose—this is linked to normal perception and normal imagery which are taken for granted. Jaspers distinguishes between the two as follows:

Normal perception		*Normal imagery*	
1	records concrete reality	1	is figurative
2	appear in external space	2	in inner subjective space
3	clear	3	unclear and vague
4	constant	4	fades; has to be recreated
5	independent of the will	5	dependent on the will; can be conjured up

The point being that hallucinations overlap between perception and imagery; they are defined therefore in a rather arbitrary way and are clinically important providing they are properly identified. The sort of problems that have arisen in clinical practice have come from the 'hearing voices = auditory hallucinosis = schizophrenia' approach.

Auditory hallucinations   These can be loud or soft, vague or definite and identifiable. They can consist of sounds, whistles, hisses or may resemble speech and consist of wordless murmurs. Hallucinatory voices may be single or multiple, recognisable or unrecognisable. Words may be repetitive or detailed. Often voices comment on the person in a derisory or contemptuous way. They may instruct or command or repeat aloud the person's thoughts. The diagnostic importance of auditory hallucinations is most fundamentally related to the presence or absence of clear consciousness since the latter implies an organic mental state. Auditory hallucinations in clear consciousness suggest either a schizophrenic or affective psychosis.

Visual hallucinations   Hallucinatory visions may occupy a small part of the visual field or may be extensive, even panoramic. An example of the former was a 42 year old alcoholic who described seeing a dog in his house. He became frightened and asked for admission. In hospital he became more frightened as he saw the dog in the ward with absolute clarity. He was in a clouded state and within hours developed full blown delirium tremens.

True visual hallucinosis is more common in organic syndromes than in schizophrenia where visual disturbance is more likely to be delusional misperception or illusion, *i.e.* a schizophrenic misinterprets what he sees. In severe organic syndromes such as delirium, visual hallucinosis commonly involves multiple small objects moving quickly across the visual field.

Tactile (haptic) hallucinations These are often indistinct and may be described as feelings of heat or cold, often interpreted as gas or poison sprayed on the skin. In schizophrenia tactile hallucinations often involve the anus or the genitals. In drug induced states, *e.g.* cocaine psychosis, the patient may complain of a feeling that these are insects in the skin ('cocaine bugs'), this is also found in amphetamine intoxication.

Olfactory and gustatory hallucinations These may be vague and described as a 'funny' smell or taste. They may dominate the clinical picture in schizophrenia where a patient may complain of a foul taste, later interpreted as poison in his food. In severe depression patients may complain of a foul smell which they interpret as the smell of their own fancied rottenness and corruption etc. In temporal lobe epilepsy olfactory hallucinations may be either part of the aura or the fit itself.

Illusions

Kraupl Taylor (1966) pointed out that the word illusion is usually defined inadequately as a 'false perception' which condenses the proper meaning which is the misconception of the properties of an object correctly identified. The most common example being the 'optical illusion' where for instance lines of equal length are seen as lines but incorrectly perceived as being of unequal length. Illusions then can be part of normal experience; typical examples include the perceptual errors made in states of fatigue or the common experience of meeting someone in the street, perceiving him as an old friend then realising he is a total stranger. The latter is a good example since when it happens there are usually at least a few milliseconds of absolute certainty which evaporates into vaguely foolish apologies such as 'I'm sorry, I thought you were someone else' prompting the surrealist reply 'Well how did you know it was me' etc.

In clinical practice morbid illusions can occur in organic cerebral syndromes such as delirium and in intoxication with alcohol or hallucinogens. They occur too in schizophrenia where the whole environment is clearly perceived but appears changed, often in a frightening way. Illusions include micropsia (everything looks small) and macropsia (everything looks big), or colours may seem altered. Illusions are reported by people as a shift in the appearance of the perceived object, this shift may be easy to describe or weird and ineffable. Subtle distortions of body shape are found, usually called 'body image disturbance' and these may be intensely distressing especially if they carry the conviction of deformity or disease.

Jaspers (1962) described illusions as being distortions of perception in which 'external stimuli unite with certain transposing (or distorting) elements so that in the end we cannot differentiate the one from the other'. He described three types of illusions: those due to inattentiveness (as in overlooking misprints in proof reading); those influenced by emotion; and those where discrete visions and develop from vague stimuli such as designs on the wallpaper etc.

The basic point about illusions then, despite these apparent quibbles, is that a person gets the wrong information from an external perception.

Obsessions

Obsessions are ideas which preoccupy the mind thus the term obsession does not always apply to the pathological. Ideas which are of interest, which cause enthusiasm in us are an important part of mental life. They become pathological when they occupy thought to a degree that seems extravagant when the ideas become overvalued. Curiously enough the term obsession derives from demonology (Brill, 1969; Kraupl Taylor, 1970). In the demonological system spirits which attacked the victim from outside produced the state of obsession, *i.e.* of being besieged from outside while spirits which entered a person possessed him.

In psychiatry the term *obsession* is used in two ways. First to describe recurrent preoccupying ideas or images which are experienced against a sense of inner resistance. Such ideas are summarised in the term obsession or obsessional idea. Obsessions may also involve acts, utterances and rituals, when this occurs they are usually referred to as compulsive acts etc. since the person carries them out against a feeling of inner resistance. Secondly the term obsession is used to describe a type of personality, the *obsessional personality*. Some prefer the term 'anankastic' meaning compulsive.

Thought and talk

Although much psychiatric writing is concerned with abnormalities of thought there is really little known about the essence of thought. In a sense 'normal thought' is taken for granted whilst at the same time psychiatry is concerned with *abnormal forms and contents of thought.*

Traditional psychiatric examination is concerned first with the form of thought, and then with thought content. This is an arbitrary approach based on the spoken word, the expression of thought. So that when we refer to the form and content of thought we are mainly referring to the form and content of speech, since spoken words tell us about thought and ideas.

The form of a person's talk may show a number of abnormalities for instance **speed**. A fast stream of talk, barely permitting interruption is usually called *pressure of talk*—a term that implies exactly what it says— *i.e.* high speed. It is mainly to the point and gives the impression that the stream of thought/talk is so intense that it can hardly be contained. On the other hand slow halting talk usually indicates *psychomotor retardation*, an important feature of severe depression.

Another speech abnormality is **perseveration** where talk is repetitive, persistent and circular. Perseveration is typically found in organic cerebral syndromes.

Circumstantiality of talk describes a tendency to wander from the point and eventually find it in a roundabout way. Actually circumstantiality is not a specific abnormality, it is found in mental subnormality, in chronic intoxications, in severe organic cerebral syndromes and in some epileptics.

Incoherent talk is incoherent, disorganised and disconnected. It is found in those chronic schizophrenics whose speech degenerates into verbal rubbish—'word salad' involving stereotyped invented words or *neologisms.*

Interruption in the flow of thought and talk is usually called *blocking*. Blocking can be part of normal experience, *e.g.* in embarrassment and at interviews or may be morbid as in anxiety, depression and in schizophrenia where 'thought block' may be caused by lost control of thought or by the interruption of thought by hallucinatory voices. Thought block is *not* peculiar to schizophrenia.

Flight of ideas is a rapid progression of thought where ideas trigger each other off in a casual way in which words are linked by puns, rhymes and trivial associations. Flight of ideas is characteristic of hypomania and mania.

Psychotic processes affecting the control of thought. These include the feeling that thoughts are controlled from outside; the feeling that thoughts are inserted into or withdrawn from the mind; and the notion that thoughts are being broadcast aloud. (German—Gedanken-lautenwerden.)

All these phenomena are generally regarded as being near enough diagnostic of schizophrenia. They may seem hard to classify and pedants may insist that they are 'delusional misinterpretation'—whatever may be the truth of this assertion it really is certain that someone in clear consciousness who says his thoughts are controlled, or inserted/withdrawn, or broadcast, is more likely than not schizophrenic. When someone says these things are happening to him this is the only way in which he can explain to himself and describe to others the nightmarish psychological dissolution of schizophrenia.

Time sense

Although people take for granted their awareness of time, this perception is important despite the fact that people rarely question the 'time bound nature of life' (Jaspers) until they grow older when time seems to slip by all too quickly. The time related phenomena of human physiology, *e.g.* bodily rhythms are currently subjects for research and study, travelling at high speed around the world and into space, have raised real problems related to physiological clocks—problems as yet partially understood and by no means solved.

In ordinary life time sense is altered by simple factors, in boredom and exhaustion time hangs heavily. In childhood the school term seems endless whilst school holidays are over in milliseconds. The anticipation of an ordeal alters the time sense as does the enjoyment of pleasure. In states of intoxication with hallucinogens such as cannabis, LSD or mescaline there is often prolongation of time sense. Strange distortions of time sense are described in schizophrenia, also prolonged time sense in psychotic depression, whilst in mania the patient finds available time insufficient. In *organic cerebral syndromes* orientation for time is impaired and this depends on the impairment of recent memory and the registration of new impressions.

Memory

Memory is the means by which the human brain records, stores and retrieves information based on experience. The ability to retain impressions and to produce them when needed, to remember and to recall, are vital functions. To study memory it is necessary to know something of the structural basis for memory and its functional nature, and also to look at some disturbances of memory, since these latter have thrown light on our understanding of the subject. When we try to discover the physiological basis of learning and memory we look for evidence of permanent change in the central nervous system, for unless there is permanent change we cannot postulate the existence of memory at all. Physiological investigations of memory attempt to explain such mechanisms. This is a fairly new area of research.

Reverberating nerve cells

In the nervous system, information is passed along neural pathways from receptor sites such as the ear, along a route that may end, say, in activity initiated in response to the sound stimulus.

It has been suggested that the central nervous system contains closed loops of neurons and that these reverberate with activity indefinitely once set off. It was said that a reverberating circuit system was a basis for memory storage but further research did not support it as a long term memory storage system, though current theory holds that they may operate in short term memory.

Some idea of the complexity of the problem is related to the fact that there are several billion cells in the brain and that it is not possible to isolate single neuronal pathways. But it is possible to speculate and hypothesise. Investigators are able to observe relatively crude phenomena, *e.g.* removal of brain substance in animals, stimulation of brain areas, and the effect of drugs.

In recent times attention has been directed to biochemical mechanisms in learning and memory, and research has looked at transmission and possible substance changes within cells. Acetylcholine is the chemical transmitter at the synapse and is inactivated by the specific enzyme cholinesterase returning the synaptic space to the resting state. Some researchers have suggested that the more efficient the synaptic transmission the more efficient the learning and memory process. The theory has been upheld in animal learning experiments.

The double helix

In recent times there has been a gradual accumulation of evidence to suggest that ribonucleic acid (RNA) and protein synthesis play a key part in information storage within the brain. DNA is present in chromosomes and carries the genetic programme of information that determines an individual's genetic inheritance. The DNA in the chromosomes is arranged in a double helical structure, and when the cell divides this provides the new cell with an identical DNA molecule. RNA occurs in the cell nucleus and around the chromosomes and exists in four types of which two types, transfer RNA and messenger RNA, are relevant here.

What is important is that DNA influences protein synthesis through RNA. In other words DNA is the site for the formation of the messenger RNA type which is produced in the cell nucleus on the DNA strand. The messenger RNA then carries the genetic information and becomes a template or pattern guide on which amino acids assemble to form protein. The second type, transfer RNA, transfers the amino acids to be assembled according to the genetic programme determined by DNA structure.

It seems likely that RNA is involved in brain information storage systems, and the evidence for this may be summarised by saying that research has shown that firstly RNA utilisation increases in nervous tissue when it is stimulated. Secondly, RNA utilisation increases in nervous tissue in experimental learning situations. Thirdly, learning can be obstructed by blocking RNA production, and fourthly learning can be accelerated by increasing RNA production. These general findings do not by any means explain the exact role of RNA in learning and memory but they do suggest that RNA is involved at a basic level in information storage.

A two stage process

A general theory of memory postulates that information is stored in the brain by producing a permanent change within brain cells as an end result of stimulation by the perception of an outside experience. The passage of the information from cell to cell could be modified by transmitter substances and the storage within cells varied by changes in the cellular storage system. Such a theory takes no account of the process of remembering and recall and the ways in which they might be modified by experience.

In general descriptions of the memory process it is customary to refer to registration, retention and recall as being three elements of memory. *Registration* is the ability to record an outside experience in the central nervous system and this might be compared to recording, say, a passage of music on tape. *Retention* means the permanence of the record and *recall* the ability to bring the recorded experience into consciousness, rather like playing the recorded tape.

The registration of an experience in memory requires first of all an undamaged brain and a state of clear alert consciousness. Someone whose consciousness is impaired by alcohol, sedative drugs or fatigue is not fit to register impressions. At the same time, adequate registration of learned material requires usually a number of repetitions. Here there are considerable variations; some people can learn and register after only a few repetitions, while others require more.

Certain people have a good visual memory and can recall things with extraordinary intensity. This is eidetic imagery and is common in childhood. It is suggested that RNA operates in registration since the memory traces produce specific changes in the RNA molecules. By this method the RNA molecules would retain a template of the recorded experience which could be reproduced as required.

During the process of remembering there is a phase of instability or lability during which the remembered impression is unstable. The hypothesis currently favoured by researchers is the consolidation hypothesis which postulates a two stage memory process. The first is a phase of instability in which short term memory traces may be formed, but which is otherwise self-limiting, but which may set off a second process in the nervous system—a phase of consolidation that is the formation of a long term memory impression. Some experimental work and certain aspects of memory disturbance in head injury tend to support the consolidation hypothesis.

Mention must be made of the relationship between emotion and memory. This is fairly straightforward. In general, incidents associated with strong feeling are likely to be remembered with intensity, though where the feeling is one of intense shame, disgust, or terror, the memory may be shut off from conscious recall by psychogenic mechanisms.

The disordered brain

Any variety of brain damage will cause memory disturbance, usually loss of memory for recent events. As mentioned earlier, in the case of recently acquired information there is a period of lability (instability) in the central nervous system immediately after exposure to the experience that is to be memorised. It seems that while the intact brain deals with this as a matter of course, the disordered brain is especially vulnerable and less able to register. The term disordered is here used in the widest possible sense, meaning a brain whose structure is affected by any process whether short or long term, so that one would include the whole range of physical processes that may cause brain damage.

A blow on the head followed by loss of consciousness will produce greater or lesser degrees of abrogation of brain function, depending on a complex interaction of factors, including the extent or presence of gross damage to brain tissue, the condition of the subject's brain blood vessels, the force and the site of the blow. All head injury involving loss of consciousness produces some loss of memory.

Minor head injuries produce states of mild concussion where there is only partial loss of consciousness, but, typically, interference with memory and learning. The sufferer may continue with the activity that led to the mild concussion, say boxing or playing football, but afterwards he will have no recollection of so doing.

The term applied to the loss of memory for events immediately preceding loss of consciousness is *retrograde amnesia*: it is characteristic of memory loss associated with head injury. It is a symptom of the brain's inability to register. It is described by the patient quite simply when he says that the last thing he remembers is, say, climbing up a ladder before he was knocked off it, or riding on his motor cycle before being struck. In other words the direct impact on the skull and brain prevents the event being recorded. Retrograde amnesia is found also in people after electroconvulsive therapy (ECT) and after prolonged repeated epileptic fits.

The term applied to the defective memory function that occurs after head injury is post-traumatic amnesia. Here the partially conscious concused patient is unable to register events until he is in clear consciousness. Therefore post-traumatic amnesia correlates with the duration of the period of disturbed consciousness though occasionally 'islands' of memory occur.

Memory worsens with age. The ageing brain is less able to retain information, it has been suggested that this fall off is due to a depletion of

RNA in ageing brain cells. In general some lessening of memory for recent events is accepted as part of the general decline that goes with ageing.

In dementia a failure of memory for recent events is usually one of the earliest signs and always one of the most persistent. The sufferer finds it increasingly hard to remember things from day to day, and may overcome this deficiency by keeping a notebook to remind him of his daily routine. However, as the destruction of brain cells becomes worse this method fails since he cannot even remember to use his notebook. New impressions are not recorded so the daily happenings pass unrecorded and unrecognised. The familiar aspects of home are recognised since this information is stored in the brain but under different circumstances even home surroundings may appear unfamiliar or even foreign. This accounts for the way in which the elderly dementing person can become completely disoriented at night when the familiar looks less familiar.

Hysterical amnesia

When a patient develops total memory loss for *all* events his condition is described as hysterical amnesia. This memory loss is quite unlike any amnesia caused by brain injury, and may be so extensive as to be global.

This is perhaps the most grotesque variety of hysterical memory disturbance. Perhaps what is more common is the selective repression of unpleasant memories. This is, in a sense, so common as to be almost a part of normal experience, but in the hysterically disabled person such memory disturbance can operate forcefully. This leads to a hysterical fugue, especially if there is an associated element of flight or wandering. Not all wanderers with lost memory are hysterics, however. Fugue states can occur in epilepsy, in severe depression and in severe psychoses such as schizophrenia. The main point is that organic memory loss is easily diagnosed as it conforms to a typical pattern, whereas other forms of memory loss do not reflect brain damage.

In everyday life, paramnesia, or distortion of recall, is found in the witness box where witnesses—each telling the truth—produce totally different accounts of an event. In normal individuals this probably has to do with the fact that the event may have been partially registered, or that painful reality may colour recall. A special variety of paramnesia is that phenomenon called *déjà vu* where a new incident is falsely recognised as being familiar, and is associated with a vaguely uneasy feeling in the individual that it has all happened before. *Déjà vu* experiences are quite normal in childhood and adolescence, and are also experienced by normal adults in states of fatigue and in certain intoxicated states. Their most important clinical association is with temporal lobe epilepsy.

Insight

Insight is a term that is not easy to define. For the layman it may mean self-knowledge or self-awareness but in psychiatry it is a word that is used in a variety of ways. Most of us assume that we have insight about our deficiencies, eccentricities etc. but if we are honest would probably be surprised, even upset, at overhearing a frank conversation about us. Presented with accurate glimpses of how we appear to others we may react in much the same way that people are often taken aback when they first hear a recording of their own speech.

In psychiatry insight is used to mean not only self-awareness in a general sense but also in a more limited sense to refer to a special type of insight, awareness of being abnormal or ill. However the use of the term extends beyond mere awarness of illness and covers awareness of the full implications of being ill or regarded as ill, *e.g.* How will being ill affect his prospects of return to work? How will being ill affect his relationships with others. To what extent has it already done so? What sort of an illness does he suppose he suffers from? What does he think might have caused it?

Thus insight is not a simple term but rather a summary under which we may include a wide range of experience. So in assessing a patient's insight into his illness it is quite meaningless to say that he has 'no insight'. This may be a polite way of saying that patient and doctor disagree. In any case denial of illness is not to be regarded as a sign of illness. Many patients with physical illnesses deny the significance of symptoms through ignorance, *e.g.* a patient might say 'I'm not ill, I've got swollen ankles and get out of breath' which means that he may have congestive cardiac failure, and even when this is put to him he may say 'there's nothing wrong with my heart'.

Psychiatric patients often make indeterminate statements such as 'I'm depressed' or 'I can't cope' which are hard to assess. In fact it is just these sort of statements that are most common and they are mainly made by patients for whom their degree of insight one way or the other may hardly seem to matter. The severely disturbed person is usually by any standards beyond reason, the normal person may complain of symptoms, but the patient who says 'Why am I here?' or 'I don't want any pills/ECT/ psychotherapy' may be perfectly correct in his judgement of the situation.

So in assessing insight the psychiatrist needs to look a good deal further than awareness of illness. Hindsight is often a more useful point to enquire about especially in patients who have apparently recovered from a psychosis. Some patients may look back on it like a bad dream from which they have awakened, others may be less certain and hint at remaining elements of the process within themselves.

5

Psychiatric history and examination

THE PSYCHIATRIC EXAMINATION

The psychiatric history is an attempt to set out an account of the patient's description of symptoms and signs that suggest illness or abnormality. If someone complains of a change in function, the person who tries to evaluate and deal with the complaint has to take a history. This is not confined to medicine. Psychologists and social workers take histories, so do garage and television mechanics and electronics engineers trying to identify a fault in a complex electronic system. History taking is therefore not peculiar to medicine, it is just that history taking is used in a special and detailed way not only to map out disorders but also to clarify problems. Parallels may seem hardly worth mentioning but can be summarised as in Table 5.1.

If we take the analogy between psychiatry and general medicine it will be recognised that 'medical' complaints may be more specific than 'psychiatric' complaints. This is not always true. Many patients go to doctors with non-specific complaints such as tiredness, vague headache, ill defined pain etc. which are only diagnosed after physical examination. Physicians can localise a relatively limited range of disorders linked to organs or systems and if, after history and examination the diagnosis is uncertain, refuge may be taken in indeterminate labels such as 'he's a hypochondriac', or 'its nerves' though this is nowadays not so common. The psychiatrist is in a different position for most psychiatric patients *have non-specific complaints and symptomatology.*

The properly equipped psychiatrist should have a greater familiarity with areas which normally are of less concern to the physician. There is nothing remarkable in this. The cardiologist has more familiarity with the significance of cardiac murmurs than has the neurologist.

Table 5.1 Types of history taking.

Person complains that:	Person complains to:	Questioning reveals that:	Suggesting possible cause
Ankles are swollen	Doctor	Person is breathless on exertion	Cardiac disease
Feels low spirited	Doctor	Has had persistent early waking feels suicidal	Depression
Can't get on with husband	Social worker	Husband is compulsive gambler and thief	Disturbed marital relations based on husband's personality disorder
TV picture constantly moves vertically	TV mechanic	Person hasn't read manual	Set needs adjusting
Car won't start	Garage mechanic	Battery not topped up. Terminals filthy	Flat battery

What puts the psychiatrist at a disadvantage is that the presenting symptoms are the least clearly understood and as if that were not enough, their universality makes them topics about which anyone can claim knowledge. This means that psychiatry is a subject which is suspect to many because it can be dismissed as 'mere commonsense' or dismissed as being so vague and ill defined as to be hardly worth consideration.

These objections should not be taken too seriously.

People do become unhappy, they do develop odd changes in behaviour, thinking and perception which may usefully be regarded as signs of illness. Not everyone who is unhappy is ill but 'unhappiness' can be a symptom of illness including depression, cerebral tumour and pernicious anaemia.

The historical method was used by the classical descriptive psychiatrists such as Kraepelin and by the founder of psychoanalysis, Sigmund Freud who said that he always began treatment by getting the patient to give him a full account of his life and illness. The *psychobiological school* of psychiatry which Adolf Meyer founded, emphasised history taking and made it so detailed as to make it less useful than expected since detail tended to obscure the essence of problems. Psychiatry should be practical and related to basic issues otherwise it is less than effective. For this reason history taking should be detailed but directed towards producing a fair assessment of the patient, the symptoms and their place as signs of pathology, and their relevance to personal and social background. Of course there *are* special areas that the psychiatrist should scrutinise carefully, *e.g.* mood change and its significance, changes in perception and thinking and the vagaries of human behaviour.

The frame of reference of psychiatry may seem unsystematic, but it is possible to look at human behaviour without dehumanising it to a set of concrete functions, and losing sight of the global view of the individual person.

THE INTERVIEW—HOW TO TAKE A HISTORY

Any fool can bully a patient and too many doctors speak loudly to patients suspected of having a psychiatric disorder, adopting the same tone used when addressing foreigners. And there is no frivolity involved in this observation. Too many doctors talk to patients in a way that barely conceals their hostility and this is still true for psychiatric patients mostly since the unhappy, the querulous, the panic stricken, the deluded patient all induce in some doctors a sense of personal uncertainty about someone whose distress is observable but not measurable, whose personal distress is hard to bear because it is too close to personal experience. This can be frightening because the patient has broken the implicit rules of being ill by suggesting to the doctor that they are both on the same side. Now acknowledging that anyone, even a doctor, can be ill is not something that should be regarded as betrayal, though some doctors still behave as if this were the case if one is to judge by the curious mixture of disapproving belligerence that they bring to the treatment of their colleagues.

A patient who has symptoms of mental disorder should be treated with the same degree of polite respect that is the due of any patient who puts his life, physical or mental, in the hands of a total stranger and trusts that stranger purely on the basis of his having passed a series of examinations several years before.

At the interview the psychiatrist should behave in a polite and sensible way, respecting always the confidentiality of the information that is given, since often it touches on highly personal areas of behaviour. These areas are *not* usually available to general discussion despite the claims of those who urge that adequate psychiatric treatment can only be based on the sharing of confidential information amongst therapeutic teams.

The interview should be conducted in a discreet way; the doctor should try to be flexible and not adhere to a too rigid scheme of examination. Above all he should not appear overintrusive, particularly at the first interview, there is always time enough to intrude, albeit in a kindly and well meaning way. The psychiatrist should not hector the patient, nor behave like a lawyer in cross examination. The patient is likely to feel unhappy or unwell, and because his disorder is strange and unusual, he may feel more than ordinarily apprehensive at the prospect of interview; particularly if mental disturbance has weakened his hold on reality or induced a state of feeling persecuted and watched.

The interview may provoke anger and hostility or the patient may be downhearted and pessimistic, symptoms may be disclaimed whilst the patient claims that he has been brought along against his will by meddlesome and interfering relatives. On other occasions the patient may try to divert attention from problems by behaving towards the doctor in a seductive and flirtatious way.

At the same time the relative who accompanies the patient may display a wide range of feeling; he or she may be on the defensive not just because of distress or shame about mental illness, but also because of guilty misgivings about rejection of the patient. The whole family may be exhausted and ill after a prolonged period of caring for a disturbed patient.

HISTORY TAKING: PRACTICAL GUIDELINES

Histories should always be written out and plenty of time allowed. The written record is not only useful for administrative purposes but also it provides a basis to organise thought and making a proper formulation of the case.

Despite the fact that the development of a psychiatric disorder may be slow and that aetiology is never precise it should always be possible to arrive at a provisional formulation in one interview. This is not to suggest that one can get to know everything about a person in one interview of say an hour or forty-five minutes; far from it.

Another important point is that wherever possible a detailed history should be obtained from an informant other than the patient. The reason for this is simple—a person's awareness of change within the self may be extensive, but awareness of what others have noticed about changes in behaviour, relationships with others and so on may be much less, in the psychoses it may be minimal; in organic cerebral disease it may be virtually absent, so that a history from someone else is always useful. Other informants include not only spouses, parents or siblings but workmates, friends and employers, in short anyone who may usefully throw some light on the patient's state. However it should also be emphasised that doing this should not mean breaking the patient's confidences. If the patient refuses to allow another informant to be interviewed the request should be respected except in very rare cases, *e.g.* where a patient presents a danger to others.

Method of history taking

There is no ideal method of history taking, nor ideal form in which the history should be set out. The patient should be permitted and encouraged to tell the story and describe symptoms in an informal and unhurried way. This does not mean permitting endless rambling; for some patients this would mean interminable interviews leading nowhere. There is an acceptable mean lying between total silence and manic pressure of talk and the interviewer should aim at eliciting a history at the same pace and same detail that one would expect from a teacher explaining something difficult. History taking is not an exact science, it can be likened to an unstructured questionnaire, most experienced historians end up by using a personal questionnaire of their own in which they include their own favourite questions.

The history should be taken in a friendly and polite manner and not in an interrogatory fashion. When a person comes to see a psychiatrist he or she is likely to be apprehensive and guarded—people have all sorts of reasons, many of them bad but some of them good, which make them uncertain and afraid about just what sort of questions they are likely to be asked by a psychiatrist. Usually the patient wants to talk about the complaint first of all so it seems only sensible to start off with the history of the present complaint.

C

Remembering that the first interview is likely to be an event of great significance for the patient the doctor should be able to assess to what extent it may actually be practical or humane to obtain a full history at the first meeting. If not the occasion can be used to go as fully as possible into the patient's account of the complaint and then perhaps interview whoever has come with the patient.

Some doctors and students at first say that they don't know what questions to ask and are surprised when a more experienced person elicits facts that they had missed. The answer to this difficulty is really quite simple and summed up in the word 'practice'. Practice involves familiarity with a range of key topics in history taking and the use of one's own personal questionnaire as already referred to. Actually this can be made more formal by the use of actual questionnaires themselves.

On the other hand it is really quite useless to sit down and have a totally unstructured interview with a patient in an attempt to get a history, such an interview dialogue will produce no information at all and possibly leave even the most well disposed patient with the uncomfortable suspicion that psychiatrists are no better than they ought to be.

The following scheme for history taking is intended as a general guide to the areas which may be relevant. It is not comprehensive in that it may not meet the requirements of the most scrupulous of doctors, on the other hand some may find it unduly intrusive. It is intended to be practical, and above all it is not necessary to take it down in this order but it is suggested that this is a good way of setting it out.

1. The complaint
2. Family history
3. Personal history
4. Past illnesses
5. Premorbid personality
6. Present illness

The complaint

This should consist of a concise expression of what it is that bothers the patient, what symptoms are troubling him—in short a statement of his problem as it appears to him. This is important, there must always be a good account of the patient's subjective experience. And if possible a verbatim account should be obtained and set down.

Family history

This should start with a family tree of parents and siblings noting age, marital status and occupation. There should be careful enquiry about the incidence of formal psychiatric illness in parents, siblings, grandparents and collaterals and direct questions about familial incidence of epilepsy, suicide and attempted suicide, alcoholism, drug use and delinquency. It is important to have accurate data about psychiatric illness in the family, so that inheritable disorders can be spotted. The incidence of formal disorder can suggest the general family climate and give clues about the patient's early years. It is important to ask about significant family events such as parental divorce or separation and also, more difficult, to form an estimate of the quality of the relationship between the parents and between the parents and children.

Personal history

This should always start with a note of the patients date of birth and age. One of the most useful bits of information about a patient is his age since youth, adolescence, middle and old age all have particular patterns of psychiatric illness, and all may produce special areas of stress and conflict. Next the personal history should cover infancy, childhood and adolescent development. This will hardly be necessary for an elderly patient but is relevant to the problems of the adolescent or young adult. The range of topics covered includes:

Infancy: Early years—health, feeding problems—easily reared or not. Developmental milestones.

Childhood: Health and emotional development. General behaviour and disposition. Schooling—difficulties in learning, school avoidance, truancy. Neurotic symptoms, temper tantrums, nightmares, sleepwalking, persistent bed wetting. Relations with parents, sibling and other children. Fears and mood. There should always be special enquiry—fits and 'blackouts'.

Adolescence: School achievement. Higher education or job training. Age when education finished. Ambitions, interests, socialisation. Relationships with others.

Occupations: Job training. Number of jobs held. Longest job held. Present job and earnings. Attitude to job and relations with colleagues and bosses.

Psychosexual: Background, *i.e.* acquisition of sexual knowledge and experience. Masturbation and variety of fantasy. General history of sexual experience and orientation. Sexual problems. Sexually acquired disease.

Marital: Date of marriage. Relationship with marital partner before and during marriage. Divorce and separation. Sexual relations in marriage.

Obstetric: Usual obstetric/menstrual history with special attention to mood or behaviour change associated with menstruation, pregnancy or childbirth.

Previous physical history: With details of any hospital admissions, treatment received etc. where possible.

Previous psychiatric history: With details of any hospital admissions, treatment received etc. where possible.

Premorbid personality: This is the most difficult part of the history and examination. It should not be a series of labels or epithets but better a word picture of the person before he became ill—his general behaviour, his mood, his attitudes, relationships with others, his sensitivity, level of drive, ambition, aspiration, energy and interest.

Past illnesses: Recorded chronologically. With details of any admissions and treatments received.

Past psychiatric illnesses: Recorded chronologically.

History of the present illness

This should be a detailed chronological account of the evolution of the patient's symptoms from their onset until the present time. The history of the illness may be regarded as an account of change—change in feeling, behaviour or perception, change in relationships with others, change in his function as husband, parent, employee or whatever. In other words the history of the illness is directed towards finding out what it is that has happened to the patient to lead him to where he is now. Clearly this is never likely to be very accurate. No one can say exactly when it was that a change of mood started unless the onset is very sudden. In general psychiatric symptoms tend to evolve slowly, in fact it is really quite common to take a history and find a notable landmark appreciated by patient and family only to discover that this was in fact preceded by other changes. On the other hand no one is totally without insight and it is interesting to note that even the most seemingly insightless patient has a better awareness of change in himself than he may at first be able to confide.

Often the symptoms of psychiatric disorder are of a different order from purely physical illnesses though there are many symptoms which overlap and commonly present difficulty in assessment. Symptoms such as nausea, abdominal pain, headache, breathlessness, dizziness, palpitations, tingling and numbness can all for instance be caused by anxiety but on the other hand any of these symptoms on their own can be the first symptoms of serious, often lethal physical illness.

Probably one of the most important things to do when taking a psychiatric history, or for that matter *any* history, is to get the history and set it down without jumping too quickly to a conclusion. Doctors often overlook the fact that diagnosis proceeds from differential diagnosis and that in making any diagnosis one is assessing probabilities. In many areas of medicine and surgery there is a better degree of accuracy in assessing probability for the simple reason that clear understanding of aetiology makes diagnosis precise.

But in psychiatry as we know this is not the case so that the clinician has to learn to assess the significance of such common symptoms as mood disturbance, loss of energy and sleep disturbance. The history of the illness given by a patient may often be dramatically different from that given by a relative.

Another important point about the history of the illness is that patients are often either unwilling or unable to tell their story in a strictly chronological order. It is not surprising for instance to find that people emphasise most the aspects of the history which are concerned with troublesome symptoms. At the same time the patient's account of his illness may be repetitive or circumstantial or so detailed that it is hard to follow the sequence of events. The way in which the patient talks will therefore determine to a large extent the way in which the interview and history taking proceeds—the silent patient needs to be encouraged in the same way that the discursive patient needs to be led. The psychiatrist should always immediately use the history taking as an opportunity to let the patient know that he, the patient, is above all accepted totally and uncritically for what he is, as he is as a real being in the world whose views and feelings he cannot share but whose view of the world remains acceptable and subject neither to criticism nor ridicule.

Another point concerns possible precipitants of illness—topics that may seem irrelevant, unacceptable or so threatening to the patient they are denied. People do tend to ignore causality. So the psychiatrist should enquire carefully about life events that may have triggered off or in any way affected the onset of the illness.

History taking—further comments

Formal psychiatric history taking should never be an exercise in the collection of minutiae. The process should be rational so that *relevant* topics and changes may be detected. Psychiatric histories can be too lengthy. This is self-defeating since histories are, after all, merely questionnaires influenced by the taker's biases and prejudices. The *guiding principle* is to aim at uncovering changes in the patient. This is taken for granted in medical or surgical histories where change can be linked to structural damage or metabolic dysfunction. In the psychiatric history it is easy to be misled by the irrelevant and to emphasise what seems to be abnormal. Therefore one should always be on the lookout for anything that indicates *change* in behaviour, mood, perception, cognition etc. A simple way of detecting change is to enquire about how the patient spends a typical day and set it out in detail. This gives a vivid account of alterations in the patient's life. Efforts to make history taking into formal screening procedures include *psychological testing* and *clinical questionnaires*.

History taking leads naturally to formal psychiatric examination in which we try to identify abnormalities in the mental state, in other words to look for psychopathology. In making the examination the psychiatrist uses eyes and ears to observe behaviour and to listen to what the patient says and tries to elicit abnormality. In some instances this may be easy since the patient may be only too eager to describe a wide range of symptomatology in great detail. In many cases it is difficult. There is no simple once off guide to interviewing. Patience is the most important attribute. Also the ability not to jump to conclusions nor be misled by first impressions.

EXAMINATION OF THE MENTAL STATE

The manifestations of psychiatric disorder *are* recognisable but they are not as measurable as physical signs. This means that any examination of or description of the mental state *must* rely heavily on self-description since objective phenomena are rarely as obvious as in physical illness. Observation and interpretation can be coloured by the doctor's own feelings and attitudes and can lead to mistakes, however if this source of error is accepted it is possible to assess the mental state without too much bias. The format of the mental state examination is conveniently set out as follows:

1　General behaviour
2　Talk
3　Emotion
4　Thought content
5　Perception
6　Cognitive function
7　Insight

General behaviour

Where this is grossly abnormal it is easy to see that something is wrong! Often the family will describe a change in behaviour which may not be obvious at interview, since the patient may conceal feelings and delusions. The student should try to assess the patient's behaviour as carefully as possible, noting such points as the facial expression, gesture and dress etc. and general activity which may be exaggerated as in states of excitement or sluggish and slow (retardation) as in severe depression. Schizophrenic patients may make poor contact and seem remote and aloof or they may display odd mannerisms (habitual expressive movements), grimace in an inappropriate way or adopt odd postures. Demented patients are likely to appear neglected and dishevelled, and make poor contact with the examiner. One starts by observing the patient's behaviour, instead of just taking it for granted. Points to note include:

1　The general level of consciousness
2　Awareness of what is going on around him
3　Level of cooperation with the examiner
4　Contact with the examiner at interview
5　Predominant facial expressions and whether they are appropriate
6　Use of gesture
7　Activity—free or constrained, continuous or interrupted
8　Presence of agitation
9　Mannerisms

Talk

It is usual to consider both the *form* and the *content* of the patient's talk. The form is the manner of talk, *i.e.* how it presents; sustained, interrupted, fast or slow etc. The simplest way to examine the content of the patient's talk is by making a verbatim sample. Content means the predominant topic. Is the patient evasive or reluctant to talk? Does he drift off into irrelevancy or stick to the point? Is the patient talkative or does the talk contain oddities such as puns, rhymes etc. (often a feature of hypomania). Gross abnormalities of speech viz. incoherence are found in organic cerebral syndromes and in schizophrenia where talk becomes fragmentary, disconnected, containing words invented by the patient (*neologisms*).

Emotions

Feelings are hard to describe; the range of words to encompass feeling is immense so that it is barely possible to sum up anyone's feelings in a single sentence. The most useful tactic is to gauge the *prevailing emotional state of the patient*.

Many psychiatric syndromes are associated with extensive mood change. Sadness, misery, dejection, pessimism and an overall feeling of unhappy wretchedness are commonplace, especially in *depression*, but they are also found in other syndromes, *e.g.* in *organic mental states* and *early schizophrenia*. It is important to assess whether the patient's emotional state is appropriate to the mental condition and whether it is constant or variable. Shallow emotional response and ability of mood are other features to look out for, they can occur in organic mental states and in schizophrenia. Some patients are apathetic and deny feelings. Others are unnaturally elated, breezy or euphoric whilst others describe states of bliss or ecstasy. These latter exalted feelings are found in mania and in schizophrenia. *Episodic ecstatic states* suggest *temporal lobe epilepsy*.

Thought content

We take it for granted that a person can control his thoughts but schizophrenics often feel that they neither possess nor control thought, they may feel that thoughts are inserted into the mind or removed from it, or that thoughts are broadcast. Sudden gaps in thinking, often called *thought block* may be pathological as in *schizophrenia*, but can occur in normal people under stress and in anxiety.

Excited patients may experience *pressure of thought*, when thoughts crowd through the mind. Difficulty in thinking clearly is a non-specific symptom which occurs in fatigue, *in depression*, in states of *intoxication* with drugs or alcohol, in *organic mental states* and in *early schizophrenia*.

Delusions   A delusion is a demonstrably false belief, held with absolute conviction which is inappropriate to the person's sociocultural background. True delusions are usually the main abnormalities in schizophrenia where they arise spontaneously and cannot be understood, as opposed to *delusional ideas* which are false beliefs that are an understandable consequence of severe mood disturbance. Persecutory and grandiose delusions of exalted status etc. are usually referred to as paranoid.

These can only be elicited by careful questioning. Some patients will talk very spontaneously about their delusions and express a wide variety of illogical ideas. Other patients will need to be questioned. Paranoid delusions are often persecutory and to elicit them requires bland questions which do not arouse the patient's suspicions too strongly. Such questions are 'Are people treating you as they should?' or 'How are people behaving towards you, do you suppose?' are often quite useful. Enquire about the patient's attitude to his own self. Ask whether he feels he has changed in any way, or whether he feels he is a good or bad person. This may help to elicit feelings of guilt and self-recrimination.

Hypochondriacal ideas   It is important to recognise that hypochondriacal concern is an extremely common finding amongst psychiatric patients. Thus the anxious patient may have a considerable amount of hypochondriacal fears surrounding bodily symptoms of anxiety such as palpitations etc. On the other hand the severely depressed patient may present with severe hypochondriasis which may well be missed by the examining doctor until he is aware of the significance of hypochondriasis in depression (see Depression). Bizarre hypochondriacal notions tend to be found in schizophrenia.

Obsessive compulsive phenomena   Here one should enquire about habits surrounding various aspects of the patient's daily life. For instance the patient with an obsessional disorder may have rituals concerned with washing and eating etc. which he feels obliged to carry out, and which occasion him much discomfort. Very often the patient will be extremely ashamed of this type of symptom and discuss it only with difficulty.

Perception

Here one records hallucinations and illusions, noting the modality of the hallucination and its content. Also the occasions in which they tend to occur. Perceptions may be heightened or dulled in certain toxic and delirious states by *hallucinogenic drugs*. Dreams are good examples of normal hallucinosis. Hallucinations may occur in *organic mental states* and in *psychoses* such as *schizophrenia* where they are *usually auditory*. False perceptions or *illusions* can occur in *fatigue, drug intoxication, organic mental states* and *schizophrenia*.

Cognitive testing

Clinical testing of cognitive ability has traditionally included:

Tests of orientation—what is the day?—where are you?—what is the date?

Tests of concentration—say the days of the week backwards—take away 7 from 100 and go on subtracting (the serial sevens test).

Tests of memory—try to remember this name and address and telephone number. (Repeat immediately and after 2 or 5 minutes.)—asking the patient to try and remember an irrelevant sentence, *e.g.* 'One thing a nation must have to be rich and great is a large secure supply of wood.'—asking the patient to try and remember a pointless story, *e.g.* A fire in New York, cowboy and his dog, a donkey loaded with salt. (Three stories which provide a good store of unintentional humour treasured by connoisseurs.)

General information—name the monarch/president/prime minister and their two predecessors—name five capitals—name five large towns—identify a combination of coins—identify famous people ranging from Wyatt Earp through Jesus Christ to Che Guevara.

These relatively simple tests have long been taken for granted as being useful but Hinton and Withers (1971) have cast doubt on this in a study designed to evaluate their reliability and usefulness. They used three forms of a general clinical test which included orientation, concentration, memory function and general information along the lines already described. They suspected that this type of test was quick, haphazard and probably rather useful but their validity was questioned. Six hypotheses were tested, *e.g.* that a high test score would correlate with high IQ, length of education and repeated tests whilst a low score would correlate with organic cerebral disease, age and affective symptoms.

Three forms of the test were administered to 24 adults and then to 57 male and 51 female consecutive admissions. The general findings were that the IQ levels significantly affected the score whilst age and length of schooling were not relevant, organic cerebral disease correlated significantly with test scores whilst repeated tests and affective symptoms were more or less neutral. The final conclusion that emerged was that the tests of orientation and general information were useful, as were serial sevens and the recall of a name and address after five minutes. The digit span and repeating the days of the week backwards were found to be relatively useless.

Insight

It is extremely difficult to assess insight. It is quite simple to regard insight as merely the expression of a patient's awareness of illness. In fact the term insight should be used to cover the patient's awareness not only of the fact that he is ill or regarded as ill, but also as a term that covers the implications of his illness as extensively as possible.

Does the patient understand the repercussions of his illness on other people? Does he appreciate that his behaviour, emotions and interpersonal relationships may have become tangled in such a way that family, friends and relatives are bewildered? Is he aware that he may be manipulating others to meet his own neurotic needs? Does the patient regard the illness as an alien experience which has appeared out of the blue or does he regard the experience as one that is totally interwoven with his whole existence? Has he any idea of the way in which the illness may leave him with some degree of social or personal handicap?

These are only a few of the questions that have to be asked in assessing insight, and it will therefore be realised that comments such as 'Patient has no insight' or 'Patient has little insight' are really without meaning.

However the examination of the mental state does not necessarily stop short with the scheme already outlined. In particular cases more detailed examination is needed, these include:

1 Patients with suspected organic cerebral disease
2 Stuporose patients

The following guidelines are intended for use in such cases:

THE PSYCHIATRIC EXAMINATION OF PATIENTS WITH SUSPECTED ORGANIC CEREBRAL DISEASE

Mayer, Gross and Guttman (1937) set out a scheme for the examination of these patients. It cannot be bettered and is now a standard in clinical psychiatry. The following section is based entirely on it though it is somewhat condensed. The object of this type of examination is to back up the basic psychiatric and neurological examination and it consists of enquiries and simple clinical tests which can detect organic cerebral impairment.

Emotional state

The patient's mood should be assessed in the course of general conversation. Special points to look for as indicators of organicity include *euphoria* —where the mood is quite out of keeping with the patient's general situation, and *lability* where the mood veers quickly and spontaneously from tears to laughter. Fatuous inane jocularity or witzelsucht is an important sign of frontal lobe damage. *Apathy and irritability* are also common in dementia.

Attention and concentration

This is an important area to examine carefully. The *clouded patient* finds it hard to focus his attention, seems abstracted and has to pull himself up to bring himself back to answer questions. The *demented* patient may seem to be striving to attend to what is going on but is unable to bring enough concentration to bear on the topic to make an adequate answer and tends to lapse into apologetic uncomfortable silences. *Rigidity* of thinking is often revealed in *perseveration* where the patient cannot shift easily from one topic to another and keeps trying to formulate a clearer answer to a question asked several minutes beforehand.

Memory

Memory disturbance is one of the key symptoms of organic cerebral disease. It is best to start by asking the patient about general topics such as how (in detail) he spent the previous day, what topics in the papers and on TV have interested him, what book he has read lately, the author's name and what the book was about. More specific tests of memory include asking the patient to listen to a name, address and telephone number, read out aloud to him, then to ask him to repeat it back immediately, to try and remember it and then five minutes later to ask him to reproduce it. But apart from this, especially where a patient has memory loss, say following head injury, it is important to find out as exactly as possible the duration of amnesia before and after the injury.

Speech

Speech disturbance includes dysarthria as well as aphasia. Aphasia is often missed and gives rise to a false impression of dementia when in fact the patient is aphasic and has no general cerebral impairment. Also it is important always to realise that speech disturbance is difficult to interpret without full knowledge of the patient's previous speech and intellectual level. So that for practical purposes the psychiatrist should be content to *recognise* aphasia and leave its clarification to the expert. Testing for aphasia involves naming, noting the patient's use of grammar and syntax, noting the use of reiterated phrases and monosyllables.

Motor behaviour

Look for anomalies of movement, gesture and expression. Find out if the patient is *apraxic, i.e.* can he carry out normal simple day-to-day activities like dressing, opening a book, folding a paper, lighting a cigarette. Also it is important to note the general level of spontaneous and purposive activity. Simple tests of writing and drawing are also useful ways to reveal diminished awareness of spatial relationships.

Body image

The patient should be asked if he can distinguish right from left, a simple test usually overlooked. After this one attempts to find out the patient's awareness of spatial relationships on his body, *e.g.* can he recognise common objects by feel and texture, has he any odd awareness or lack of awareness of any part of his body?

Visual

Apart from assessing the patient's basic function such as visual acuity and colour sense it is important to find out if his visual attention and recollection are correct, *e.g.* to describe familiar objects, to recognise various objects, tell the time and be aware of perspective and distance. *Note:* This type of test *presumes* normal speech function.

Reading tests are used here too but again their interpretation is an expert matter if aphasia is present and gives a false impression of dyslexia.

Summary

The general examination of these patients described here is to be used as a clinical screening procedure which will need to be backed up by expert neurological and psychological examination.

EXAMINATION OF STUPOROSE PATIENTS

The examination of non-cooperative and stuporose patients has been set out by authors such as Kirby (1921) who directs the clinician towards noting:

1 The patients degree of reactivity to the situation being examined, *i.e.* Is he passive or voluntary, awkward or natural in posture? How does he behave towards those who try to interview or examine him? What degree of spontaneous behaviour does he show? Has he control over bowels or bladder?

2 Expression. Does he react facially to what is said? Does he resist examination?

3 Cooperation. How does he follow instructions, requests or commands?

4 Muscular reactions. Are there any disturbances of muscle tone? Are there any disturbances of facial expression?

5 Emotional reaction. How does he react to references to personal topics?

6 Speech and writing. What disorders are detectable?

CONCLUSION

Examining the mental state is difficult and essential. Too many psychiatric records are rendered illusory by comments such as " ?Schiz R/ inj ———".

Careful description of the mental state in as detailed form as possible remains the nub of good clinical psychiatry. After the history and mental state have been described the careful clinician should always write out a concise *formulation of the provisional diagnosis* and back it up with a prognosis and plans for treatment.

PSYCHOLOGY AND PSYCHIATRY—THE USES OF PSYCHOLOGICAL TESTING

Most doctors are suspicious of psychology to the extent of reacting to the word in an uncertain and often hostile way that cloaks the dim remains of undergraduate experience in which 'psychology' was covered in a small number of lectures given in a rather sneering manner by an academic physiologist. *Psychology* is not only a highly complex study but also it is a subject that many doctors approach in a way that resembles the theological concept of 'invincible ignorance'. This is an interesting point since it might be thought that a 'rounded' medical education would equip doctors with at least an adequate appreciation of the vagaries and normalities of human behaviour. Unhappily, despite the attempts of well intentioned and progressive medical schools this is still not the case. Worse still the 'psychologically aware' medical student tends too easily to wear his awareness like a supporters club scarf and negates the usefulness of what he has been taught in self-righteous overconfidence.

Doctors, are too often encouraged to be insensitive and moralistic and trained in a way that banishes commonsense, replacing it with omniscience and ratty timidity disguised as knowledgeable concern. This probably leads to a barely concealed antipathy between doctors and psychologists. Doctors however, despite these handicaps, do cure the physically ill, use improved medical technology, save lives and generally behave in a way that defies the comment 'I don't like him/her, but he/she is a good doctor'. Psychology is a discipline that encompasses science and art in much the same way that medicine does. The doctor relies on clinical experience, the psychologist relies on statistics and in so doing knows that this is a subject that can make even the most trendily educated doctor break out into a cold sweat.

In psychiatry this often leads to conflict since the psychiatrist values hunches and carries the approval of society in so doing even to the extent of recommending brain surgery, whilst the clinical psychologist, armed with valid and reliable knowledge of human behaviour, is not permitted to take responsibility for anything or anyone without the approval of a doctor who may have been qualified for only a year but has official sanction for an authority that must seem illusory. When this is backed up by a tendency to regard psychology as a sort of mental Path. Lab. service it is hardly surprising that there are tensions between the two disciplines.

For these reasons it is not possible, nor even permissible to do more than refer briefly to some of the uses of psychological testing. Proper understanding of psychology—what it is about, what are its practical uses are best available to the psychiatrist in consultation with a professional colleague in a relationship of sensible parity.

Psychological testing—psychometry

The term psychometry is anathema to some since it seems to imply an attempt to measure the immeasurable—nevertheless, like psychiatry, it is a term and a professional activity that we are, so to speak, stuck with. There is a store of measurements of human behaviour, perception and feeling that is now generally acceptable. These measurements are relative, *i.e.* people are compared one with another in the absence of absolute measurements of 'normal' behaviour. This is something that is often criticised with the question 'how can you tell what or who is abnormal?' The pedant would point out that in science there are no absolute units of measurement—all measurement is relative. A more relevant point is that psychological measurement is a way of finding out an individual's distance from the average. Thus statistical techniques amplify psychological measurements since statistics measure probabilities (*i.e.* 'have I backed the right horse?') and distribution about the mean. In psychological terms 'normal' and 'abnormal' are *entirely statistical* in that a person is placed in relation to the mean and compared to it by *standard deviation* from it, *i.e.* 'how far is he/she from the mean?'

Tests are standardised, *i.e.* everyone gets the same test that is given to properly stratified samples of the population in the expectation that the test will be valid, *i.e.* it should measure what it is meant to measure, and reliable, *i.e.* it should measure the attribute in a consistent fashion.

Psychological testing is most commonly used to measure ability (*i.e.* by intelligence tests) and to assess personality in terms of dominant characteristics (*i.e.* typology).

Having established that psychometric testing is only a minimal part of psychology we may arbitrarily select *those aspects of* psychometry that interweave with clinical psychiatry.

These include:

1 Tests of ability—these are mainly concerned with the measurement of intellectual function, *e.g. intelligence tests*

- Tests aimed at revealing organic cerebral impairment

3 Tests aimed at investigating personality attributes and traits
4 Tests aimed at detecting specific psychological abnormalities

Intelligence tests

The definition of intelligence and the concept of the intelligence quotient is referred to in the chapter on subnormality. In essence it can be said that intelligence has never been satisfactorily defined in contrast to the enormous industry that goes into giving people IQ tests. Certainly in the English-speaking world the average person is more likely to have his intelligence tested than to be vaccinated against smallpox. Some regard intelligence as an ability to learn, others as a capacity to adapt, others as the ability to deal with the abstract, to form concepts, to think, one might almost say. Great weight is attached to IQ scores; they can influence a child's educational chances, or a man's chance of job training or promotion, and yet intelligence remains undefined beyond the somewhat dubious assumption that it is something that is successfully measured by intelligence tests.

In general the tests used assess a person's verbal and arithmetical ability as well as his ability to see relationships between objects and make concepts out of them and his ability to manipulate objects in a mechanical sense. The most popular tests are the *Wechsler* (WAIS) and the *Stanford Binet*. The former is undoubtedly the most widely used, is well standardised and appears to be valid and reliable. The other advantage it has is that it is said to measure the IQ regardless of any educational influences.

In England the *Raven Progressive Matrices* and the *Mill Hill Vocabulary Scale* are also used and remain of particular interest to psychiatrists since they can be administered by psychiatrists and give good results and thus save the time of clinical psychologists for more relevant work.

Tests of organic cerebral impairment

Testing for organic cerebral impairment consists usually in employing a variety of tests which can detect such organic defects as:
1 Aphasia
2 Dyslexia
3 Defects in visual motor coordination
4 Defects in memory and concentration

5 Organic thinking disturbance, *e.g.* defective handling of concepts, inability to move from the concrete to the abstract
6 Perceptual disturbance, *i.e.* inability to see size, space and perspective relationships, to see shapes and groupings, to assemble objects by colour and shape, to draw and reproduce shapes and designs
7 Visual memory tests
Organic impairment may be revealed by characteristic performances in IQ tests such as the WAIS. Other tests used include the
1 Bender Gestalt test—the patient is required to copy designs
2 Goldstein Scheerer—a test to elicit defects in concrete and abstract thinking, consisting of five sets (colour sorting, object sorting, colour form sorting, object sorting, stick test)
3 Benton Visual Retention test—a test of visual memory
It should be emphasised that *testing for organic impairment*, like all psychological testing, produces the best results when a wide range of tests is employed rather than one or two.

Personality tests

Many clinical psychologists would concede that tests designed to reveal personality traits or even to measure them are the most contentious and equivocal test procedures that are available. Yet despite this, psychiatrists tend to ask for this type of test to be carried out usually in the hope of clarifying diagnostic doubt and therapeutic uncertainty. Personality tests fall into two main categories: *projective tests* which are designed to reveal unconscious psychological processes and tendencies and *objective tests* which are designed to reveal personality characteristics or traits, *i.e.* a test which may quantify personality.

The projective test is in principle simple since it is a standardised test situation where the patient is required to give his interpretation of an *ambiguous stimulus*. The two most popular are the *Rorschach* and the *Thematic Apperception Test* (*TAT*). In the former the patient is required to describe what he sees in a series of patterns. The literature on the Rorschach is enormous, the methods of scoring responses is by any standards obscure and the results are on the whole hardly to be taken seriously.

In the *TAT* the patient is given a series of ambiguous inartistic illustrations and asked to describe the situations that they represent. In both instances current opinion is that these projective tests are probably the best of a pretty unhelpful series.

Objective tests of personality traits suggest by their category a style of brisk scientific efficiency contrasting strongly with the seeming mythology of projective testing.

Unfortunately *objective tests of personality* have not proved as credible and useful as all that, though they have in some instances been accepted as more useful than projective tests.

Many objective tests are based on questionnaires—the theory being that if a sufficiently extensive questionnaire is designed to cover every conceivable type of psychological abnormality then careful statistical analysis of answers to questionnaires given by large numbers of respondents will reveal clusters of answers which will suggest statistically significant factors A, B, C, D, etc., each of which may be related by association, *i.e.* by statistical correlation with a previously defined psychological abnormality. The abnormality may be indicated by the presence of the respondent along a continuum that extends from intraversion → extraversion, nice → nasty, or even croquet player → Millwall F.C. supporter.

On the other hand the factors extracted may suggest the respondent's place in a general category, *e.g.* psychotic/neurotic/normal/uncertain or hysteric/depressed/paranoid/psychopath, etc.

Actually it is as usual not quite as simple as that.

The idea of *trait personality* is seductive, especially to doctors whose education is based on a reductionist philosophy where the whole is broken down into a functional series. This is an excellent approach to human physiology in which we may separate respiration from reproduction and reproduction from alimentary function, although anyone who has experienced sexual desire or even love must have noticed that the reproductive drive seems to affect respiration now and again, also the heart rate at times and appetite some of the time.

Trait psychology is an interesting school which started with the observations of those psychologists who suspected that human behaviour could be measured by using a methodology based on a philosophical concept of human behaviour (or as some might say humanity—not to say being a real person) that assumed that a reductionist principle should be applied to the understanding of being. Now there is good scientific evidence to support reductionism as a philosophical construct which can be sensibly used to examine the functions of the cardiovascular system, the alimentary system, but when it comes to the *mind* we are really in difficulties because we don't know what the word mind means and this makes a reductionist approach superfluous, or in contemporary jargon irrelevant. And yet the reductionist approach to psychological problems, like an ever rolling steam roller, rolls on and with about as much effectiveness as a steam roller employed as a butterfly catcher. Reductionism *is* attractive—there ought to be ways of splintering human experience into measurable dimensions but really there does not seem to be any credible evidence to support such a concept of human existence. Professor H. J. Eysenck is probably the most influential experimental psychologist in the world. His views and findings are stated with enviable clarity and represent reductionism at its most absolute. Yet some have demonstrated inconsistencies in 'Eysenckian' theory and express doubts about a reductionistic philosophy that relates eye-blink conditioning to conditionability and a whole theory of personality typology. (Christie, 1956; Storms & Sigal, 1958; Hamilton, 1959; Lykenn, 1959; Becker, 1960; Champion, 1961; Foulds, 1961.)

Many tests of personality are designed to uncover dominant traits and characteristics. There are many such tests but in practice there are two that are the most widely used: they are the EPI (Eysenck Personality Inventory) and the MMPI (Minnesota Multiphasic Personality Inventory). The EPI employs a short series of questions that have been shown to correlate well with the concepts of intraversion–extraversion thus placing the respondent in an identifiable scale of neuroticism.

MMPI (Minnesota Multiphasic Personality Inventory) This questionnaire consists of over 500 items. The questions are designed in such a way as to tap attitudes in the respondent which may be construed as indicating in the personality the presence of elements going to make up a personality structure and also to reveal the presence of elements resembling certain clinical psychiatric syndromes.

6

Causes of psychiatric disorder

The causes of psychiatric disorder are generally regarded as 'multi-factorial'. Some features of aetiology are now reviewed under this general heading.

PSYCHOANALYTIC THEORY, PSYCHOANALYSIS AND RELATED SCHOOLS

It is impossible to consider the history of psychiatry in the 20th Century without acknowledging the extent of the influence of psychoanalytic theory. As we have seen Freud's earliest observations were set out in a period when psychiatry seemed to have reached an impasse since the work of the descriptive psychiatrists of the 19th Century had led seemingly to psychiatric practice being regarded as the differential diagnosis of untreatable disease, with apparently no basic discoveries in the offing. So it is not surprising that a doctor who advanced an articulate and credible theory of psychiatric illness and human behaviour soon found support after initial hostility.

As events have turned out the most lasting influence of psychoanalytic theory has occurred in America where it has coloured not only psychiatry but has extended into popular attitudes towards the understanding of human behaviour. In Europe and in the United Kingdom the influence of psychoanalytic theory has been implicit rather than explicit and many psychoanalytic concepts have been adopted in a covert fashion. In the

United Kingdom psychiatry has been influenced by the traditions of empiricism and eclectism rather than by dogma, nevertheless many British psychiatrists use a Freudian-psychodynamic orientation without admitting that they do so in any formal sense. For most psychiatrists Freudian theory is faulted in its methodology—the theories and hypotheses remain untested and, some would suspect untestable.

And for many the main faults of Freudian theory have been centred around its excessive preoccupation with the individual when it seems likely that any scientific examination of human behaviour is most rigorously derived from data drawn from large numbers.

But for the outsider Freudian theory attracts by its basic simplicity, an approach that has influenced many social scientists, in particular those concerned with the dynamics of interpersonal and family relationships. The basis of psychoanalytic theory as proposed by Freud was derived from his clinical observations on patients and the mechanisms of their illnesses and led to his theories of libido, instinct and ego psychology, all of which were based on his basic contention that unconscious drive and motivation provided the springs of behaviour—a theory which is strongly deterministic in tone. No one would deny that unconscious forces *are* important but many reject the notion that they dominate human behaviour totally.

Freud's whole outlook was scientific. He and his contemporaries were a new breed of psychiatrists influenced by Darwin and Helmholtz rather than by the mysticism and metaphysics of earlier years but the weakness of Freudian theory was that it was based on highly selected cases. Thus a combination of biased sampling and biased observation led to deductions that negate the validity of the theoretical system.

Freud's first psychiatric investigations started when he began to treat cases of hysteria in collaboration with Breuer; in particular with the treatment of Anna O. a 21 year old girl with multiple hysterical manifestations. Under hypnosis she revealed to Breuer forgotten and unconscious fantasies which seemed relevant to her condition and this stimulated Freud's curiosity about her, and other cases and led him to theorise about the psychological causes of hysteria in general and about the role of repressed sexuality as a force in the aetiology of neurosis. To appreciate the real strength of such an idea it should always be realised that Freud brought out his theories at a time when sexual life was a forbidden topic obscured by guilt—at least for middle class people. The upper classes were not accessible to study and the working classes were regarded as rather dull people anyway.

Freud was impressed by the role of strong emotion, concealed sexuality and concealed aggression as background factors in neurosis and found that his patients were more able to talk about disturbing topics if they were encouraged to lie down and talk about *anything* that came into their head without fear of disapproval or hope of encouragement. This became known as *free association* and was the foundation of psychoanalysis. In time this relatively simple technique was modified; the theory was expanded by Freud and his followers but the intelligent humanity of the concept remains unchanged—the psychiatrist should always be someone to whom the patient can talk freely and without prejudice either way. Freudian theory has become an area of study in its own right; the literature is enormous, the varieties of influence of Freudian Theory in psychiatry, psychology and sociology extensive but there are a number of basic concepts and statements that are part of the language of psychiatry— whether or not their theoretical basis is acceptable.

Freud's early *theory of the mind* was topographical—mental activity is represented in three regions, the preconscious, the conscious and the unconscious. The *preconscious* is said to develop in childhood, is accessible to the conscious and the unconscious but functions mainly as a control over the unconscious bringing the child nearer to an adult mode of existence. The *unconscious* is regarded as a store of repressed feelings and thoughts, inaccessible to consciousness from which they are excluded by *censorship* or *repression*. The content of the unconscious is tied to instinct and wish fulfilment; both represented in 'primary process thinking' where wishes are seen as already fulfilled with no checks on the gratification of immediate and urgent desires. Thus primary process thinking is said to be manifest in psychosis. The *conscious* is regarded as the monitor of aware behaviour. Freud regarded conscious mental life as mainly an attentive and perceptive type of central nervous activity, but, he suggested the *bulk* of mental activity was at an unconscious level.

It is hard to quarrel with the idea of a simple tiered array of mental activity as stated by Freud. It is in line with what is known of brain/mind activity and has an admirable parsimony to it. For example conscious awareness is necessarily relatively constricted in being limited to the person's attempts to make sense of the massive information flow that is the essence of the waking state. Unless there was a way of selecting the relevant for the scrutiny of consciousness the brain/mind system would be overrun by an overload of information. There is already considerable evidence, for instance, that in schizophrenic psychoses the patient is unable to discriminate the irrelevant from the relevant and so is left in a state of bewildered muddled thinking where casual trivia obscure his ability to construe accurately what is going on around him. Freud also pointed out that conflicting motives and drives in the unconscious could spill over into consciousness in a revealing way that illuminated their concealed reality, *e.g.* in slips of the tongue, in forgetting to carry out unwanted acts, in revealing unconscious hostility etc.

Psychological mechanisms

Freud suggested that the personality was essentially a dynamic flexible unity in which function was modified by a process of dynamic interaction. This led to his concept of a structural model of the personality based on the interactions between the *Id*, the *Ego* and the *Superego*. This theory has been modified by many including Anna Freud and Hartmann.

The Id   This is a generic name given to a reservoir of instinctual drive based on physiological needs such as sex, hunger, thirst etc. and psychological needs, *e.g.* rage, aggression etc. The Id is regarded as instinctual and innate.

The Ego   This is the conscious self, the conglomerate of the personality that is presented to others. The Ego perceives, directs behaviour, is involved in problem solving and is concerned with the preservation of the integrity of the personality via various defence mechanisms. Ego activity is concerned with *reality* and, according to Freud, is guided by the *reality principle*, another way of describing the homeostatic tendencies of human behaviour, in contrast to the primitive biological strivings of the Id. This was described by Freud as the *pleasure principle*.

In Freudian theory the integrated effectiveness of the personality is summarised in the concept of *ego strength*—in other words the capability of the personality to be stable, resilient and flexible in its ways of dealing with stress and change and in its capacity to deal with threats to its integrity without reacting with rigid terror or overreacting with neurotic defence mechanisms.

The Superego   This is the controller of ego activity, it monitors and assesses the acceptability of ego performance. Thus superego activity is moral in tone since the superego constantly compares ego activity to the needs and value systems of society in general and in particular to approved and established behaviour in infancy which conforms to the expectations of basic authority figures such as parents. Superego function is based on values conceptualised in childhood as the result of the child identifying with the parents. If the parents are rigid and punitive the child becomes influenced by censorious attitudes.

Thus the superego develops the function of modulating and checking ill directed ego behaviour. This is thought to be its normal operation but it is recognised that where the superego is overactive, rigid or irrational then this will cause psychological handicap.

Freud's theory of personality and ego structure is attractive but really hardly goes beyond assertion. Hence though the neatness of the theory is accepted, the lack of proof of its validity remains as the weak point in a whole system of belief that has influenced not only a whole concept of treatment but has influenced 20th Century culture in diverse ways.

We are entitled to question the Freudian concept of normality and this question becomes more urgent if the theory influences a society's definitions of normality. Examples of the latter have included the fact that large organisations particularly in America have specified the desirable 'normal' attributes of 'good corporation men', based almost entirely on Freudian speculative hypotheses. The individual needs to be protected from the arbitrary and intensive activities of large organisations who operate in this way. Behaviour can hardly be given approval or condemnation purely on the say so of a school of psychiatry. Furthermore there is an essentially sinister absurdity about well meaning desires to mould personalities to meet the norms of society.

Personality development

In Freud's theory personality development is based on three stages of infantile maturation and infantile sexuality. Infantile sexuality turned out to be Freud's most effective bombshell since for a century or more before childhood was regarded as a time of unblemished sexual innocence. The view was in contrast to the realities of life say in Victorian England where child brothels and child prostitutes were common, children were exploited sexually and on the labour market.

19th Century childish sexual innocence may well have been a comforting middle class fantasy which bore no relation to the brutality of life of a working class that had no articulate voice. It is to Freud's great credit that he challenged the certainty of many of the comforting platitudes of the day and tried to encourage man to take a long cool look at himself.

The phases of infantile sexuality start with the oral phase in which sexual pleasure is centred on oral satisfaction by eating, sucking etc. Failure of maturation beyond this stage is shown in the oral character, *i.e.* one who is passive, overdependent and overinvolved in eating, drinking and talking etc. The anal phase extends into the second and third years and is directed towards the control of bowel action. Having regular bowel action and clean pants is a way of pleasing parents and allaying their fears of faecal soiling, a badge of failure which makes them feel incompetent if not neglectful parents. The 'anal' character fixed at this level of psychological development is said to be rigid, stubborn, overconscientious and overscrupulous.

The genital (phallic) phase brings the child to the discovery of the pleasures of masturbation—a topic that has caused doctors and psychiatrists in the past to behave in a fashion which combined cruelty with total absurdity. Masturbation was thought to cause psychosis and even such eminent men as Henry Maudsley wrote about the stigmata of the secret and chronic masturbator. This sort of thing led to the ultimate in medical nonsense namely the antimasturbation garment (male and female) some of which were still catalogued by a Surgical Appliance Maker in England in 1938. Faced with a profession who regarded masturbation as a disease, Freud's comments on its normality brought down on his head the wrath of the antimasturbators. And yet now no one is bothered about masturbation, attitudes have gradually become more sensible. Entry into the genital phase leads the child towards adult sexuality, passing on the way the Oedipal situation where the child competes for parental sexual partnership at a level below consciousness, but given appropriate parental affection, emerges unscathed.

Neurotic defences and the Ego defence system

A central feature of psychoanalytic theory is the concept of an array of mechanisms, usually called *mental mechanisms* used by the ego to protect its integrity against the threat of anxiety. They include *repression*. In repression unacceptable desires and motives are buried below consciousness and are thus out of reach of ego activity. This mechanism is a basic way of dealing with anxiety provoking impulses and conflict by as it were pushing them out of sight. *Compensation* is a mechanism by which the individual's self-esteem is bolstered in the face of apparent personal deficiency typical examples of this include the promiscuous sexuality of the man haunted by fears of impotence, and in psychosis the erotic delusions of the ageing unloved spinster and in everyday life the belligerent pomposity of little men. *Regression* is a process in which an individual returns to an infantile role. This removes him from the necessity of facing problems let alone solve them and by ensuring him a dependent role reduces anxiety and enables him to be treated as a sick, dependent, helpless person.

Reaction formation is a mechanism by which strong impulses are converted into their opposite in order to conceal their reality. Thus hatred becomes solicitous concern and a sense of fear and inadequacy becomes cocky belligerence. *Rationalisation* is not a Freudian term but is in line with Freudian dogma. This is the means by which our conduct, our failures and mistakes are justified by reason. 'I didn't get the prize because I didn't really want it and so I didn't bother to try.' *Projection*, is a handy mechanism by which one's own more tiresome characteristics are attributed to others, *e.g.* 'If you weren't so unreasonable, rigid and paranoid you would be able to see that I am right.' *Displacement*, here a highly charged idea or feeling is relieved of its traumatic potential by shifting the charge to an idea that resembles it.

Intellectualisation, like rationalisation this mechanism diffuses intense emotion by giving it an intellectual detachment thus maintaining a hold on reality already threatened by the strength of the feeling concerned. *Denial* is straightforward negation of what is obviously true, especially if the truth provokes anxiety. *Sublimation* is the diversion of unacceptable impulses into acceptable activity. *Acting out* is a way of avoiding the unacceptable or painful by aggressive or impulsive but basically uncontrolled behaviour. Thus a conflict may be relieved by an explosive discharge. In the Acting Out situation the person is so overwhelmed by unconscious conflict that he resorts to action which depicts it, often physical or explosive—to divert the threat posed by the conflict. Some also use the term to cover any substituted activity produced by a person to avoid painful ideas, but this is, strictly speaking, not accurate. It is therefore not a catch all phrase used to describe any violent display but should be used to describe behaviour in which the person literally acts out the conflict.

The list of mechanisms is larger than this but these examples have been included to illustrate some basic psychoanalytical propositions. Psycho-analytic theory really stands or falls by the testability of these hypotheses. Clearly experience gives many examples of the ways in which psycho-analytic theory fits, and psychiatrists, being doctors, tend to value their own clinical experience with the saying 'I can only speak from my own experience'.

But in fact medicine has gone beyond mere clinical anecdote though it should be acknowledged that clinical experience is a start in the process of understanding the patient and his problems.

Summary

The psychoanalytic theories of neurosis and psychosis are beyond the scope of this volume. They do not readily lend themselves to a convenient summary and any attempt to do so is a travesty of the extensive writing and theorising on the topics that have appeared over the years. A common thread that runs through the theory of neurosis and psychosis is one which emphasises conflict, and in particular sexual conflict relating to unacceptable sexual impulses.

Conflict is viewed as a dynamic state which can be worked through, *i.e.* accepted, examined and resolved without self-deception, given an adequate state of emotional maturity. Conflict which is not worked through but which is dealt with by stratagems and defence is a likely source of neurotic disturbance. Inevitably regression is crucial in the genesis of neurosis by concealing and smothering drives below con-sciousness and leading into further unconscious conflict. Specific examples include hysteria in which the dynamic mechanism is one where intolerable stress whether real, fantasised or distorted is rendered harmless by trans-forming the psychic response to stress into functional loss and immobility. Thus painful stresses are rendered harmless by switching out the response. Again in obsessional disorder the obsessions and compulsions etc. are seen as defences against painful impulses. The obsessional act is dis-sociated from feeling and the anxiety provoking nature of the stimulus becomes lost. Similarly phobic states are seen as expressions of symbolic fears.

Psychiatrists and others may disagree about the ultimate value of psychoanalytic theory, but many psychiatrists use its basic concepts in trying to explain psychiatric disorders. Above all psychoanalytic theory has emphasised the importance of the individual as a person who has a right to his own thoughts and feelings—it has been a humanising influence in an inhuman time where the individual has become devalued by materialism, rapid growth technology and loss of value systems.

Alfred Adler

Alfred Adler was a psychiatrist who saw the concepts of mind and body as totally interrelated. Early in his career he was a colleague of Freud but separated from him since he was interested in the *aims* of neurosis and psychosis whilst Freud was more interested in their fuel sources. Adler developed his own theory of personality in which he emphasised and stressed human activity as purposeful and introduced two terms, 'life goal' and 'life style'. The latter has become part of contemporary jargon but for Adler it had meaning since he viewed human behaviour as a constant struggle in which the individual starts life with generalised feelings of dependence and inadequacy. The 'inferiority complex' Adler saw as a prime influence in personality development straining towards a 'life goal' —a stage of idealised superiority and independence and the 'life style'—a person's mode of coping with the world and being involved but a mode selected on the basis of childhood and adolescent development—leading to a way of living that has meaning and consistency.

Adler's theory of neurosis was based on feelings of failure, psychosis was viewed as the breakthrough of fantasy overriding any drive the person might have. The Adlerian school eschewed conventional diagnosis in favour of special consideration of every individual. Adlerian theory is oversimple and may be criticised in the same way as Freudian and Jungian theory since they are unverifiable assertions rather than testable hypotheses.

Carl Jung

Jung's contributions to psychiatry are mainly to do with his theories of mental life, in particular with his theory of the unconscious. Freud saw the unconscious as a driving force which somehow derived its energy from the repressed material that it contained; a turbulent ferment of fantasy and feeling. Jung saw the unconscious as a template of behaviour which became more intense and obvious and more effective with age—the unconscious is a true 'psyche' in the sense that it is a primary force present from birth which drives the individual on but never reaches total conscious awareness. It follows from this assumption that fantasies and dreams are not distorted images that symbolise the unacceptable but are in fact a programme of the individual's drives and experience.

Jung's theories are beyond the scope of this work, they can only be appreciated by studying his writings and those of the Jungian school. It is hard to estimate the extent of Jung's influence although he left behind words such as archetype which are hard to understand. However it is never wise to dismiss a topic merely because the language describing it is hard to follow. Jung stressed the importance of the unconscious in a different way than Freud. Freud emphasised its personal relevance, Jung emphasised its collective, *i.e.* general relevance. In other words the unconscious mental processes were not regarded as being the personal property of the individual but rather as a fragment of a pool of unconscious mental life built up not only from personal–instinctual drives but also from the inherited unconscious drives of the human race. And it was essentially this view of the unconscious that formed the basis of Jung's concept of *analytical psychology*.

Jung was also very concerned with *personality typology* in terms of introversion–extroversion. For Jung the term *libido* had an entirely different meaning than the Freudian meaning which stressed sexual energy as a basic motive force. In Jungian terms the *libido* was a life force; a drive to exist and to survive. Jung had earlier been a contemporary of Freud who had at first agreed with his ideas but later not only disagreed with him publicly but also privately in correspondence which did little beyond confirming the suspicions of many that psychiatrists are an embittered quarrelsome set of naive meddlers with the minds of others.

Jung's *analytical psychology* is mystical rather than personal and, as such defies any attempt to derive any heuristic merit. However, at the same time it does provide a fascinating store of speculation about the potential collective varieties of dynamic forces that may shape the individual's psychological drives and life experience. His early references to the collective unconscious (objective psyche) postulate the independent existence of a person's subjective experience in terms of memory traces and mystic forces that lend to each person a separate individuality based on ineffable metaphysical influences and drives.

The *archetype*, a nebulous conglomerate of instinctual drives, furnishes a basis for the *self*, the *persona* and *complexes*. The *self* strives towards ideal existence, the *persona* is the outward display by which a person identifies himself to the world and the *complexes* refer to groups of associations of ideas and instincts that may lead, psychopathologically either to neurosis or psychosis. Jung's strength lay in his perceptions of general roots of behaviour, his weakness lay in his failure adequately to define them.

Thus the study of a person's problems becomes highly individualised in terms of understanding their general and collective origins which makes paramount the special description of dreams, fantasies and wishes in terms that have more of the flavour of classical texts of metaphysics than of the objective description of an understanding of personal drives coloured by psychosocial influences. For these reasons Jungian theory has a special quality that serves to illuminate for some, but leaves the majority in some degree of perplexed falure to understand just exactly what it is that Jungian theory is really all about.

THE BRAIN AND BEHAVIOUR

It is commonly said that the brain is the organ of the mind. This is a simple statement but like many simple statements it needs careful consideration since simplicity does not imply absolute truth. In fact all we can really infer from it is that the brain is an organ of indeterminate function since the word 'mind' is used to encompass a range of activity assumed to be based on an intact 'normal' brain. We may apply a reductionist principle to the concept 'mind' and break it down into a series of recognisable characteristics including consciousness, perception, emotion, thought and learning etc. or summarise functions as general abilities or characteristics such as 'intelligence' or 'personality' but we are left with the realisation that the word 'mind' is indefinable since it is hard to avoid becoming entangled with questions about the relation of psyche to soma—classical problems that have produced much philosophy but no adequate scientific answers.

The dilemma of mind–body relations pervades psychiatry, often the issues seem impractical since most psychiatric disorders occur in the absence of demonstrable somatic correlates. Even in organic mental disorders there is often a considerable disparity between organic damage and the extent of mental disturbance. The gap between the two may seem narrow but at the end of it we are left with philosophical speculations as guide lines. We may accept the hierarchical monism of Aristotle and Aquinas or we may accept the dualism of Descartes or we may accept an existential formulation which gives primacy to psychic events, but which-ever way we turn we are left with a philosophical dilemma.

However, the psychiatrist has to be practical so that while the philo-sophical dilemma is acknowledged, it is reasonable to accept the statement 'the brain is the organ of the mind' with reservations and try and make use of a model of brain activity that seems to make sense. The brain is a highly complex system (ten billion cells) in which information is accepted, coded, stored and retrieved and which maintains the living organism in a homeo-static state in relation to the internal and external environment. Informa-tion is monitored in such a way that appropriate responses can be made, in short leading to purposive and economical behaviour.

The basic control system of the brain and central nervous system is thought to be based on simple feed back loops where input modulates output and thus maintains stability. The basic cortical apparatus of the human brain: frontal, parietal, temporal and occipital lobes are at the highest level of evolutionary development and are most advanced in man. Localisation of cerebral function is partially understood but the circuitry is not except in hypothetical terms.

In recent years interest has centred on the hypothalamus and its links with the limbic and reticular systems. The reticular system and the medullary centres are thought to be the site of the central nervous system servomechanisms. The reticular system, extending downwards from the pons, is essentially a long column of cells whose physiology is unclear but which appears to serve internal homeostasis and at the same time pass on information upwards. The role of the reticular system is seen as one of maintaining and balance between 'arousal' and 'rest', the two states being represented by sympathetic and parasympathetic activity respectively, thus maintaining alert consciousness or sleep according to the demands of the environment and the needs of the individual.

The reticular system receives information about cardiovascular and respiratory activity, transmits its output to higher levels, *i.e.* the cortex, on which it exerts a negative feedback effect. In other words it modulates cortical impulses in a simple servomechanism fashion, *e.g.* if muscular exertion requires a higher blood pressure and pulse rate, this information is relayed to the cortex via the hypothalamus. Presumably the cortex scans the signals and the hypothalamus/reticular system modulates the response.

In recent years also there has been much attention directed at the limbic system (cingulate gyrus, hippocampus, indusium griseum, amygda-loid and septa) as a modulator of emotion. Both these models of brain activity are based on electronic circuitry and the information processing of computers, and are regarded by some as a dehumanised way of looking at human behaviour—this is less than fair. They are merely ways of trying to explain the activity of a complex system in as simple a way as possible and the idea of a servomechanism *is* attractive *and* simple, though of course it may be as simple as saying 'the brain is the organ of the mind'. However, it is known that the basic element of the central nervous system, the neurone, is a conduction system that operates firstly by impulse transmission; a sinusoidal wave pattern carried by sequential electrical depolarisation along the nerve fibre, and secondly by on/off conduction between neurones at the synaptic level.

Having recognised a simple transmission mechanism it is reasonable to theorise that there must be essentially simple methods of processing the vast streams of impulses, all representing information that can only be encoded in the central nervous system in terms of numbers and frequency of stimuli. For instance, although seeing is different to hearing the conduction of visual impulses is identical with the conduction of auditory impulses, each causes the same type of neuronal activity, yet the interpretation of the two sets of signals is associated with wildly different subjective experience. All this makes the brain's scanning and selecting system serve highly complex requirements since modulation is needed to sharpen the image or direct attention to relevant stimuli in the environment. It is suggested that the limbic system may intensify or dissipate emotional experience and thus play a central role in human behaviour since it may present data to the cortex and transmit responses via the reticular system, altering arousal levels in response to external stimuli.

The study of brain activity has come a long way since the early days of the neuroanatomists Gall and Spurzheim, the first cerebral localisers and founders of phrenology—a 'science' that localised 'faith, firmness, love' etc. in definite areas of the brain. Clearly there *are* localised areas of function in the brain but at the same time it is increasingly realised that cerebral function is poorly understood and that it is a dynamic highly complex system based on simple elements.

Brain biochemistry and psychiatry

Interest in disordered brain biochemistry and its role in mental illness goes back a long way. Though it has been given considerable impetus since psychoactive drugs are so commonly used. Treatment has led to the

D

relatively new science of psychopharmacology. Many of the early observations were concerned with opium, for example *The Mysteries of Opium Revealed* by Dr. John Jones (1700) physician and cleric whose slightly zany writings remain an intriguing source work. He described the benefits of opium almost ecstatically.

'Therefore people do commonly call it a heavenly condition as if no worldly pleasure were to be compared with it . . . it has been compared (not without good cause) to a permanent gentle degree of that pleasure which modesty forbids the naming of. . . .'

Albrecht von Haller described the psychic effects of opium in more scientific fashion (1773) after having to take opium for urinary symptoms, but perhaps one of the earliest scientific works on psychopharmacology was Moreau de Tours (1845) book on *Hashish and Mental Illness* (1973).

Moreau belonged to the classic era of French descriptive psychiatry and clinical medicine. In *Hashish and Mental Illness* he described the use of hashish and its varied physiological and psychological effects based on his own experiences which led him to enquire further since he suspected that hashish might give clues to the understanding of mental illness since the substance produced striking effects on perception, feeling and behaviour. He was ahead of his time, so far ahead that he has been overlooked in recent reviews of cannabis effects—which mention Moreau only in passing. He listed eight main symptoms caused by hashish. These include euphoria, excitement and increased sensitivity, distortion of space/time perception, increased musical appreciation, paranoid ideas, mental disturbance, irresistible impulses and hallucinations. It is interesting to note his observations (1845) about chronic hashish use. One quote should suffice:

'A state of constant drowsiness, hebetude, mental apathy, and, as a consequence thereof, disappearance of spontaneity of action, willpower and the ability to make decisions. These psychic anomalies are visible by an expressionless physiognomy, a depressed, lax and languid countenance, dull eyes rolling unsteadily in the orbits, or with a robot-like immobility, drooping lips, slow movements without energy, etc. Such are some of the symptoms characteristic of the excessive use of hashish. We have had occasions to observe several examples of this.'

Then in 1892 Emil Kraepelin published a book on the psychic effects of morphia, tea, alcohol, chloral, ether and paraldehyde, and became the first systematic writer on the science he termed pharmacopsychology.

The important point made both by Moreau and Kraepelin is that we may learn about psychic processes from the examination of the effects on psychic processes produced by drugs.

Nowadays the basic hypotheses of brain biochemistry studies have to do with predicting a biochemical substrate for behaviour and also with searching for abnormal biochemistry in mental illness; a typical example being the abnormal transmitter hypothesis, first stated in 1952 by Osmond and Smythies, who proposed that schizophrenia could be caused by the intervention of an abnormal metabolite such as adrenochrome. However, brain biochemical studies are difficult because measurement and identification of metabolites depend on relatively crude methods. The diagnostic criteria, say, in schizophrenia are muddled, and above all the environment of the experimental subjects has to be held constant so that biochemical monitoring can yield useful data rather than a ragbag of biochemical guesswork.

In the case of schizophrenia biochemical study was given straight-forward impetus by Connell's (1957) clinical description of amphetamine psychosis, and also by the work of Slater and Beard (1969) on psychosis associated with epilepsy.

There are two main methods used in studying biochemistry and psychiatric disorder. The first is to compare patients with controls, the second is to carry out serial studies on individual patients looking at specific biochemical measurements during illness and recovery in the hope of finding a phasic variation in biochemistry exclusive of diet, exercise, medication etc. (Gibbons, 1968).

In schizophrenia an abnormal transmitting substance produced by faulty methylation was originally suggested in 1952 by Osmond and Smythies. Later it was postulated that this might be DMPE (dimethoxy phenyl ethylamine) a mescaline-like substance which could conceivably be derived from dopamine, a known CNS transmitter. The hypothesis in this case had four statements (Smythies 1967):

1   Schizophrenia is related to the production of a mescaline-like substance
2   The biochemical abnormality is stress related
3   Transmethylation is involved
4   The normal metabolite is a central transmitter

This will be considered further under Schizophrenia but is here re-corded to hint at the real methodological problems involved in studying biochemistry and psychiatric disorder. It should also be noted that no one would now seriously put forward biochemical theories of psychiatric disorder as excluding social and personal factors but at the end of the scale of causality there are generally determined biochemical and metabolic errors that cause psychiatric disorders, *e.g.* porphyria, phenylketonuria, classic examples of biochemistry altering behaviour.

Electroencephalography

Relatively few psychiatrists really understand electroencephalography, most are content to request EEGs and more or less hope for the best. However, although the EEG is not of great value in clinical psychiatric practice it is an important investigation which has important implications in psychiatry since epilepsy is relatively common amongst psychiatric patients. Although many regard the EEG as a complicated procedure, it is basically simple, in principle being a record of surface changes of electrical activity on the scalp which reflect cerebral electrical activity. The changes are low voltage and need considerable amplification which leads to the inclusion of electrical artefacts from muscles in the face, scalp and eyes. The complexity of the records is increased by the use of up to sixteen recording channels, this means that brain electrical activity has to be distinguished from artefacts before the significance of brain based electrical potentials can be discriminated. This can be done by eye but is made a simpler task by using scanning devices which analyse the frequency distribution pattern of the signals. The frequency patterns of the EEG which reflect brain activity include:

Alpha — 8–13 cps
Beta — 14 cps and above
Delta — below 4 cps
Theta — 4–7 cps

which have been agreed as constant findings as electroencephalography has increased in scope and sophistication.

Thus EEG records are concerned with rhythm, wave form and cerebral location of disturbed patterns. The most fundamental EEG changes relate to frequency changes, electrical activity below 7 cps is usually abnormal whether diffuse or focal. Voltage changes, especially low voltage diffuse activity, is found in extensive organic cerebral damage. Paroxysmal activity is generally found in epilepsy where spike and wave activity occurs in temporal lobe epilepsy, focal epilepsy and generalised epilepsy.

The EEG is and never should be a routine investigation. It should be used to clarify diagnosis when epilepsy is in question, especially temporal lobe epilepsy where serial recordings are usually necessary and in the investigation of focal epilepsy—particularly if there is suspicion of a space occupying lesion. It is of little use in the investigation of generalised cerebral disease such as dementia or general paresis. Above all it should not be used as the lazy man's way of diagnosing epilepsy, unhappily EEG departments still expend too much time in dealing with requests such as 'Faints? Fits? ?Epilepsy. EEG please?'.

Sleeping and dreaming

Of all vital functions sleep is probably the least well understood, yet for the psychiatrist's patients, sleep disturbance is one of the most common symptoms. It is so common that hypnotics are amongst the most frequently prescribed medications and the most avidly consumed, yet though there are about 30 million prescriptions written every year for insomnia there is growing evidence that hypnotic drugs tend in general to reinforce insomnia and not only that but their effects persist well into the following day causing headache, irritability and poor concentration with worse insomnia on the following night.

Most of the scientific knowledge of the nature of sleep has been discovered in the last 15 years. Until then sleep was regarded as a uniform resting state with certain characteristic disturbances but sleep was revealed as a much more complex phenomenon when neurophysiological studies including eye and bodily movements and continuous EEG records revealed it as a phasic phenomenon in which two types of sleep were identified (Dement, 1965; Kleitman, 1963; Oswald, 1962). The first type, sometimes called classical, orthodox or light sleep, is characterised by slow ocular movement and slow wave EEG activity whilst the second type, REM (rapid eye movement) sleep, first described in 1953 is characterised by rapid eye movements, increased cerebral blood flow and temperature and fast, low voltage EEG activity. REM sleep is more prevalent in infancy—some newborn animals for instance show about 80% of REM sleep. Infants sleep more than middle aged and elderly people and their increased sleep and higher proportion of REM sleep may be related to growth, in terms of increased growth hormone secretion and increased tissue turnover.

REM sleep occurs in bursts throughout the sleeping period, about 20 minutes every 90 minutes is the usual distribution. In addition to this in human beings certain phases of sleep have been described.

Phase 1 No rapid eye movements (NREM) sleep. The person feels drowsy and sleepy.

Phase 2 Easily awakened but looks deeply asleep.

Phase 3 Slow wave EEG activity appears.

Phase 4 Deepest sleep. Increase slow wave EEG activity.

REM sleep Rapid eye movements and fast EEG activity.

It was originally thought that REM sleep was 'dreaming' sleep but this theory has not been confirmed; however, the consensus of opinion so far suggests that REM sleep is physiologically *necessary*. Others suggest that sleep disturbances in affective disorders such as depression and anxiety may be linked to the disorder at a physiological level so that the psychiatric disorder may ultimately turn out to be a syndrome based on a disorder of sleep mechanism (Jouvet, 1970). Others have taken this idea further and suggest that 'psychosis' is really the emergence of dreaming into wakefulness. Dreaming is badly understood, the psychoanalytic school emphasises the importance of dreaming as an activity in which unfulfilled desires, emotional conflict and drive are all immersed in a pool in which the unacceptable and inexplicable become at least tolerable and their more unpleasant elements are soon repressed below consciousness. Neurophysiologists suspect that dreams may be purposive in the sense that perceived and learned experience is run through in an apparently random but actually useful fashion.

Commonsense tells most of us that what we seem to remember of dreams is usually a mixture of immediate previous experience, usually somewhat garbled, about equally mixed with the symbols and realities of fears, wishes, desires and plain nonsense.

Patients frequently complain of bad dreams and very frequently complain of insomnia. It is not possible to be precise about the clinical significance of dreaming beyond recognising bad dreams as being common in *depressive states* and as being early signs in *acute and subacute delirious states*.

Sleep disturbance is another matter. Insomnia is a common symptom, more often than not hastily evaluated and badly treated.

In psychiatric practice the most common severe sleep disorders are associated with affective disorder. The *anxious* patient complains of delay in getting to sleep; the *severe depressive* notices *early waking*, a symptom often assigned diagnostic importance as meaning 'endogenous' depression. In fact the significance of early waking is hard to establish beyond its association with *severe depression* and its persistence. At all events insomnia is distressing, although its ill effects are only severe where a person is artificially deprived of sleep.

Manic patients are often sleepless, or at least they go to bed late and rise early. Patients with delirious and subacute delirious states tend to spend the whole 24 hours in a mixed state of wakefulness and drowsiness.

Sleep depends on a biological clock mechanism that may be hard to define but is common experience for anyone who crosses the Atlantic by air. Many drugs interfere with sleep by suppressing REM sleep, these include alcohol, the barbiturates and most non-barbiturate hypnotics. This means in practice that over 90% of sleep inducing drugs prescribed by doctors are not only useless but in fact make the insomnia worse by causing increased wakefulness on withdrawal. Even the benzodiazepines such as diazepam and nitrazepam are involved in this criticism.

Yet the doctor is constantly asked for hypnotics and advised to prescribe them by manufacturers. There is no simple answer. All that can be said is that barbiturates should be used only rarely, that non-barbiturates such as methaqualone and glutethemide are useless and dangerous and that the best thing to do is use benzodiazepines reluctantly. No one has ever died of insomnia and it is likely that people have been encouraged to be hypochondriacal about sleep.

PSYCHIATRY AND EPIDEMIOLOGY

Epidemiology is the study of the incidence and prevalence of illness in a population, so that treatment and prevention may be organised. This is a limited definition of epidemiology which, in a wider sense can be regarded as *medical ecology*, that is the study of the relationships between the environment and the illness.

In the case of incidence/prevalence surveys, the 'bread and butter' of epidemiology, these started with truly epidemic illnesses such as the observations of John Snow in 1849 on cholera in London culminating in his removal of the handle of the water pump. This belongs to medical history, it tends to overshadow later observations on epidemiology made by Florence Nightingale who seems to have been one of the first to emphasise the importance of incidence and prevalence studies, but being a nurse and a woman her observations *do* tend to be overlooked!

In psychiatry the epidemiological method is used first of all to study prevalence since this is a sad deficiency in psychiatry; morbidity risks have been guessed at for too long. Early studies on the prevalence of mental illness were limited by being hospital bound, *i.e.* tied to admission rates which gave a biased picture of general population incidence and prevalence.

Early psychiatric prevalence studies were limited by hospital admission figures since in general there were no other psychiatric treatment facilities. This might suggest that earlier hospital admission figures must on this account have been accurate, but this is offset by the fact that hospitals only catered for the most severely ill and therefore missed out the 'not-so-ill' but still incapacitated.

Early attempts at psychiatric prevalence studies in this country go back to 1733 when Cheyne suggested that nervous disorders accounted for one third of the illness in England, and related their causes to climate, rich food, soil, bad weather, sedentary work etc. In 1842 Cowan found that of all cases seen in a year 10% had diseases of the nervous system and 10·7% had 'diseases of uncertain seat', a thoughtful observation by a doctor who was ahead of his time.

Early 20th Century surveys such as that of Rosanoff (1916) in Nassau County NY set out prevalence rates for mental illness, while in 1929 in England the Wood Report gave detailed figures for the incidence and prevalence of mental subnormality. Since then community surveys have increased in number and accuracy. An intriguing example was carried out in Norway by Bremer in World War II when he was a doctor looking after 1000 people cut off by distance and hostile invaders. He found that 25% of his population had psychiatric symptoms over a five-year period. In contemporary psychiatry the narrower aspects of epidemiology have revealed harder data about the prevalence of illnesses such as schizophrenia Wing (1970, 1972) whilst in general epidemiological studies have highlighted family influences in schizophrenia and general environmental factors which can antedate illnesses such as schizophrenia. Cooper and Shepherd (1970) reviewed the usefulness of an ecological approach to psychiatry, *i.e.* how to relate 'life change and stress' to mental illness, noting historical antecedents such as early beliefs that plague had been spread by water contaminated by Jews, beliefs which had far reaching effects in terms of human misery and persecution.

Other epidemiological surveys have tried to relate mental illness to war service, mass disaster and social change or the effects of specific incidents in mental health of a population, *e.g.* after the evacuation of Tristan da Cunha (Rawnsley & Loudon, 1964). They examined the epidemiology of mental illness in the people of Tristan da Cunha after they were evacuated following volcanic eruption. The population (264 indigenous, 29 temporary) came to England and all but 14 returned 2 years later in 1963.

The population is descended from five couples who settled there in the early 19th Century. It is a closed community. Rawnsley and Loudon found a prevalence rate of psychosis which was no higher than expected, a current incidence of 22% with asthma (mainly unrelated to emotional factors) but most interesting of all an outbreak of hysteria in 1937 reported by Cristopherson (1946). Twenty-one islanders had been affected with convulsions, globus hystericus and aggression plus 'fainting'. Symptoms were group related; one patient 'set another off'. Rawnsley and Loudon examined 14 of the original 21 and found that convulsive attacks, 'spells' had continued since 1938. The 19 survivors had a higher rate of doctor consultation rate, but an extremely interesting finding was the high prevalence rate of psychogenic headache, most common in the 1937 epidemic survivors. The community regarded the headache as a special endemic disorder peculiar to islanders.

The Tristan da Cunha study is a good example of a survey of psychiatric disorders in a small community—larger scale studies that need to be considered include:

1 The Hollingshead and Redlich Study 1958—United States (Hollingshead & Redlich, 1958)
2 The Midtown Manhattan Study 1962 United States (Srole *et al*, 1962)
3 Psychiatric Illness in General Practice—United Kingdom (Shepherd *et al*, 1966)
4 The Camberwell Case Register

These surveys are selected because they are not only relevant to the study of psychiatric epidemiology but also because there is a useful detectable progression between the methods used and also a valuable and educative interplay of the findings—despite transcultural differences.

Social class and mental illness

This survey (Hollingshead & Redlich, 1958) is an important piece of psychiatric epidemiology which looked at prevalence rates, psychiatric practice, also a general demographic and case study.

The basic hypotheses of the survey were that social class would influence:

1 Prevalence rates of psychiatric disorder
2 Diagnoses of psychiatric disorder
3 Treatment of psychiatric disorder
4 Psychiatric aetiology
5 That social class mobility would somehow influence the aetiology of psychiatric disorder

The study was carried out in 1951 in and around New Haven, Connecticut. Prevalence rates were based on the numbers who had started psychiatric treatment in the last half of 1950. This part of the study is hard to evaluate since in the US, even in Connecticut, the health services appear to have been poorly organised. Hollingshead and Redlich however were confident that they had missed only 2% of the total prevalence rate, they discovered 1891 cases. However the study did confirm that the major hypotheses were correct.

Using a social class scale of I to V which is something like the Registrar General's scale in the United Kingdom the authors found that schizophrenia was more prevalent in social class V, the lowest. Did this mean a higher prevalence rate in the lowest social class, or diagnosis by socially biased psychiatrists, or did it mean that the lowest social classes get the least competent psychiatrists? The study is in a sense non-committal about this except for the interesting discovery that local psychiatrists could be classified into two main groups:

1 A–P—analytic/psychologically oriented psychiatrists—mainly in private practice, using psychotherapy.
2 D–O—directive/organic psychiatrists, *i.e.* working in state mental hospitals, not in private practice, tending to use drugs and ECT and not use psychotherapy.

Also D–O psychiatrists tended to wear white coats, earn less than A–P psychiatrists and were more prone to diagnose schizophrenia in their predominantly lower class patients while their more affluent A–P colleagues used psychotherapy, earned more and diagnosed schizophrenia less often in their upper class patients.

As to diagnosis and treatment the hypotheses were proved without question: neurosis was more likely to be diagnosed by A–P psychiatrists in upper class patients who earned more for doing so.

The A–P psychiatrists spent more time with their patients. Social class determined treatment more than did diagnosis: upper class schizophrenics received psychotherapy; lower class schizophrenics ECT and drugs.

The study pointed out very clearly that percepts and concepts of psychiatric illness are class related: upper class private patients tend to be regarded as neurotic or having personality disorders by appropriately trained psychiatrists who use class oriented treatments. This, it seems was true of a specific community in the USA in 1951. No one has, to date, estimated how true this may be in the UK. The author suspects that class bias operates just as forcefully here despite the NHS. The study suggests, by implication, that the health of a community is too serious a matter to be left to the private sector.

The best feature of the study is that the authors partially recognised the class oriented deficiencies of the time despite their barely stated but implied assertion that people get better treatment from high earning analysts as opposed to white coated non-intellectual doctors who use ECT and label the lower classes as mad. Somewhere in this study someone is being criticised.

The Midtown Manhattan Study

This was an intensive epidemiological research study in which psychiatric morbidity was surveyed in a densely populated urban area, Midtown Manhattan, which at the time of the study had a population of 172 000 people. The area was, and is, special by being a residential quarter close to the central business area of Manhattan and is unique in its mix of people who range from the highly affluent to slum dwellers. Family earnings ranged from $300 to $50 weekly and the main group of workers were 'white collar' office employees ranging from top executives to lowly clerks. About 30% were native New Yorkers, 30% came from other American towns and the rest were foreign born: a fairly good American urban ethnic mix. The area is noisy, competitive and by most standards socially and emotionally hard to tolerate. Rapid social change and social mobility are endemic and the environment is uncompromisingly urban, *i.e.* a distressingly ideal area for sociological enquiry directed at establishing the prevalence of psychiatric disorders, identifying symptomatology and relating prevalence to socioeconomic status.

The sociocultural milieu of Midtown Manhattan is an ethnic/religious mix—50% Catholic (lower class) with the remaining 50% one-third

Protestant, and one-sixth Jewish (both mainly middle and upper class people).

The community structure is residential with village-type shops, single people and childless couples. It proved to be a socially disorganised area as shown by a high infant mortality rate, high death rate from alcoholism and a rate of active pulmonary tuberculosis that was twice as high as expected and a high juvenile delinquency rate—in short an area that is full of surprises, not least of which is that its inhabitants make pitifully ineffective use of available social and medical services. The mental health survey (Srole & Langner, 1962) covered the 20 to 59 age group cutting the available subjects to 110 000 of whom 1660 were randomly selected and held to be truly representative.

Three social groups were defined:

1 Wealthy upper class
2 Middle 'white collar' class
3 Lower class (manual workers 'blue collar')

All subjects were interviewed for 2 hours which included a 100 symptom check list based on the MMPI, an Army symptom list and clinical examination.

This was reduced to a scale:

1 Severe symptoms
   a marked
   b severe
   c incapacitating
2 Moderate symptoms
3 Mild symptoms
4 No symptoms, *i.e.* 'well'

This was backed up by psychiatric assessment on a 7-point impairment scale. The main findings were at first negative, there was no relationship between psychiatric symptoms and being town or country bred, but what did emerge quite unequivocally was that 'socioeconomic status' is the most important criterion in mental health and mental illness; it was associated with mental illness more closely than any other factor. 'The socioeconomic status of the parents as determined by the father's occupation and education is a definite correlation to their mental health . . .' and 'The physical and mental health of the parents also are contributing influences upon the mental health of the residents.' Many a Marxist might here be permitted a nod of assent.

The main clinical psychiatric findings showed a high prevalence rate of psychiatric disturbance as based on symptom ratings (see Table 6.1).

Table 6.1   Symptom ratings.

Symptom	%
Well	18·5
Mild symptoms	36·3
Moderate symptoms	21·8
Impaired function	23·4
(*i.e.* 23·4% of the sample showed 'personal impairment'	
a marked	13·2
b severe	7·5
c incapacitated	2·7

The most striking finding was the 23·4% who showed 'some personal impairment', which later we should compare with similar English findings. The authors did not and never have overstated their case—they merely pointed out poverty and poor social status as crucial influences.

The Camberwell Case Register Study

This began in 1964 and its varied findings have been described in a number of papers culminating in a comprehensive review (Wing & Hailey, 1972), not only of findings to date but also of its implications for the planning and evaluation of mental health services for the community.

The particular value of the Camberwell Survey has been that careful data collection about prevalence and morbidity in psychiatry are the only basis on which services can be based—since hitherto planning has been ad hoc, at times inspired but rarely based on hard data. Camberwell is a densely populated area, 304 000 in 1966 (43 people per acre) making it the eighth highest in population density of 32 London boroughs.

A large collection of demographic data shows that, in common with most urban areas there are few obvious social correlates with psychiatric extremes such as a severely raised admission rate for schizophrenia though socioeconomic status, is, as ever suspect.

In general although Dickens dismissed Camberwell via Samuel Weller senior ('but he vos only a Cambervell man Sammy') it is an area that comes across from the Case Register Study as a pretty stable area of mainly working class people (57% are skilled or semi-skilled). Social morbidity, social isolation and poverty are not extreme and its rates of suicide, schizophrenia, and delinquency are about average. Wing and Hailey comment 'It is no paradise and it is definitely not the most exciting part of the conurban London scene (one might even call it dull), but in certain places and on a sunny day, its residents might reflect that they could do very much worse than stay where they are.'

The Case Register is a data linkage system which has identified psychiatric morbidity more effectively than any similar studies to date. All available contacts with treatment services in the area are identified and followed up so that since 1969 it has been possible to form a data bank of admission rates, treatment services, after care facilities in such detail that not only can conclusions be drawn but also predictions can be made about future treatment/rehabilitation needs.

The Register began with a straight census of all people living in the area who were either psychiatric in-patients or day patients, or who had been in out-patient treatment on the first day, *i.e.* 31 December 1964. Since then all psychiatric treatment involving Camberwell residents has been recorded covering not only adults but also children and also mental handicap whether the contact is with hospital or local authority services. Thus the register provides an on-going monitoring process which identifies the type of diagnosis, treatment or rehabilitation. The Register has built in reliability checks and is linked to computer based recording systems, though it may be added the whole effort represents an immense coordination of individual case finding etc., *i.e.* pure 'leg work' of such a conscientious and laborious nature that its persistent diligence in terms of real scientific effort cannot be too highly emphasised or praised.

From this data bank there emerges a scientific instrument which analyses information about admission and readmission—the continuities and discontinuities of the process of patient care which is a model of scientific enquiry nourished by high quality—British empiricism, a tribute which is stated here without any trace of chauvinism.

The Camberwell Register is exemplary on three counts, first its lack of bias, secondly its relation to all identified population and thirdly because it is cumulative. The workers are modest in their statements and argue carefully the limitations of the Register.

Basically the Register is used to try and answer a number of questions based on certain simple principles. The principles are that health care services should be responsible for a defined area and to that end, aim to provide a range of services, essentially comprehensive but always linked to the concept of flexibility in the face of changing treatment methods and population needs. The services should be integrated and have pragmatic aims based on the limitations of present knowledge of the aetiology and natural history and treatment of psychiatric disorders, so that a primary aim is 'containment' or decrease in psychiatric morbidity in the patient, the patient's family and the community. The varying roles, methods and attitudes of services be they medically based, socially oriented or aimed at prevention are all recognised and their relative values by implication accepted. Thus the system is one in which there are no assumptions, no prejudgements and above all no airy theorising, fancied data or inspired guesswork.

The evaluation of services is construed as clear answers to six questions which may be paraphrased thus:

1   How many people are in treatment, how did they get there and are there trends in the rate of contact with treatment agencies?
2   What are the needs of those to be 'treated'?
3   Are current services being deployed effectively and in every sense economically.
4   Who are the people who need treatment but who do not get it and are their needs the same as those in treatment?
5   What services are likely to be needed for people whose treatment needs are at present unknown?
6   Do new treatments reduce the demands for treatment?

These six questions are paradigms of psychiatric treatment and the ways in which it may be planned for a community and they are questions which, if left unanswered, can only leave psychiatric services in a state of fragmented groping and disorganised uncertainty.

Measuring psychiatric morbidity was and is never easy, as we have seen there is enough basic disagreement about what psychiatric illness is all about. But if we leave the academic discussions about who or who is not ill and look at patients as they present themselves or are referred, only a person of absolute unsympathetic detachment could fail to be impressed by the fact that people do become psychotic, do become depressed, do have personality difficulties, are born mentally handicapped and do develop brain damage despite the assertions of those who say that they are really the victims of a vague societal conspiracy. At the end of it all we are left with numbers of people that we can only regard as ill because they suffer from symptoms that distress them and because their social functioning falls away and more than that, that they vastly exceed in numbers those patients who come into psychiatric treatment because they offend society or are dangerous to themselves and others—it is as simple as that. Measuring the efficacy of treatment and rehabilitation is difficult since our understanding of aetiology is poor.

The Camberwell Case Register study has suggested many topics which have been examined, these range from reasons for admission, reasons for increase in admissions, reasons for compulsory admission, to the use of long term support, industrial rehabilitation, poverty, mental handicap, the planning of services; in short a comprehensive overview of the ways in which a community tries to deal with psychiatric illness. It is here neither desirable nor reasonable to examine all of these in detail but one area is selected because of its high relevance for the clinical psychiatrist and this is in *Reasons for admission to hospital* (Gleisner *et al* in Wing & Hailey, 1972).

This section of the research sets out a detailed study of all Camberwell people who had a first contact with a psychiatric service in the first 6 months of 1971. People who were under 15 or over 64 were excluded as were addicts and people with organic cerebral syndromes. Information was produced concerning 50 new admissions, 40 patients who might have been admitted and 10 who were day patients.

Reasons for admission were itemised, the mental state was examined using the PSE (Present State Examination) and the patient's personal and social behaviour was carefully checked. The three groups of patients were examined in this way and the significant clinical finding was that psychosis, particularly schizophrenia was most likely to lead to admission. And the other findings were that there were four main reasons for admission, viz. psychotic behaviour, pressures from relatives, doctors and social workers, bed availability and lack of other types of care. Now to some these may seem self-evident but anyone who thinks this is missing the point. The point is that anything to do with planning psychiatric services needs groundwork of this sort even though the example chosen had to do with a relatively small sample.

Reasons for long term stay were similarly examined (6 months to 3 years) and it was found that one quarter of the cases needed further treatment, one third needed supervision because they were unpredictable, in fact there were valid reasons for long term stay in over 65% of cases. For the rest the reasons had to do with lack of alternative facilities but the question remains unanswered as to what the best alternative facilities may be.

This reference to the Camberwell Case Register is intentionally kept brief in the hope that it will stimulate the interest of the reader in a classic piece of research in social psychiatry which pays close attention to methodology and sampling, indeed all the scientific tools of applied social psychiatric research. For without such research, talking about planning psychiatric services becomes a monologue which can be only of value to the person who is delivering the monologue.

PSYCHIATRIC DISORDERS IN GENERAL PRACTICE

The prevalence of psychiatric disorders in general practice is an important area of study since it should give a clearer idea of what the real extent of population psychiatric problems may be. An important recent study is that of Shepherd *et al* (1966). This research aimed to determine reliable prevalence figures and also to find out what factors might influence general practitioners to diagnose and treat psychiatric disorders, also the research team aimed to determine how extensive the burden of psychiatric morbidity might be on individual doctors and also what criteria were used to decide that patients needed psychiatric treatment.

The first task of the research team was to get a representative practice series, *e.g.* it is no good sampling Kensington and assuming that the findings will be the same as Stepney. Secondly there had to be a simple classification of psychiatric disorders, standard ways of measuring morbidity and finally proper sampling and adequate follow up, *i.e.* good design. The first target was forty to fifty practices sampling every eighth patient in the practice list thus leading to a 12·5% random sample. The researchers used the Cornell Medical Index as a screening questionnaire plus a standard interview on a subsample of identified cases. Another aim of the study was to explore possible pathology in non-attenders in the practices and also an attempt at exploring possible relationships between psychiatric and general illness, *i.e.* how ill are 'neurotics' as opposed to people with 'physical' illnesses?

First of all a pilot study on three practices (21 000 patients, 9 doctors) over 2 months revealed 2176 patients at risk with a diagnosis rate of

12% for psychiatric disorder (16% women, 7% men). Major psychoses were rare, the main problems were neuroses, psychosomatic illness and organic illness with overlay.

After this the main part of the study involved 27 practices (51 doctors) but half the doctors refused to participate so the study focused on 12 practices. The illnesses were classified as in Table 6.2.

Table 6.2 Classification of illnesses

Physical	Psychiatric
1 Cardiac	**a Formal psychiatric illness**
2 Respiratory	1 Psychosis
3 Orthopaedic	2 Mental subnormality
4 Gastrointestinal	3 Dementia
5 Neurology	4 Neurosis
6 Genitourinary and Gynaecology	(anxiety, depressive, hysterical,
7 Skin	phobic, neurasthenia)
8 Cancer	5 Personality disorder
9 Endocrine	**b Psychiatric associated conditions**
10 Acute infective	6 Physical illness ⎫ where psychic
11 Other	7 Physical symptoms ⎭ mechanisms were aetiological
	8 Physical illness ⎫ where psychic
	9 Physical symptoms ⎭ factors aggravate
	10 Other psychological or social problems

Morbidity was estimated by consultation and consultation rate per 1000, prevalence rate per 1000, new psychiatric case rate per 1000 and chronicity.

General findings

The most relevant findings from the point of psychiatric morbidity that emerged from the study were as shown in Table 6.3.

Now in fact the study went a good deal further into detail than mere crude morbidity rates but prevalence rates and distribution of morbidity were obviously a central part of the research. The rates were broken down by age and sex and in addition there was a careful examination of patients' symptoms using the Cornell Medical Index (CMI).

Table 6.3 Patient consulting rates per 1000 at risk for psychiatric morbidity, by sex and diagnostic group

Diagnostic group	Male	Female	Both sexes
Psychoses	2·7	8·6	5·9
Mental subnormality	1·6	2·9	2·3
Dementia	1·2	1·6	1·4
Neuroses	55·7	116·6	88·5
Personality disorder	7·2	4·0	5·5
Formal psychiatric illness*	67·2	131·9	102·1
Psychosomatic conditions	24·5	34·5	29·9
Organic illness with psychiatric overlay	13·1	16·6	15·0
Psychosocial problems	4·6	10·0	7·5
Psychiatric-associated conditions*	38·6	57·2	48·6
Total psychiatric morbidity*	97·9	175·0	139·4
Number of patients at risk	6783	7914	14 697

* These totals cannot be obtained by adding the rates for the relevant diagnostic groups because while a patient may be included in more than one diagnostic group, he will be included only once in the total.

Among the general conclusions found by the study was a 'total prevalence rate of 140 per 1000 persons at risk and an inception rate of 52 per 1000 at risk, for all types of psychiatric disorder combined'; thus placing psychiatric illness among the commoner causes of consultation. As to psychiatric diagnosis despite the various differences in diagnoses well known to psychiatry the London study compared pretty well with the Baltimore study of Passamanick *et al* (see Table 6.4).

Examination of these figures shows a great difference from hospital type statistics, also the study revealed a good deal about doctors' attitudes and treatment options. Above all it revealed how important will be the psychosocial aspects of medicine in the proper training of doctors and also that a proper awareness of psychosocial factors in illness and their treatment *are* in fact consistent with a scientific approach to medicine—despite the misgivings of those who see sociology and psychiatry as wordy waffle.

General morbidity rates for psychiatric disorders in general practice

Table 6.4 Psychiatric diagnosis in London and
Baltimore

	per 1000	
Diagnosis	*London*	*Baltimore*
Psychoses	5·9	4·3
Psychoneuroses	88·8	52·6
Psychophysiological	45·7	36·5
All psychiatric disorders	140·4	93·4
No. at risk	15 000	12 000

summarised by Kessel and Shepherd (1962) are tabulated (Table 6.5)
merely to amplify the basic observation that if we want accurate data about
prevalence of psychiatric disorders it can really only be obtained from
general practice surveys of the community.

Table 6.5 Psychiatric morbidity rates reported from a number of general practice
surveys

Surveys of patients registered	*Number at risk*	*Period of survey*	*Conditions specified*	*Percentage of patients at risk*
Ryle, 1959 (139)	2 400	1 year	neuroses	4·1
Logan, 1953 (102)	27 000	1 year	mental and psychoneurotic disorders	4·7
Logan & Cushion, 1958 (104)	380 000	1 year	mental and psychoneurotic disorders	5·0
Martin *et al*, 1957 (109)	3700	1 year	mental and psychoneurotic disorders	5·6
McGregor, 1950 (105)	2500	1 year	anxiety states and hysteria	6·8
Kessel, 1960 (90)	900	1 year	'conspicuous psychiatric morbidity'	9·4
Primrose, 1962 (129)	1700	1 year	psychiatric morbidity	13·2

Surveys of Patients	Number consulting	Period of survey	Conditions specified	Percentage of Patients consulting
Davies, 1958 (36)	2700	1 year	psychoneuroses	6·4
Fry, 1957 (57)	4000	5 years	psychoneuroses	8·5
Hopkins, 1955 (76)	650	6 months	psychiatric illness, stress disorders	11·1 31·7
Hewetson *et al*, 1963 (72)	650	1 month	psychiatric disorders	23·2
Paulett, 1956 (119)	—	5 years	neuroses	65

Survey of illnesses	Number of complaints or episodes	Period of survey	Conditions specified	Percentage of complaints or episodes
Handfield-Jones, 1959 (69)	2700	1 year	mental and psychoneurotic disorders	3·7
Davies, 1958 (36)	3400	1 year	psychoneuroses	5·2
Pemberton, 1949 (121)	4800	2 weeks	mental and psychological ill health	6·5
Perth, 1957 (122)	150	1 month	'non-organic'	53·7

Surveys of consultations	Number of consultations	Period of survey	Conditions specified	Percentage of consultations
Logan & Cushion, 1958 (104)	1400 000	1 year	mental and psychoneurotic disorders	5·0
Horder & Horder, 1954 (78)	2000	consecutive series	psychiatric disorder	7·7
Finlay *et al*, 1954 (52)	—	4 months	stress disorders	20
Pougher, 1955 (127)	500	consecutive series	neurosis	47·6

7

Organic cerebral syndromes

INTRODUCTION

All organic cerebral syndromes are, by definition, caused by brain dysfunction at cellular level. This holds true whether the syndrome is caused
by toxins, inflammation, tumour, vascular or degenerative disease.
Organic syndromes are a more coherent and consistent group than the
functional psychoses; the manifestations are reliable and predictable, thus
producing a high degree of diagnostic agreement, *i.e.* validity and reliability. This is an important point, central to clinical psychiatry, about
which there is no disagreement. Even writers such as Szasz who has
criticised psychiatric nosology on the grounds that terms such as psychosis,
alcoholism, personality disorder etc., are really medical misrepresentations
of 'Problems in Living' concedes that the recognition of organic cerebral
syndromes is an important psychiatric skill that should be taught to the
medical student.

The *classification of organic syndromes* presents little difficulty; organic
cerebral disease causes three basic types of syndrome:

1 a delirium
  b subacute delirium (confusional state) } clouded states
These are syndromes mainly characterised by *clouded consciousness.*
2 the dysmnesic syndrome (amnestic syndrome)
3 dementia

The diagnosis of organic cerebral syndromes is a two stage process, *i.e.*

1 recognition of the organic syndrome, *e.g.* dementia
2 identifying the cause, *e.g.* arteriosclerosis

The medical model is universally acceptable here—a 'disease of the mind' caused by a physical disease process.

ORGANIC SYNDROMES—GENERAL COMMENTS

In organic mental disorders the most important symptoms reflect impairment of consciousness and cognition—the damaged brain is diminished intellectually. These manifestations are *primary*. In addition to this there are relatively specific symptoms and signs related to damage to certain *areas*, *e.g.* frontal lobe syndrome, parietal lobe syndrome. Also there are '*release*' effects, *i.e.* symptoms caused through loss of control of higher cerebral activity. Finally, emotional symptoms are always *secondary* to the organic damage. At all times it should be remembered that the overall clinical picture is inevitably *coloured* by the patient's *premorbid personality* and his social and cultural background—the collected information store of his lifetime.

Proper evaluation of an organic mental state should always include careful physical and neurological examination. These usually require to be backed up by investigations. For example an elderly patient admitted in a subacute delirious state (confusional state) will suggest a list of possible medical causes. The list includes infections, such as bronchopneumonia and urinary tract infection; metabolic causes such as uraemia; toxic causes such as medication and alcohol; hypoxic such as anaemia and cardiovascular disease. The list is large, in fact a comprehensive list of organic mental states includes over 60 possible causes, many are rare, and a few are common but all can be recognised by a doctor who has sensible awareness of the range of possibilities.

Symptomatology

The most striking symptoms of organic syndromes are often those related to disturbances of *consciousness and awareness* since accurate perception of the environment based on constant monitoring of sense data is a primary function performed by the intact conscious brain via sensory input channels, the reticular system and its associated integrative mechanisms.

Changes of consciousness and awareness are to be found in *attention* which becomes *narrow, fluctuant and drifting*. With this goes a *loss of grasp* of what is going on, of awareness of the surroundings and of what is being said etc. This disorganisation of the monitoring of sensory input is mirrored in *incoherence of thinking, talk and activity* since coherent thought, talk and motor response depend to a large extent on an organised input system. The incoherent thinking etc. is recognised as a tendency to muddle and perplexity. Often the severely brain damaged patient loses mental flexibility and becomes rigid and repetitive, even to the extent of rigidly repeating sayings and acts.

Memory is affected: this may be a consequence of inattention which prevents recognition and registration of sensory impressions. The most common type of memory disturbance in organic syndromes is a loss of memory for recently acquired information (see memory). *Thinking* may become muddled and incoherent. Delusions, when they occur, tend to be ill formulated and transient. *Perceptual disturbance* is probably a consequence of narrowed attention. Perceptual errors (illusions) and misinterpretations are common though *hallucinosis* occurs in delirium.

The emotional state in organic syndromes is usually shallow and labile. The feelings are as capricious and distractible as is attention. Anxiety and fear are common in delirium and are probably a consequence of the uncertainty and bewilderment that follow perceptual misinformation. In severe delirium a patient may be terrified and respond to his frightening environment with aggression.

Motor activity is ill directed and disorganised in delirium where purposeless overactivity is common. In dementia activity tends to fall off and be punctuated by patchy perseveration. Consider the following case.

The confused old man must get out of bed and try to catch a bus to visit his daughter. He gets out of bed, mutters to himself and may become angry if someone tries to prevent him. He tries to get dressed but cannot get his trousers on and may be found wandering about with them half off. In severe organic dementia the patient is tired and languid, he seems weary and apathetic.

Insight may be impaired to the extent that the patient has fluctuating or at best limited awareness of how ill he is. In acute states, *e.g.* delirium, this is striking, and when the patient recovers he has little clear recollection of the episode and can look back on it as an experience that seems like a dream.

THE ORGANIC SYNDROMES

Clouded states

These occur in subacute delirium, and delirium.

Subacute delirium

This is often called 'confusional state'. In this state clouded consciousness is *not* severe, nor are symptoms, in fact the absence of severity is an important aid to recognition. Subacutely delirious patients have a changing level of awareness and grasp. Often they seem weary and rouse themselves from doziness in a way that can pass for normal amid the dry tedium of an afternoon in a medical ward.

Incoherence is pervasive, involving not only perception and thought but also responsiveness and emotional display which is fleeting, labile and irritable. These states are often missed and this is important because recognition and treatment can prevent development of full blown delirium which is both psychologically and physically exhausting. Mr. X. the elderly patient in the end bed who is unexpectedly abrupt and vaguely difficult at tea time, causing a tart response from the nurses, may be wildly excited and drinking from his urine bottle at 2 a.m.

Delirium

In delirium consciousness is badly clouded, attention is narrow, fleeting and distractible; perception, interpretation of sense data are incorrect. The bedside table becomes a monster, the door a prison gate and bedside conversation a conspiratorial plot.

Acute severe mental disturbance is the rule; being delirious is a nightmarish experience. The extent of misinterpretation and illusory fantasy is so bad that the patient can barely hold on to reality. This disorganization affects feeling and behaviour. The total experience is fearful, even terrifying and provokes a motor-behaviour response, superficially purposeful but usually including indecisive angry searching and attempts to flee fancied persecutors. In the early stages sleep is light and fitful, the patient wakes up suddenly in terror and it is hard to reassure him. By day, periods of seemingly breezy chattiness evaporate into disorganised muttering. Fits may occur, usually in fever and no doubt caused by cortical instability.

Delirium ends in sleep and is followed by exhaustion with, at best, patchy recollection of the experience.

Woolf and Curran (1935) reviewed 108 patients with various symptomatic psychoses, including alcohol (23), myocardial disease (9), postoperative states (9) bromides (9) and various infections. They examined the phenomenology of delirium and also looked for specific relationships between the causal agent and the type of syndrome. Their main finding was that clinical pictures were variable though impaired grasp, incoherent thinking, suspicion, hallucinosis and restlessness were dominant features. There was no evidence to link causal agents with the form and content of syndromes. Symptoms were found to be worse at night, aggravated by activity and on waking. Rapid changes in environment were found to be bad for patients but in general patients' mental states were improved by simple, neutral and undemanding environmental conditions. This is important since the study was carried out before antibiotics and tranquillisers were available for the treatment of delirium. The authors also found that delirious content often reflected the patient's past experience and personality and that patients who had repeated delirious states tended to have repeatedly similar content.

Romano and Engel (1944), and Engel (1959, 1969) carried out extensive EEG studies in delirium and have commented on the unsuspected frequency of clouded states, noting the frequency of delirium in most patients with severe anaemia, high fever, peripheral circulatory failure, pulmonary insufficiency, renal and hepatic failure, acidosis or alkalosis, electrolyte imbalance and infection. In fact Engel had shown that 10 to 15% of patients in medical and surgical wards 'show some degree of delirium'. As to the aetiology of delirium, Engel commented that it is related to metabolic malfunction involving not only obvious causes such as oxygen and glucose lack but also disturbances of enzyme systems, interruption of synaptic transmission and altered cell membrane permeability. EEG recordings are good non-specific investigations in delirium and correlate well with levels of consciousness and cognitive impairment and particularly well with awareness and attention; this is in contrast to the relative non-specific EEG changes found in the functional psychoses. In delirium the most common EEG finding is diffuse slowing below 8 cp/s. In severe delirium general slowing to below 6 cp/s. is common.

Dysmnesic syndrome (amnestic syndrome)

This syndrome may be caused by a number of disorders. It may follow infective delirium or may occur with diffuse chronic brain disease such as arteriosclerosis or neurosyphilis. The main symptom is severe loss of memory for immediate events. The patient is also unable to retain impressions of what is going on around him, or recall them. With this goes total disorientation for time and place. The patient tries to cover up his defect by inventing answers, confabulating, *e.g.* the doctor introduces himself to the patient who then identifies him with a totally different name. The emotional state is flat, emotional responses are diminished and the patient is usually bland and euphoric. The basic defect of retaining recently perceived impressions and the associated symptoms are most striking in Korsakov's syndrome when alcoholism and peripheral neuropathy plus thiamin deficiency cause damage to the dorso medial nuclei of the thalamus.

Dementia

Dementia is a syndrome in which diffuse brain cell destruction causes a general deterioration in mental function. By definition dementia is irreversible since dead brain cells cannot be replaced although in certain cases a *dementing process* may be one that can be halted by treatment as in general paresis, or in dementia limited by head injury. These points are worth mentioning since there is a general tendency to equate dementia with a process that is always progressive and irreversible. Now in general this *is* true but not inevitably so; any valid definition of dementia must always be qualified. Dementia, then, is a *generic term* which encompasses a variety of aetiologies and does not imply prognosis until the cause of dementia is known.

Clinical features of dementia

The clinical features of dementia include cognitive impairment and memory loss which develop gradually, converting the patient into a bedridden, lost, helpless shell of his former self, a bitter caricature of how he used to be and later incontinent and wasting. Of all syndromes dementia is the most shattering.

The early symptoms of dementia start with loss of memory for recent events. At first this is a nuisance for the patient, something that he can hold off with a note book and carefully ordered routine. With failure of brain function, understanding slackens and life is too much for the patient. Thought content is diminished and talk becomes rigid and repetitive. Delusions are fleeting and ill formulated and emotional responses are shallow; they are replaced by the foolish lability that follows loss of emotional control.

Manifestations of dementia

Memory disturbance Progressive loss of memory for recent events is a specific symptom of dementia and goes on to total memory loss where the patient has no recollection of what happened in the preceding 24 hours. Disorientation for time and place go with amnesia and contribute further to the ultimate lost state of fragmented vacuity that is the end point of the disorder.

Intellectual disturbance Loss of flexibility of thought is an early sign and may pass unrecognised in elderly people in whom a progressive rigidity of thinking is part of a biological process. Abstract thinking becomes poor, the concrete cannot be related to the abstract. Change cannot be appreciated, new faces, new situations cannot be absorbed or comprehended; there is a general weakening of grasp. Thought content diminishes, half forgotten ideas may be recalled and discussed in a vague uncomprehending way. Delusions are loose, held with little conviction and unformulated.

Emotional disturbance Depression is often said to be an early symptom of dementia, usually chronic depression which fails to respond to anti-depressant treatment. In fact this sort of depression is unlikely to be caused by dementia, far more likely is *labile depressive mood* which is really quite unlike the unrelenting gloom and despondency that accompanies and determines severe affective disorder. Another important feature is that in dementia depressive content is totally unrelated to life events. Apathy, loss of feeling and the 'feeling of having lost feeling' are probably more important features than apparent depression in the development of dementia. In the late stages of dementia emotional control is lost, responses may be violent but soon subside into emptiness and apathy. Irritability and flashes of anger and resentment are as quickly replaced by tears and fatuous laughter.

Personality disturbance   Early personality change in dementia may be hard to spot, often with hindsight others recognise in the patient a general hardening of attitudes and responses that mirror the previously described rigidity in thinking. Dominant personality traits tend to be exaggerated— mild hypochondriasis for instance, hardens into total absorption with fancied illness, financial prudence becomes miserliness, the gourmet becomes an unsightly glutton. Dementia often releases socially unacceptable behaviour such as sexual exhibitionism, shop-lifting etc. in a previously law-abiding person; probably frontal lobe damage causes this.

Memory loss, muddled thinking and disorientation can land the dementing person in distressing and embarrassing situations—for instance the patient may pick up goods in a supermarket—genuinely unaware of what is happening, and end up arrested, charged and appearing in court with attendant anguish and distress, though usually the basis of the offence is soon recognised. The elderly dementing patient is in hazard crossing the road, particularly at night, *e.g.* a 73 year old man was found in shock after being knocked over by a car. He walked into the road in the dark. The inquest revealed a typical story of dementia, memory loss, self-neglect and isolation. Dementia may 'blow up' in to acute delirium particularly if intercurrent infection or an emergency operation causes hospital admission. The patient appears muddled, a state that can easily change into severe clouding.

In severe dementia patients often show a surprising survival capability until a simple crisis such as wandering off and getting lost causes family or neighbourly concern, usually at night, when ordinary sensory cues are less available. But dementing people *do* get lost by day as well.

Organicity

'Organicity', a bad term, is often used to summarise psychological changes associated with brain damage. Many of the most important psychiatric observations on 'organic behaviour' were made by Kurt Goldstein in the light of his extensive experience of the sequelae of head injury. Goldstein emphasised the total activity of the brain which could be regarded as a complex system responding to various stimuli quite apart from specific functional areas and stimulus—response arcs. Goldstein moved away from a topographical theory of brain action and suggested that functional loss could show itself in a general style of behaviour that could be identified as 'brain damaged'—a response system that he supposed represented the patient's strivings to overcome the handicap imposed on him by brain damage. Goldstein's main observations were as follows.

Organic cerebral damage lowers the response and threshold so that a brain damaged patient cannot hold his attention and shifts easily from one percept to another, thus showing 'distractibility'.

There is also a paradoxical change in that a brain damaged person may need a higher intensity of stimulation for a response to be evoked. The brain damaged patient is often unaware of the disability—it seems to be suppressed from consciousness but whether or not this is a hysterical shunting out or anosognosia is not clearly stated.

Brain damaged patients become excessively tidy and concerned about their possessions, so called 'organic orderliness'. Goldstein regarded this as the patient's attempt to impose order on a shifting, dissolving environment which becomes progressively harder to monitor as brain function fails. When a brain damaged patient is given a task which is beyond his ability he may break down into anger, tears, rage and shifty attempts at avoidance. This goes beyond mere realisation that a task is too difficult but is actually a specific response to a situation which erupts with the attempt to complete the task and is quite unrelated to any degree of difficulty, or any setting of failure. The patient finds it all inexplicable and breaks down.

Goldstein's most important contribution relates to the concepts of the 'concrete' and 'abstract' attitudes to the environment. Concrete thinking and the concrete attitude are limited to the immediate and are inflexible and rigid; the brain damaged person cannot draw general conclusions from particular observations, as exemplified in the severe organic defect where a person is unable to find a general meaning in a general statement such as a proverb. Abstract thinking is regarded as a more sophisticated response, thinking is flexible, comprehensive and includes a ready ability to select relevant information from a mass of apparently irrelevant information, and an ability to detach the general from the particular, in short to deal in the abstract as opposed to the concrete. Goldstein's general observations are practical but tend to skim over the practical possibilities of at least a certain degree of cerebral localisation which should not be dismissed.

In summary it can be said that there is a basic differential between acute and chronic organic cerebral syndromes which may be summarised as in Table 7.1.

Table 7.1 Acute and chronic organic cerebral syndromes

	Acute organic cerebral syndromes	*Chronic organic cerebral syndromes*
Causal agent	a may be diffuse b may be exogenous reaction *i.e.* symptomatic psychosis	a diffuse damage
Duration	Transient	Long term
Onset	Rapid	Slow and insidious
Course	Reversible	Irreversible but *can be* halted in some cases
Symptoms	Attention Consciousness Perception	Memory Orientation Intellect
Duration	Weeks	Years
Known aetiology	Physical illness *e.g.* infection CVS Trauma Endocrine Renal	Degenerative disorders Arteriosclerosis
Treatment	To primary cause	Supportive

The diagnosis of dementia

Diagnosing dementia and organic syndromes remains one of the most important tasks of the psychiatrist. The psychiatric syndromes associated with physical illness were taken for granted by 19th Century physicians who expected severe infection to be associated with delirium, recognising it as a symptom that was part of a clinical picture and not something that needed the attention of a psychiatrist. Increased specialisation has diverted psychiatric interest away from organic syndromes and the physician is less prepared for delirium since it is less common than it used to be (Roth, 1969; Stengel, 1969; Mayer Gross *et al*, 1969). This is important. Many psychiatrists act as if organic brain disorder is of no interest to psychiatry yet organic dementias numerically form a large group of psychiatric syndromes in the developed countries. And just because senile and arteriosclerotic dementia are progressive and untreatable at present it does not mean that this will always be the case.

Investigating dementia

In many instances an adequate assessment of dementia may be possible using the history and clinical examination backed up by relatively few investigations. There are no hard and fast rules about how extensive the investigations should be, this is something that is influenced largely by clinical findings, clearly there is no justification for putting every patient through a rigid formula of investigations. This is especially true in the case of uncomfortable and distressing investigations, it is less than kind to investigate without some positive reason, *i.e.* if failure to continue the investigations leaves the extent and nature of the underlying disorder unknown.

Physical examination should reveal disease processes that might cause a dementia-like picture, in elderly people vitamin deficiency such as scurvy, should not be overlooked, rarities such as pellagra hardly ever occur in England but they *do* occur and can present with a clinical picture of apparent dementia. Severe anaemia, particularly pernicious anaemia may present with a confusional state. Neurological examination may reveal a wide range of diagnostic possibilities—dementia complicated by strokes, thrombosis of the internal carotid artery being every day clinical examples —space occupying lesions such as cerebral tumour and subdural haematoma are also important conditions which are in practice missed more often than they ought to be. A basic list of investigations includes: **WR; blood picture and ESR; chest X-ray; skull X-ray; urine examination; and psychological testing.**

WR Syphilis is still overlooked despite the resurgence of venereal disease. *E.g.* A 32 year old man was admitted with depression and paranoid ideas. Further examination of his mental state revealed slight memory loss, poor concentration and puzzled perplexity. The examining doctor noted 'odd' pupils and an otherwise normal central nervous system but failed to recognise the possible significance of the findings. The patient had small unequal irregular pupils. The WR was positive and the CSF showed a meningitic type Lange-curve.

Blood picture and ESR Anaemia and an organic mental state should always suggest possible pernicious anaemia or folate deficiency until proved otherwise. It has been shown that psychoses associated with B_{12} deficiency are more common in psychiatric patients than had formerly been suspected.

E

Though the ESR is a non-specific investigation it remains a useful indicator of previously unsuspected chronic inflammatory and malignant disease and as such is used as a routine investigation in organic syndromes.

Chest X-ray   The chest X-ray is one of the most important investigations in organic syndromes, it may for instance reveal a 'silent' broncho-pneumonia which may cause an apparently inexplicable subacute delirious state in an elderly patient with previously minimal evidence of dementia. The other important condition which a chest X-ray reveals is carcinoma of the bronchus which can present either with a peripheral neuropathy or with an organic syndrome caused by cerebral secondary deposits.

Skull X-ray   Skull X-ray may show up midline structure deviation caused by tumour or bony alterations caused by Paget's disease.

Urine examination   Drugs, particularly barbiturates are important since they can cause subacute delirious states whose origins frequently remain unrecognised. Glycosuria may occur in cerebral tumour and late onset diabetes may present with confusion. Porphyrinuria is rare but is an important cause of inexplicable episodic organic cerebral syndromes.

Thyroid function   In myxoedema the protein bound iodine is low, below 4·8 µg, also a raised serum cholesterol (above 300 mgm%).

Further investigations in organic syndromes

Further investigations include **lumbar puncture; EEG; echogram; brain scan; air encephalogram; and cerebral arteriography.**

Lumbar puncture   Lumbar puncture is not a *routine* investigation, it is uncomfortable for patients and is not essential unless it is called for by neurological deficit or some other indication such as a positive WR. Cerebral tumour, if suspected, is a contraindication.

Electroencephalography   In dementia the EEG is likely to be normal though in Alzheimer's and Pick's disease high voltage slow waves are found. However a dementia caused by tumour or subdural haematoma usually produces an asymmetrical EEG record.

Echogram The echogram can reveal midline structure shift caused by tumour or subdural haematoma. The echogram works by comparing the reflection of ultrasound from midline structures.

Brain scan Brain scan employs intravenously administered short life radioactive drugs. The technique is used for finding vascular abnormalities, subdural haematomata and tumours.

Air encephalography Air encephalography is usually carried out on the recommendation of a neurologist. The great value of the AEG is that it shows up gross damage, ventricular enlargement or dilatation and flattening of cerebral sulci, as in cerebral atrophy. The limitation of the air encephalogram is in those cases where it appears to display minimal ventricular dilatation, *i.e.* it is not as sensitive an investigation as has sometimes been thought: a study of apparent brain damage in drug users was confidently backed up with AEG studies and received much critical attention until the limitations of AEG interpretation were definitively stated. Fleminger (1973) has commented on the relative unreliability of the AEG in the diagnosis of cerebral atrophy. In a follow-up study of 100 patients with the label 'diagnosis uncertain' Fleminger found that presenile dementias diagnosed provisionally and apparently backed up by AEG studies were not reliably confirmed on a 5 year follow-up.

Cerebral angiography Cerebral angiography is a valuable method of localising cerebral tumour and showing up vascular abnormalities. In straightforward dementia cerebral angiography is not a routine investigation except for dementia caused by thrombosis of the internal carotid artery. Dementia in old age should be investigated carefully and always with regard for the comfort of the patient. What is there to be gained by air studies on an old lady with straightforward senile dementia? In all dementia at all ages, investigation should be aimed energetically at the discovery of a treatable cause, and investigations should be used thoughtfully and not as mere routine.

Differential diagnosis of dementia

Before considering the many diseases that can cause dementia it is first necessary to differentiate dementia from other organic syndromes and other psychiatric disorders which may resemble it.

OTHER ORGANIC CEREBRAL SYNDROMES

Delirious states

In delirious states as we have seen clouding of consciousness is the predominant symptom, this and the associated perceptual disorders make delirium a more fantastic experience than dementia. The delirious patient if anything has a crowded psychotic experience and one that comes on quickly in contrast to the failure and poverty of experience that is the hallmark of dementia. There are numerous causes of delirium, the most important include:

1   Fevers
2   Unrecognised pneumonia
3   Urinary tract infection
4   Renal failure
5   Hepatic failure
6   Vitamin deficiencies
7   Cardiovascular disease
8   Trauma
9   Epilepsy
10 Coexisting dementia, *e.g.* in tumour and cerebral arteriosclerotis.

Amnestic syndrome

Here the predominant symptoms are amnesia and confabulation, again mental content is profuse as opposed to the emptiness and apathy of dementia.

Schizophrenia

Memory defect and clouding of consciousness do not occur in schizophrenia. Fall off in interest and drive can be clearly related to a typical progressive schizophrenic history and such features as delusions and thought disorder. Delusions in schizophrenia are elaborate and well formulated unlike the loose vague delusions of the demented patient. Also, schizophrenia starts at an earlier age.

Depression

In old age depression is often mistaken for dementia, too many doctors readily assume that self-neglect, apathy and general debility in old age are inevitably caused by dementia. This is not so. The apparent organic picture of a depressive is often compounded by a real organic mental state caused by starvation, avitaminosis etc. Since depression is treatable it is urgent always to diagnose it in elderly people, a depressed patient may do poorly on memory and IQ tests but his performance is not one of global failure, his defects are patchy. This should always be remembered when the 'atypical depressive' who fails to respond to treatment is re-considered as a possible organic dementia. In fact follow-up studies (Fleminger, 1973) suggest that chronic depression is often too easily regarded as dementia. True depressive mood is deeper than organic mood disturbance which is labile and fleeting. Response to antidepressant therapy is a diagnostic aid.

Personality disorder

People with personality disorders tend to mature and get into less difficulties as they grow older but this is not always true, and an eccentric person may develop a behaviour disorder that suggests dementia but is really an extension of their personality disorder. This should not be overlooked, especially in elderly patients where dementia is called into question, e.g. a 75 year old lady was said to have a confusional state and underlying dementia. The confusional state cleared when her lifelong alcohol and barbiturate abuse were recognised and she was found not to be dementing but her normal self, a difficult eccentric and cantankerous personality for whom time had produced no improvement.

Neurosis

Neurotic symptoms, like depression, can obscure the diagnosis of dementia by diverting attention from symptoms of dementia or suggest dementia where it does not exist. The sudden onset of anxiety in someone over the age of 50 should alert to possible dementia. It is for question whether such anxiety is organically caused or whether it is symptomatic of the patient's awareness of his own disability.

The **organic cerebral syndromes** may be listed as follows:

1 Syndromes following *infection*; here the most important is neurosyphilis.
2 Syndromes associated with *cerebral tumour*.
3 *Cerebral trauma*.

4 Syndromes associated with *vascular and degenerative disorders*, e.g. cerebral arteriosclerosis; senile dementia; and the presenile dementias.
5 Syndromes associated with *deficiency diseases*: pellagra; B_{12} deficiency; Wernicke's encephalopathy; and Korsakov's syndrome.
6 Syndromes associated with *endocrine and metabolic disturbance*: Addison's disease; acromegaly; Cushing's syndrome; hypoglycaemia; myxoedema; porphyria; and Wilson's disease (hepato-lenticular degeneration).
7 Syndromes associated with *genetic inheritance*: Huntington's chorea; and Tay-Sachs disease.
8 *Toxic causes*, e.g. industrial poisons, drugs, etc.
9 Syndromes associated with *epilepsy*.

Organic syndromes *following infection* are in general fairly uncommon since infective disorders are themselves uncommon. Nevertheless their possible occurrence should never be overlooked, particularly since nowadays people travel so much more freely and may develop odd behaviour etc. which at first may be supposed to be psychosis but which turns out to be for instance a manifestation of cerebral trypanosomiasis, which unrecognised and untreated will cause death. Other infections such as *meningococcal meningitis* have cropped up again in recent years. Usually recovery is complete but the patient may be left with organic impairment or a general sense of lassitude with persistent headache. Probably the most well known sequelae of infective cerebral disease are the personality changes of Parkinsonism following *encephalitis lethargica*. Here patients, particularly those of the 1920 epidemic, often ended up as chronic mental hospital patients. Interest was reawakened in their seemingly untreatable plight by the comments of Sacks (1975) on the way in which L-dopa awakened such patients after years of inaccessible withdrawn physical and mental handicap.

The range of infections that may leave behind organic cerebral impairment is large and covers a number of rarities. However, one ever important condition is neurosyphilis.

Neurosyphilis

Neurosyphilis is less common than it used to be. Its historical relationship to the development of psychiatry is important and has been reviewed by many including Hordern (1968), Hunter and MacAlpine (1963) and Jacobowsky (1965).

Syphilis was common in the 16th Century but the first description of general paresis was not until 1822. Hunter and MacAlpine (1963) suggested that the recognition of neurosyphilis was stimulated by the beginnings of neuropathology so that general paresis, a common 19th Century 'mental disorder', was found to be a physical illness—bringing psychiatry closer to general medicine and the 'medical model'. The discovery of *T. pallidum* in the brain and the development of malarial therapy by Von Jaurreg gave psychiatry its first successful physical treatment—no trifling achievement at a time when 20% of mental hospital beds were occupied by general paretics who progressed from early facetious insightlessness along a hideous clinical journey through fits, paralysis and dementia into stinking incontinent hebetude.

The story of malarial therapy is interesting. Many clinicians had noticed that patients who had had high fevers, smallpox, typhus etc., did not seem to develop GPI despite earlier syphilis. Jacobowsky (1965) noted that in 1904 Matteuschek and Pilcz had followed up 4134 syphilitic Austrian Army Officers of whom 4 to 6% developed GPI except for 241 who had had acute infections including malaria, erysipelas and typhoid, years after primary syphilis.

Von Jaurreg was inspired to try malarial inoculation on the basis of this and other observations and the treatment stopped the progress of the disease in 9 patients. Eventually he received the Nobel Prize for his discovery. In modern times early antibiotic treatment of syphilis is the rule so there has been a fall in the incidence of neurosyphilis. On the other hand venereal diseases are more prevalent than they were even 10 years ago so there is no need for complacency. Venereologists are faced with the unknowing confidence of patients who suppose that non-specific urethritis is the worst they have to fear.

Syphilis can still be overlooked, it remains a protean and remarkable disease, all doctors agree on this and yet the tendency to miss it recalls G. K. Chesterton's observation that a man could look at something for 999 times but when he looked at it for the 1000th time he was in danger of seeing it for the first!

Clinical types

There are three types:

1 *General paresis* (GPI—general paralysis of the insane), *i.e.* parenchymatous neurosyphilis where brain cells are directly affected.

2 *Meningovascular syphilis*—a gummatous basal meningitis.
3 *Tabes dorsalis*—where there is sclerosis of sensory pathways leading to sensory ataxia.

Pathology

Though the details of pathology are best described in appropriate texts a brief reference is necessary.

In *general paresis* there is generalised cerebral atrophy, usually most marked in the anterior and middle parts of the cerebral hemispheres. Destruction of cortical ganglion cells is extensive. *Treponema pallidum* is found in brain tissue and the ventricles are dilated and the meninges thickened. Since syphilis is basically a vascular disease the characteristic perivascular cuffing and endothelial proliferation are widespread.

In *meningovascular syphilis* there is extensive basal meningitis with associated hydrocephalus. The subarachnoid space is choked with exudate and this causes ocular palsies since the 3rd, 4th and 6th cranial nerves pass through the subarachnoid space where they become involved in the basal meningitis.

In *tabes dorsalis* the syphilitic lesions affect the posterior columns and nerve roots thus leading to loss of position sense and sensory ataxia and the 'lightning pains'.

Clinical manifestations of neurosyphilis

General paresis In the past the 'classical' descriptions of general paresis covered 'expansive', 'simple' and 'paraphrenic' types but these terms really describe dominant symptoms in an organic syndrome—the basic features of GPI, that are personality change and memory defect which start slowly from 8 to 30 years after primary infection. Acute onset, *i.e.* clouded states, are described but are rare. Grandiose and persecutory content are related to the patient's premorbid personality.

The usual history is of gradual deterioration in a middle aged man, there is an unaccountable sex differential in GPI, males are affected more than females in the ratio 5:1. The deterioration shows itself in a gradual blunting and coarsening of behaviour, probably caused by frontal lobe damage. Sometimes this is first recognised when a previously impeccable person behaves strangely; washing his hands in the soup or urinating on the carpet at a public function are the examples usually quoted. Such behaviour calls for medical investigation which reveals memory disturbance etc. pointing to unrecognised dementia. The *pupils are abnormal*, small, sluggish and unequal: the full blown *Argyll-Robertson* pupil is a late sign. Insomnia and headache are common early symptoms, also lack of energy and a general lack of self control leading to irritable quarrelsome outbursts and a general indifference to other people's feelings. Ability, interest and persistence fall away and the patient becomes abstracted, inept and forgetful.

After these early symptoms a typical clinical picture of dementia appears with increasing paresis and tremor affecting limbs, face, tongue and lips. The arms are often affected worst so that the patient's writing becomes smaller and indecipherable while dysarthria causes his speech to be incomprehensible. Fits, strokes and total incapability complete the picture.

Meningovascular syphilis   Here the clinical picture includes a general failure of mental ability with *severe headache*, loss of energy and insomnia. Episodes of clouding and stupor are common; focal syndromes are particularly common.

Tabes dorsalis   The posterior column damage causes sensory ataxia and loss of pain sense, later 'lightning' and 'girdle' pains occur, these are agonising, inexplicable and episodic. Tingling and paraesthesiae are also commonly found. Ankle and knee jerks are absent and the limbs are hypotonic. Optic atrophy and loss of vibration sense are relatively late signs.

Severe crises, 'tabetic crises', can occur; these take the form of severe bouts of pain, abdominal, bladder and renal pain, no doubt rare nowadays but a possibility not to be neglected.

Diagnosis of neurosyphilis

The diagnosis of neurosyphilis is not difficult providing it is remembered as a possibility; the following cases are exemplary.

1   A 35 year old ex-naval rating was admitted for investigation of depression. He was depressed, phobic, unable to work and had severe headaches and insomnia. He had memory loss and was disorientated in time and place. His pupils were unequal and sluggish. His Lange curve was paretic. He responded well to antibiotics.

2   A 31 year old Puerto Rican was admitted for investigation of headache

and suicidal impulses. He was depressed but was also forgetful and lacked interest, complaining of severe headache. He showed clouded consciousness, poor comprehension and gross memory defect. His pupils were abnormal and the Lange curve was meningitic.

Dewhurst (1969) reviewed neurosyphilis and traced 91 cases (62 male, 29 female) diagnosed between 1950–65 in three English counties. Frequent symptoms were: *headache, mild depression, memory loss, insomnia* and *irritability*. Fits were uncommon.

The modes of onset were different; 46 cases came on slowly but 45 came on suddenly: 13, following arrest for antisocial behaviour; 8, following amnesia; 7, following violence; 3, following indecent exposure; 6, following fits; and 5, following attempted suicide.

Initial diagnoses varied considerably: 24 were diagnosed with neurosyphilis; 28 with depression; 13 with dementia; 8 with confusional state; 6 with schizophrenia; 6 with hypomania; and 3 with epilepsy. In other words the initial diagnosis was wrong in 70% of cases. The types of neurosyphilis eventually diagnosed were 19 with simple dementia; 25 as simple depressive type (organic syndrome plus depression); 16 with taboparesis; 10 with grandiose; 5 with manic; 6 with senile; 4 with protracted; and there were 6 others.

Most of the patients were unskilled workers; military service was the chief occupational risk. Dewhurst concluded that the early descriptions of expansive types etc. were no longer true, this was in line with the observations of Power (1930) and Hart (1959). There is, in short, no 'classical' type of general paresis; the most important thing is to look out for an organic mental state and odd, eccentric, antisocial or unexpected behaviour. This should always raise the suspicion of GPI or tumour.

In fact, the proof of the diagnosis of neurosyphilis is entirely a matter of serology—a positive CSF, WR and the typical changes in the Lange colloidal gold test.

Treatment

The treatment is simple: 1 million units of penicillin daily for 10 days to destroy the organisms. No other treatment is necessary. *Differential diagnosis* is from other organic mental states, *e.g.* presenile dementia, tumour, arterioslerotic and senile dementia.

Cerebral tumour

Psychiatric disturbance is common in cerebral tumour. This clinical fact should always be remembered especially when the patient is middle aged and presents with unexpected change in behaviour. Tumour and GPI are easily overlooked. There are few ground rules for the diagnosis of cerebral tumour, like most serious illnesses cerebral tumour does not play fair. Tumours are hard to diagnose and in many cases it is easy to be wise after the event, but many studies of cerebral tumour emphasise first of all the high prevalence rate of psychiatric symptoms and secondly basic data about cerebral tumour. Two-thirds of cerebral tumours occur between the ages 20 and 50, peaking between 40 to 50 (Cushing 1932); gliomata account for 40%, meningiomata for 20% and secondary growths for 20%.

The clinical picture produced by cerebral tumours is related to the type and site of the growth, the rate of growth and to raised intracranial pressure. There are many 'classic' publications on cerebral tumour, Cushing (1932), Bleuler (1951) Walther (1951) and Cox (1934). And what emerges from all of these and others is that there is no *typical cerebral tumour syndrome* of psychiatric disturbance but that there are general associated focal, physical and psychiatric symptoms. General symptoms include those caused by raised intracranial pressure, *e.g.* headache, nausea, vertigo, papilloedema and fits.

Usually the *headache* is described as 'bursting' and is worse in the morning and aggravated by coughing and bending; nausea and vomiting are also worse in the morning. *Papilloedema* is diagnosed by examining the optic fundi, but *visual disturbance* may be glossed over and mentioned only in passing by patients as 'a bit of eye trouble' or blurred vision. *Fits* are common and are *the first symptom in 30% of cases. Dizziness and vertigo* are always hard to evaluate and are often early signs of raised intracranial pressure.

General psychiatric manifestations

There are no isolated psychiatric symptoms which indicate the site of a tumour, on the other hand most large series reported include a high incidence of psychiatric symptoms. Walter (1951) found that 70% of cases had some psychiatric symptoms whilst Waggoner (1954) reporting a statistical analysis of 326 cases of supratentorial tumours found mental changes in 58%, the highest incidence in glioblastomata 71%, with 53% in the astrocytoma and oligodendroglioma group.

The important point to note is that gliomata are the commonest cerebral tumours and that they are most likely to develop in the frontal and temporal areas, two 'silent' areas where non-specific and vague psychiatric symptoms may conceal widespread organic disease. In Bleuler's (1951) series 37% of cases had clouded states and 38% had a dysmnesic syndrome.

General symptoms such as headache, vague mood disturbance, apathy, insomnia and anorexia, a picture of being generally unwell are common enough in medical practice, and this merits more than mere passing mention for many patients have symptoms like this but only a few turn out to have a cerebral tumour. It would be impossible for every doctor to carry out a full neurological examination when confronted with such indefinite symptoms every time, yet using the methods presently available, in the absence of a serological test for cancer, early signs of cerebral tumour are easily missed. Consider the following case. A 19 year old man developed acute gastroenteritis. Six weeks previously he had stopped work, upset his parents by his preference for cannabis and undesirable companions. His diarrhoea persisted for two weeks and he stayed in bed complaining of vague nausea.

Three months after he still tended to spend mornings in bed and was thought to be 'work shy' since he got up late and spent his evenings drinking alcohol and smoking cannabis. When examined he was morose and apathetic and said 'I'm inclined to be sick'. He had severe vomiting and headache in the morning. His fundi showed early papilloedema, investigation revealed an extensive fronto-temporal glioma. He had minimised important symptoms, as had his family who were more concerned about his 'idleness'.

General psychiatric symptoms in tumour include clouded states, memory disturbance, dementia and personality change. *States of clouded consciousness* are common and are episodic rather than persistent. A picture of frank '*typical*' dementia is uncommon: there is intellectual deterioration, the patient finds it hard to think clearly, his concentration and grasp are poor. He tires easily, has no energy and is mentally slow, all general signs of organic cerebral disease not peculiar to tumour. Personality change may be patchy and its significance not recognised, so that while there is general agreement that psychiatric changes are common in cerebral tumour it is also true that there is no simple 'once off' symptom cluster. As in all clinical diagnosis, there is no substitute for adequate history taking. In addition to symptoms of raised intracranial pressure or one of the recognisable organic cerebral syndromes patients often develop second order symptoms caused by their partial realisation of what is wrong and these symptoms can mask the organic symptoms. For instance a patient may be depressed because he is aware that his brain function is failing, though in fact depression and neurosis are uncommon presenting symptoms in tumour (less than 5% in Bleuler's series).

Early diagnosis then is difficult; a good basic rule is to be suspicious of a first psychiatric illness in the 40 to 50 age group, particularly if there is even a faint suggestion of clouding or of memory loss (early symptoms in 40% of cerebral tumours).

Waggoner and Bagchi (1954) reviewed the many ways in which organic brain damage could be hidden in the early stages by psychological symptoms. They noted that 40% to 100% of patients with cerebral tumour tended to show psychological symptoms at some stage in the disease process, supporting this observation with eleven references to the literature covering the years 1897 to 1943. They found that the incidence of cerebral tumour is the same in general hospital and in mental hospital populations though the incidence figure has shown a wide range, *i.e.* from 0.2% to 6% (Davidoff, 1930). This review describes 6 patients with cerebral tumours in whom psychiatric symptoms were the primary presentation and in each case a focal lesion was revealed by EEG examination. Later (Freedman & Kaplan, 1967) Waggoner reported a statistical analysis of 326 patients with supratentorial tumours. The survey was designed to discover causal or significant relationships between psychiatric symptoms, fits, raised intracranial pressure and the site and type of tumour.

The study was inconclusive except as a general warning to psychiatrists that patients with cerebral tumours may present with a wide range of symptoms, many of them psychiatric and few of them diagnostic.

Mental changes occurred in 58% of the series, but bore no relation to the level of intracranial pressure nor to the tumour location, although frontal lobe and temporal lobe tumours caused more psychiatric symptomatology than others. Fits occurred in 48% of cases, this is in line with previous studies, and were associated with slowly developing benign growths. Common symptoms included confusion, disorientation, cognitive impairment, personality change and lethargy, although they were less prevalent than described by Bleuler (1951). Waggoner also noted that the highest incidence of psychiatric symptoms was in the gliomata, 71% contrasted with the meningioma and pituitary group (52%).

The important clinical finding from this and many other studies is that cerebral tumours often cause altered mental states, but these are rarely specially recognisable syndromes. Even the fatuous inane euphoria (Witzelsucht) of a frontal lobe lesion tells us that there is frontal lobe damage and no more.

Remington and Rubert (1962) reported on 34 tumour patients admitted to psychiatric hospitals over a 30 year period. Ten were known to have a tumour: the remaining 24 were admitted as 'psychotic'. Symptoms included depression (8), memory loss (7), aggression (5), personality change (2), paranoid ideas (2), agitation (2), obsession (1), epilepsy (1), and schizophrenia (2). The authors warned against expecting vomiting, headache and papilloedema as early symptoms. They suggested that tumour should always be considered as a possibility in cases of presenile dementia, arteriosclerotic dementia, encephalitis, Parkinsonism, cerebrovascular accident, multiple sclerosis and subdural haematoma.

They also noted that psychotics can develop tumour, and that psychotic symptoms, though rare, can be released by tumour. Also they commented that brain damaged people may develop say a depression, related to their own awareness of a worsening degree of handicap and also that a brain damaged person, as is now more fully realised, may develop cognitive impairment, or at least worsening cognitive impairment as a result of the wrong treatment, *e.g.* ECT or plain unsympathetic and unheeding and unaware treatment.

It is not within the scope of this work to describe the pathology and focal neurological aspects of cerebral tumour, on the other hand it is necessary to list and describe the most important focal signs and clinical syndromes. Such a complicated system as the brain functions as a whole and a purely topographical concept of brain function is no longer accepted. On the other hand certain brain areas can be functionally identified and are represented as aspects of lost or impaired function when the brain is damaged.

There is no need to labour this point, the common causes of hemiplegia are well known but when we examine more subtle types of loss of brain and mental function, it is not so easy. For a start, there are large areas of the brain, *i.e.* the frontal and temporal lobes that are 'silent' in the sense that widespread destruction can be compatible with apparently normal function, as in patients who have a frontal lobe removed and show little personality change. The other important point is that our descriptions of subtle types of brain function are really very crude. It is easy to describe motor and sensory function but when we come to perception, memory and orientation we are in difficulty; a problem that becomes trifling when we examine words like 'aphasia' which have been classified in many different ways, none of them entirely satisfactory and some of them contradictory.

If we add to these two very large areas of uncertainty the important anatomical fact that frequently a space occupying lesion in the brain causes functional loss not so much in the areas of immediate cell destruction as in areas adjacent to the lesion because of pressure, interference with blood supply etc. the reasons why it is frequently difficult to relate symptom to tumour hardly need emphasising. And the whole difficult process is compounded by the type and degree of malignancy of the tumour and its speed of growth. Bearing all these points in mind it is possible briefly to summarise various syndromes without assigning to them high reliability and constantly recognising the prevalence of non-specific symptoms in cerebral tumour.

Frontal lobe

Though the frontal lobes are 'silent' areas it is well known that they are associated in an undetermined way with the regulation of behaviour. The use of lobotomy and leucotomy operations as crude methods of reducing agitated behaviour is now a part of medical history, also these operations, particularly when excessive drew attention to the role of the frontal lobes in higher control over social behaviour and integration of the personality.

Frontal lobe tumours cause personality change, usually recognisable as unacceptable and unself-critical social behaviour, at first episodic, or trifling but later inevitably rude and inappropriate to the person's previous behaviour to the extent of being grotesque. It is a sad but absolute fact that some of the most accurate clinical descriptions of the consequences of the loss of frontal lobe function have come from observations in patients who had been subjected to overgenerous prefrontal leucotomies. Early signs of frontal lobe damage include a certain ebullient abrupt rudeness which soon merges into socially unacceptable coarseness, a blunting of emotional response and sensitivity, an indifference to the reactions of others that is both unthinking and unfeeling. This progresses on to a state of emotional lability with a general background of apathetic indifference and silly euphoria that is called Witzelsucht in German.

Temporal lobe tumours

Temporal lobe lesions are most easily recognised if the patient develops temporal lobe epilepsy. Temporal lobe epilepsy is referred to in the section on epilepsy: suffice it here to recall that it is characterised by clouded states often coloured or followed by experiences of heightened familiarity with the environment, states of having been through the experience before, *déjà vu*, or else accompanied by and followed by feelings of increased reality of the self, or loss of personal reality (depersonalisation) or of the environment (derealisation). Vivid changes in perception, auditory and visual, may be very detailed, and so impress the patient that he strives but rarely succeeds in conveying to the doctor the ineffable complexity of it all. The emotional state may be blissful, even ecstatic: or again fearful, so fearful that the whole experience is episodic and always occurs in clouded consciousness, even dreaminess. These temporal lobe fits or psychomotor fits are usually interspersed with classic grand mal epilepsy. Clearly the sudden onset of temporal lobe epilepsy in a middle aged man would raise the suspicion of tumour, as indeed would the sudden onset of uncinate fits where gustatory hallucinosis appears suddenly and is followed by altered perception while the patient seems far away and dreamy. *Déjà vu* experiences can occur as can the most detailed recollections of past events. The patient is rather vacant, is not properly aware of his surroundings and his talk is sparse and repetitive.

Now the point about these two syndromes is that clinically they are very suggestive of epilepsy and above all their onset in middle age is a very alarming sign. But in fact these presentations of temporal lobe tumour are not common. As ever, the signs are likely to be non-specific since most temporal tumours are diffuse and not so likely to set off fits. So we fall back on personality change as a key sign in temporal lobe lesions, just as in frontal lobe lesions. Yet another example of the general non-specificity of psychiatric symptoms in cerebral tumour. The personality change can be insidious or may show itself in irritability, merging into violent outbursts.

Other defects such as aphasia can occur but these after all, are or should be, easily recognised as organic signs.

Parietal lobe tumours

Here we enter the borderlands of neurology and psychiatry, for the parietal lobes are above all the brain areas that are concerned with recognition, discrimination and scanning of the environment in a much more complex way than can be accomplished by phased array radar. Radar it will be recalled is a method of investigating the presence of objects in the environment by picking up interruptions in electromagnetic transmissions based on the observation that since EM waves travel at the speed of light, the interval between signal emission and echo if halved and multiplied by the speed of light will reveal the range of the object. Phased array radar though it is the basis of international defence against missiles and anti-ballistic missiles happens to be an interesting process in that whereas 'simple' radar uses a single beam, phased array radar uses millions of beams per second, and the emission of these beams is phased on a time base, predicted and monitored by a computer. Thus a complex equipment system is able to detect, identify, count and size and even range on to objects in its environment.

Now we are not suggesting that the parietal lobes operate in this way but what they do achieve, or appear to achieve is a highly accurate presentation to the cortical communication system of a complex set of data about the position of the body and its parts in space, their relationship to each other, a method of identifying objects by touch which can display their shape to the cortex. In other words the parietal lobes are intimately concerned with information sorting, appreciation and integration of the highest degree. Therefore when the parietal lobes are damaged there is loss of complex functions as shown by manifestations such as *apraxia*, inability to carry out familiar acts such as dressing; *acalculia*, inability to calculate; and *agraphia*, inability to write.

One of the most important disturbances in parietal lobe disorders involves loss of the ability to tell right from left and to appreciate simple spatial relationships. This type of disturbance may easily be detected by asking the patient to draw an outline of a familiar object such as a house. Parietal lobe damage strikes at basic integrative functions of the brain and can be detected by a variety of tests which are described in neurological and psychological texts. The important clinical point lies in the recognition of the fact that parietal lobe damage leads to diminished awareness of spatial relationships in the body and in the environment. At their most severe parietal lesions can cause unawareness of one half of the body or unawareness of disease on one side of the body (anosognosia). As far as the rest of the brain is concerned, focal signs are the concern of neurological texts to which the reader is referred. Third ventricle and mid brain tumours often cause odd changes in consciousness, episodic or prolonged, and occipital lobe tumours often cause visual changes, *e.g.* flashes, hallucinosis etc.

It cannot be too often reiterated that most cerebral tumours occur in 'silent' areas, develop slowly and present organic mental states which must always be regarded as organic mental states in which tumour must be excluded. If the doctor is not tumour sensitive he will miss them. It is also important to know that although a neurotic or affective picture is rare as a mode of presentation, that it can occur, *e.g.* a 35 year old woman had been treated for 'depression', 'psychoneurosis', 'vague symptoms', 'hysteria' for two years, with tranquillisers, psychotherapy and antidepressants. Her symptoms did not improve until a meningioma was removed.

Cerebral trauma

Head injury whether closed or open can cause a wide range of brain damage. Damage may be minimal after what seems to be a serious accident, or extensive after an apparently trifling injury. This latter is especially true in elderly people. Loss of brain function may be transitory as in concussion where unconsciousness is thought to be caused by acceleration–deceleration or very severe following large scale cell destruction as in post-traumatic dementia—a syndrome of non-progressive dementia where a patient is left with learning deficit and intellectual impairment, with in many cases quite severe personality change. Though there are no hard and fast dividing lines of diagnostic classification, certain syndromes are recognisable. In all cases it should be remembered that functional loss represents not only the quantitative effect of cell death but that it is always coloured by the patient's premorbid personality, and intellectual level.

A simple classification includes:

1 Acute syndromes: a, coma; b, delirium; c, Korsakov syndrome (dysmnesic syndrome); and d, concussion.
2 Chronic syndromes: e, post-traumatic dementia and personality change; f, subdural haematoma; g, post-traumatic epilepsy; h, focal syndromes; i, psychoses; and j, post-concussional syndrome.

Acute syndromes

Coma Coma after head injury is common and is usually directly related to large scale cell destruction either by solid material or by blood tearing through brain tissue. On the other hand coma can follow injury in which tissue damage is relatively limited, *e.g.* in injuries to the brain stem. The diagnosis and management of traumatic coma is not a common task for psychiatrists but familiarity with traumatic coma is essential for the psychiatrist who is asked for advice about the management of post-traumatic delirium and dysmnesic syndromes.

Post-traumatic delirium Post-traumatic delirium is clinically the same as any other delirium but it may be more prolonged. It occurs in recovery from coma in a head injury and where brief is taken for granted but if prolonged the psychiatrist may be asked to advise on management, *e.g.* a 21 year old university graduate was thrown through the windscreen of his car and was in a coma for six weeks. As consciousness lightened he became noisy and violent and developed a typical delirious state. He failed to settle in a few days and was transferred to a psychiatric unit where he remained hallucinated and overactive for six weeks and gradually settled into a dysmnesic state. One year later his measured IQ was 90. Two years later the main abnormalities were emotional lability, perseveration and lack of awareness of the extent of his disability. He joined a religious order with the object of becoming a priest but was unsuccessful. His persistence was low, he tired easily and he was unduly irritable and suffered from fitful depressive spells, headache and fatigue. Three years after injury he was able to work at a simple clerical job.

Dysmnesic syndrome A Korsakov syndrome may follow head injury. The usual features are present; *e.g.* severe memory disturbance, disorientation and confabulation. A simple psychiatric example is the short lived syndrome that can follow ECT.

Concussion Concussion is an acute, transient and reversible syndrome following closed head injury, *i.e.* sudden acceleration and deceleration after a blow on the head which stuns the patient. Usually the concussed patient has a headache for a day or two. In mild cases, familiar to games players, a man is hit on the head, seems dizzy and may fall down with transient loss of consciousness. After this he may get up and score a goal or a try, and have no recollection of what happened. Recovery is complete.

Summary

The acute mental disturbances of head injury may be slight and transient, however the most severe head injuries cause prolonged loss of consciousness and coma, often followed by delirium and dysmnesic syndromes during recovery. From a prognostic point of view the convalescent stage is important since it is here that the clinician can begin to assess the extent of permanent damage. The most reliable clinical index of traumatic disability is post-traumatic amnesia as described by Russell (1959).

Often recovery from head injury is complicated by anxiety and histrionic (hysterical) symptoms. Where compensation is involved hysteria is hard to distinguish from frank malingering.

Post-traumatic amnesia   Post-traumatic amnesia includes retrograde and anterograde amnesia (post-traumatic amnesia).

Retrograde amnesia occurs in head injury, after ECT, status epilepticus, indeed any acute loss of consciousness (Russell, 1959). The amnesia covers events just before the injury, *i.e.* the injury and loss of consciousness prevent registration and retention of information.

Anterograde amnesia covers events following head injury (*i.e.* post-traumatic amnesia) and describes memory defect during the recovery phase during which the patient recovering from unconsciousness is unable to register impressions of what occurs during his state of altered consciousness, he only becomes able to register when clear consciousness is present.

General psychiatric aspects of acute head injury

1   It is not easy to correlate macroscopic brain damage with clinical disturbance, this makes separate syndromes somewhat artificial since one often merges into another in time. In recovery from head injury, time is the great factor and prognosis is never easy.

2   The psychiatrist is rarely involved with the care of the comatose patient. But there is much for the psychiatrist to learn in these cases. The comatose patient is the focus of professional and family concern, he is usually young and otherwise healthy. His chances of survival are the subject of great anxiety and concern so the relatives need support and reassurance that go beyond platitudes. Doctors experienced in this field take great care of this aspect.

Chronic syndromes

Post-traumatic dementia and personality change   Dementia following head injury is non-progressive. It is comparatively rare, typical examples being patients who survive severe head injury and gunshot wounds. The powers of recovery of the brain are extensive though dead cells cannot be re-generated and it is important to realise just how good a degree of recovery may be attained by someone who survives quite extensive injury. In practice post-traumatic dementia is most commonly found in patients whose brain function is already impaired by old age or vascular disease.

Personality change is uncommon and most striking where there is exten-sive frontal lobe damage. Where severe personality change occurs the important point is that the patient's personality is transformed. Minor degrees of personality change are harder to detect and may remain sus-pected rather than confirmed. This is especially true of patients who develop persistent neurotic or hysterical symptoms.

The *post-contusional syndrome* is the best example of this. In this state the patient remains ill and anergic to a degree that exceeds the extent of the brain injury which may be comparatively slight. Headache, lack of energy, anxiety and labile mood disturbance are common symptoms as are irritability and a hypochondriacal attitude often amounting to preoccupa-tion with symptoms centring around the head. This is understandable since human beings are naturally very afraid of head injury in the same way that they are easily terrified by heart disease. It is for question whether the postcontusional syndrome is a type of personality change or a reaction to injury.

Post-traumatic epilepsy is unpredictable and not directly related to the extent of injury, but is directly related to penetrating injury.

The incidence of *psychosis following head injury* is hard to evaluate. It is generally regarded as rare and as something that occurs in people who are susceptible to psychosis.

The occurrence of *subdural haematoma* still presents diagnostic problems usually because it happens to people with either repeated minor head injuries or to patients with damaged cerebral vessels or in chronic states of intoxication with alcohol or barbiturates.

Assessment of chronic syndromes following head injury The important clinical problem here is to assess the relative importance of symptoms caused by organic damage and symptoms related to the patient's basic personality and by psychological reaction to injury and awareness of disability. This is not a simple task and is best achieved by collaboration between neurologist and psychiatrist from the clinical point of view, and by the psychologist from the standpoint of measurements of functional capacity. There are no simple rules to follow: in severe cases any history of blood in the CSF external bleeding, prolonged coma, focal signs and fits are definitely relevant. Other symptoms and signs are less definite and need to be taken into account collectively, *e.g.* fatigue, lassitude and headache.

Vascular and degenerative disorders

Cerebral arteriosclerosis

In cerebral arteriosclerosis there is an organic syndrome with cognitive, affective and behavioural symptoms caused by generalised and focal deficiencies in the cerebral circulation. Arteriosclerosis is usually diagnosed in the fifties and sixties though often it starts much earlier, definite signs of cerebral arteriosclerosis may be found as early as age 45.

Apart from focal syndromes where there may be recognisable neurological defect, *e.g.* transitory paresis, generalised cerebral arteriosclerosis usually causes dementia with a picture of intellectual failure coloured by the patient's premorbid personality.

The onset is usually slow and the progress episodic, seemingly halted or slowed by short lived improvement. There may be a period of up to two years while symptoms are vague and which is recognised with hindsight as the start of the disease, but it is always possible to pick up a history of *decline*, at first obscure but later obvious.

Close relatives confirm a history of failing intellectual function which they suspected but tended to dismiss because of the episodes of apparent recovery.

Manifestations   Early signs and symptoms include headache, dizzy spells and faintness with fleeting episodes of focal brain damage which improve quickly, leaving the patient apparently fully recovered. *Failure of recent memory* appears with indecisiveness and failure to make sensible judgements.

Neurotic symptoms   Anxiety and empty persistent hypochondriasis come in and often cause the patient to visit his doctor more frequently than before, this may lead to fruitless investigations which miss the real diagnosis.

Paranoid or eccentric personality tendencies are likely to become prominent as brain function is less controlled leading to *unexpected and antisocial acts in previously seemingly stable personalities*, *e.g.* pilfering, feeble and incongruous sexuality etc. which leads to court appearance, public disgrace and failure by others to recognise that the offender needs treatment and not condemnation. An *acute onset* is said to occur in up to 50% of cases who first present with *a subacute delirious state* but this is probably a matter of recognition rather than a mode of onset.

Differential diagnosis The main differential of cerebral arteriosclerosis is from senile dementia, the essential features of cerebral arteriosclerosis have been summarised by Bergmann (1972) as follows:

1 A history of strokes
2 Symptomatic epilepsy
3 Hypertension
4 Stepwise course with plateaus of preservation
5 Relatively good preservation of the personality and appropriate affective responses up to a late stage in the illness

Pathology The pathological findings in cerebral arteriosclerosis include widespread infarcts and diffuse and variable areas of cerebral softening.

Prognosis The short term prognosis is better than in senile dementia (Roth, 1955) after 6 months a significantly higher percentage of cerebral arteriosclerotics survive than do patients with senile dementia. At 2 years there is no difference in survival rate.

Treatment Treatment is symptomatic and supportive.

Presenile dementia

Presenile dementia is a generic term applied to dementia starting between the ages 40 and 60. The presenile dementias may be considered under the categories of primary (*i.e.* idiopathic) and secondary, where the cause is known. The primary presenile dementias include Pick's disease; Alzheimer's disease; and Jakob-Creutzfeldt disease (strictly speaking Huntington's chorea should really be included but somehow never is!).

The secondary presenile dementias include dementia in the age group 40 to 60 caused by known primary agents such as neurosyphilis, tumour, alcoholism, myxoedema, cerebral vascular disease and B_{12} deficiency. Therefore the clinical descriptions of presenile dementias usually cover the three named idiopathic dementias.

Pick's disease   Though first described in 1892 by Pick who thought it was a special type of senile dementia with aphasia, it is now realised that it is a presenile dementia of unknown aetiology. It is a rare presenile dementia which does show specific familial incidence in some cases though this does not account for all. The dementia predominantly affects the frontal lobes with minimal temporal lobe involvement.

The clinical picture is one of slow dementia with a high incidence of aphasia, agnosia and apraxia. The patient tires easily and is distractible. Memory loss is a late symptom. The frontal lobe changes and aphasia etc. are characteristic early changes and the full blown dementing picture appears relatively late. The duration may be prolonged as far as 10 years and the end is total hebetude. There is no treatment other than palliation and support.

Alzheimer's disease   Was first described in 1906 and is a presenile dementia clinically indistinguishable from senile dementia, some regard it as a variant of senile dementia. It is the most frequent of the presenile dementias.

Clinically the disease tends to start in the mid-fifties with memory disturbance as an early symptom. Gait disorders, aphasia and parietal lobe symptoms are also common early findings and fits are very common (up to 30%). Later the picture of generalised dementia comes on. The duration rarely goes beyond 6 or 7 years. The cerebral pathology is similar to senile dementia and there are neurofibrillary changes in brain cells, similar to those found in postencephalitic Parkinsonism, and repeated head injuries etc.

It all adds up to an untreatable early onset dementia of unknown cause though a hereditary influence is found in about 10 to 15% of patients with Alzheimer's disease. Treatment is palliative and supportive, and the end point, like all dementias, is appalling.

Jakob-Creutzfeldt disease   This is a rare untreatable disease of totally unknown aetiology where there is random cell destruction in the CNS, in the cortex, basalganglia, thalamus, cerebellum, substantia nigra and anterior horn cells.

The clinical signs include indefinite prodroma such as tiredness, lack of energy and more obvious organic symptoms such as memory disturbance and ataxia. Odd and eccentric behaviour causes worry to relatives and dysarthria is often striking.

The progress of the disease is rapid, 3 months to 3 years are the usual limits described, spastic paralysing dementia is the ultimate end point. Occasionally lower motor neurone destruction causes confusion with amyotropic lateral sclerosis. Either way the prognosis is bad. Amyotrophic lateral sclerosis lasts longer, supposed by some no doubt to be a consolation.

Antiparkinsonian medication in high doses is often recommended but makes no difference to the outcome.

Deficiency disorders

Pellagra

Pellagra is a deficiency syndrome, rarely found in developed countries except in severely undernourished alcoholics. It was first described in Spain in the 18th Century where the skin lesions caused it to be called 'mal de la rosa'. It is a multiple deficiency syndrome caused by lack of *niacin* and *tryptophan*. The lesions of skin, gut and brain are summed up in the triad 'diarrhoea, dermatitis and dementia', though dementia is a late stage manifestation. The disease usually starts slowly and hence may be missed. Early symptoms include weakness, poor memory and concentration and headache. The clinical picture can suggest personality disorder or neurosis but an organic mental state supervenes; usually subacute delirium. Neurological signs such as paresis and fits come on later in the disease, when dementia is obvious. Untreated it ends in coma and death. Treatment is with parenteral niacin 100 mg hourly for 10 hours, followed by oral niacin.

Vitamin B$_{12}$ deficiency

The neurological complications of B$_{12}$ deficiency are well known mainly in subacute combined degeneration of the cord involving damage to the posterior and lateral columns. The usual history is of numbness and paraethesiae in hands and feet plus associated ataxia. Diagnosis is made by measuring the serum B$_{12}$ level which distinguishes it from other causes of similar neurological deficit such as cervical spondylosis and multiple sclerosis. The mental changes are not specific and this has led to the suggestion that all psychiatric patients, particularly the elderly should be screened for B_{12} deficiency (Edwin *et al*, 1965; Hunter R. Matthew D.M., 1965).

A wide range of psychiatric syndromes are described in B_{12} deficiency; affective psychoses, confusional states, paranoid psychoses and dementia. Shulman (1967) surveyed 117 elderly psychiatric patients of whom $8 \cdot 5\%$ had serum B_{12} levels below 150 $\mu g\%$, but when compared with B_{12} levels in 100 elderly medical patients there was no significant difference. Shulman (1967) reported on 10 psychiatric patients with low B_{12} levels, five had senile dementia, three were depressed, one was hypomanic and one had an acute confusional state.

The four patients with affective symptoms improved without B_{12} therapy, one patient died and the five demented patients showed no improvement with B_{12} therapy. Shulman concluded that B_{12} deficiency does not have a general psychiatric aetiological role, in his view routine B_{12} investigations are not justified in all patients but that careful haematological screening should be carried out in patients with obscure organic cerebral syndromes. In the past there have been a number of assertions to the effect that nutritional deficiencies, anaemia and disordered mental states might be common in mental hospital patients with B_{12} deficiency. This does not appear to be the case. It was formerly asserted that there were special psychoses associated with B_{12} deficiency, in fact affective and schizophrenic pictures are rare, the association is quite clearly with organic syndromes.

Early B_{12} therapy may avert irreversible organic cerebral damage, depressive symptoms were common in Shulman's series but occurred only in B_{12} deficient patients with a previous history of depression.

Psychiatric symptoms associated with B_{12} deficiency are not easy to spot and are often missed, this is hardly surprising since pernicious anaemia usually comes on slowly with glossitis, weakness, and abdominal pains which often follow neurological or psychiatric symptoms. Management of psychiatric syndromes associated with pernicious anaemia consists of B_{12} therapy (100 μg daily for 3 weeks and thereafter maintenance doses).

Wernicke's encephalopathy

Wernicke's encephalopathy is the result of thiamine deficiency and is found in chronic alcoholics and in patients suffering from any condition that can cause severe malnutrition, conditions such as gastric carcinoma, pernicious anaemia, hyperemesis gravidarum and starvation.

There is usually a sudden onset of delirium or a change of consciousness; nystagmus, pupillary abnormalities and opthalmoplegia. The latter reflect the neuropathological changes in the mid brain and corpora mamillaria. Confabulation and disorientation are common, also fits. There is a considerable overlap with the Korsakov syndrome, and polyneuritis is commonly found. Response to parenteral thiamine (100 mg daily) is dramatic but complete recovery does not necessarily occur, but the recovery rate is said to be better than Korsakov's syndrome.

Korsakov's syndrome

In 1887 Korsakov published a dissertation *On Alcoholic Paralysis* in which he described polyneuritis and a severe confusional state associated with confabulation. The syndrome is a non-specific manifestation of a variety of conditions, cerebral trauma, nutritional deficiency and metabolic abnormalities such as cerebral arteriosclerosis. In alcoholism the syndrome is caused by poor diet and thiamine deficiency. It was formerly held that there was a specific anatomical lesion affecting the mamillary bodies and dorso medial thalamic nuclei, but it now seems likely that there is no specific lesion in the CNS. In alcoholics the syndrome usually follows an attack of delirium tremens.

The manifestations are:

1 Severe memory impairment
2 Disorientation
3 A tendency to manufacture answers—confabulation
4 Euphoria

The patient is usually breezy and insouciant though the euphoria is rather empty. He answers questions confidently, apparently unaware of how wrong he is. Full recovery is uncommon and the response to treatment with thiamine and vitamin B is never complete. Consider the following case.

A 57 year old man was admitted having been found unconscious, smelling of alcohol with an empty whisky bottle in his pocket. Twenty-four hours after admission he said 'Oh yes, Doctor, I've been here for six weeks. My job is in the hospital so every one around me here is hospitalised. The date today? Well I'm not quite on the spot—I suspect it is April 23rd, 1924—well Tuesday of course—that is my best day as you well know Dr. Wilson, I'm sorry I mean Baker. This hospital? Well, it's

Guyson isn't it. Where do I live? Well, Dr. Butcher fancy asking me that—in the surrounds—they still exist, well don't they Sir. Visitors—of course, they pop in and do clerical work? Do I drink—well, yes not purely and simply for drink—it gets topside of you.'

Endocrine and metabolic diseases

Adrenal insufficiency—Addison's disease

In Addison's original description he stressed the presence of anergia, apathy and depressed mood. And this is continually reflected in clinical experience. Mental changes may precede the appearance of physical symptoms by months and may prevent recognition by being atypical and the picture may be complicated by odd episodic behaviour caused by hypoglycaemic attacks.

Addison's disease is uncommon, more common in men than women between the ages 20 and 40. The onset is usually insidious and although the classic picture of pigmentation, anergia and low cardiac output clinches the diagnosis, missing it can be near fatal if Addisonian crises occurs. The onset may be so insidious that patient and doctor may overlook it together. E.g. A 25 year old patient was the acquaintance of a doctor whom he occasionally met. The patient told his doctor acquaintance that he always felt ill though all his friends constantly remarked on his suntan. He felt weak and thirsty all the time. His suntan was Addisonian pigmentation.

Cushing's syndrome

Cushing's syndrome, osteoporosis, hypertension, wasting and striae, can be caused not only by basophil adenoma of the pituitary but also by steroid therapy, lung and ovarian tumours. There are no specific psychiatric syndromes though depression and organic syndromes are the most common, mainly clouded states and dementia. The appropriate treatment while halting the Cushing syndrome, does not of course, reverse any dementia that may have occurred.

Acromegaly

The onset is insidious. Often there are persistent complaints of weakness, sweatiness and vague depression. All non-specific complaints and a good reminder of the unhelpful diagnostic quality of non-specific symptoms. More specific symptoms include headache and visual loss.

Late symptoms include more severe depression, loss of libido and impotence. Again these are all symptoms which are found in any middle aged depressive.

Hypoglycaemia

The relationship between glucose metabolism and the mental state are poorly understood, despite investigation. Psychiatric interest in insulin induction was intensified when insulin coma became the first apparently effective physical treatment in schizophrenia, following Sakel's discovery that hypoglycaemia was an effective sedation in narcotic withdrawal. Insulin coma treatment remained standard in schizophrenia until Ackner *et al* (1954) showed it to be no more effective than barbiturate induced coma. Until then it was thought that the insulin effect was specific but this view is now discarded, first in view of Ackner's findings and secondly because of the better results achieved using neuroleptic drugs.

On the other hand it is interesting to note that schizophrenic patients recovering from coma used to make better contact, lost their delusional preoccupation and seemed more 'normal' until they reached clear consciousness in the same way that psychotic patients often improved during recovery from anaesthetics. Possibly this improvement in lightened consciousness has not been studied enough.

In ordinary life hypoglycaemia often causes vivid effects on feeling and behaviour. The early morning sluggishness and irritability of many is relieved by tea and toast. Episodic hypoglycaemia in the unstable diabetic is a well known cause of anger and odd behaviour before loss of consciousness.

In insulin secreting tumours the symptoms are often severe though these episodic changes are often missed until the combination of rage and facial flushing suggest that the blood sugar and glucose tolerance curves should be measured. Pathological changes can be severe including visual and auditory hallucinosis.

Thyrotoxicosis

Thyrotoxicosis is said to be more common in colder climates and is more common in women than men in the ratio of 4:1. Excess thyroid hormone secretion and diffuse thyroid enlargement are usual, rarely hyperplasia is localised as in toxic nodular goitre. The symptomatology of thyroid over-activity is familiar; restlessness, anxiety, irritability with raised pulse and cardiac arrhythmias, weight loss and eye signs.

The psychiatric picture may be hard to distinguish from anxiety—in severe cases psychosis occurs—either affective or schizophrenic, related to the patient's premorbid personality. Some have suggested that certain personalities are more prone to thyrotoxicosis than others, this has not been proved.

Myxoedema

The original description of hypothyroidism in adults was made by William Gull (1873) in a paper discussing female cases: he mentioned mental symptoms and this was reinforced by Ord (1878) and Savage (1880) who completed the early contribution of the physicians of Guy's Hospital—by describing a myxoedematous patient in a mental hospital. The psychiatric aspects of myxoedema were reviewed by Asher (1949) Browning *et al* (1954) and Tonks (1964). There has been some disagreement as to whether or not there is a specific psychosis associated with myxoedema. Apathy and depression are common symptoms in myxoedema where physical sluggishness and inertia are typical well known findings, whose significance can easily be missed. Myxoedema can also cause organic mental states, subacute delirium and dementia, the end point of untreated myxoedema before coma and death.

Porphyria

The porphyrias are important for the psychiatrist since one group, the *acute intermittent porphyrias*, often mimic 'pure' psychiatric disorders and the diagnosis may be missed.

Porphyrias are inborn metabolic disorders which occur in two main forms, *congenital porphyria* and *acute intermittent porphyria*; the former affects men more than women and is thought to be a marrow disorder. Inheritance is Mendelian recessive. Acute intermittent porphyria is more common in women than men, inherited as a Mendelian dominant trait and often presents psychiatric symptoms. Associated manifestations include dermatitis, fits and peripheral neuropathy. Psychiatric symptoms may be very misleading suggesting neurosis or personality disturbance but a common presentation is a subacute delirious state or sometimes inexplicable anti-social behaviour. A psychotic picture can also occur, in other words the whole gamut of psychiatric symptomatology. The subacute delirious state with hallucinosis is said to be the most common.

Precipitants Attacks of acute intermittent porphyria can be set off by alcohol and barbiturates, also sulphonamides and chloroquin.

Hepatolenticular degeneration (Wilson's disease)

This rare disease is caused by chronic copper poisoning which produces liver damage and extrapyramidal syndromes. It is a hereditary metabolic disorder, transmitted by excessive inheritance of abnormal copper metabolism based on ceruloplasmin deficiency.

The pathological changes are degeneration of the putamen and caudate nuclei, plus cortical and cerebellar damage. There are excessive copper deposits in brain and liver.

Manifestations

1 Acute syndromes, usually an early onset with rapid deterioration. Neurological signs tend to be prominent and the psychiatric picture is mainly one of severe emotional lability.
2 Late onset cases presenting with psychiatric symptoms which may mimic psychosis or a personality disorder. Fits and aggressive outbursts are common.
3 The most common picture is dementia and severe speech disturbance.

Diagnosis The diagnosis is clinched by the triad of extrapyramidal disorder, hepatic cirrhosis and a green yellow pigment on the lower corneal margin, the Kayser-Fleischer ring. Urinary copper excretion is increased and the serum ceruloplasmin is under 20 mg%.

Treatment Treatment aims at encouraging copper excretion by using chelating agents such as penicillamine (1–4 g/daily) or BAL (2–3 dimer-capto propanol).

Genetically determined disorders

Huntington's chorea

Every doctor knows that Huntington's chorea is a hereditary degenerative brain disease with involuntary movements but most have never seen a case although the prevalence rate has been estimated as 9 per 100 000, *i.e.* in Britain it is about twice as common as heroin addiction. It was described in simple 19th Century prose by George Huntington, a physician of East Hampton, Long Island. His father and grandfather had observed cases for over 70 years in their practice and suspected it was hereditary. Despite its tragic outcome it remains a fascinating disorder because it produces not only dementia and involuntary movements, but also a wide range of psychiatric disturbance, including personality disorders and suicide. The cases described by Huntington were traced to two brothers who went to America in 1630 from Bures in Suffolk. It is found all over the world, is transmitted by dominant inheritance thus affecting 50% of children in the family. The disease never skips a generation and is never found in un-affected families though unexplained sporadic cases have been described. Pathological changes include atrophy in the basal ganglia, cortical atrophy, mainly frontal, and basal meningitis.

Clinical picture   The first symptoms usually start insidiously between ages 30 and 50. Choreiform movements are not necessarily the first symptoms, personality change often precedes them. The typical personality disorder suggests frontal lobe impairment with changes in ethical standards, irritability, generally 'difficult' behaviour, sometimes with outbursts of aggression and violence. Other personality changes include suspiciousness and hypersensitivity which can develop into a full blown paranoid psychosis with delusions and hallucinations. Choreiform movements affect face, neck and arms at first, later affecting the whole body. As the chorea and ataxia get worse, the mental state becomes more obviously that of dementia, with, as might be expected, a depressive mood.

In Huntington families there is also an associated significant incidence of alcoholism, mental subnormality and criminality. Minski and Guttman (1938) noted the interesting finding that affected family members resembled affected parents more closely than did non-affected. Suicidal tendencies are common and involve affected and non-affected family members alike. Psychosis is common, diagnostic difficulty arises if a person from a

Huntington family becomes psychotic without involuntary movements. Consider the following case.

A 48 year old woman was admitted from a railway terminus where she had been wandering around in a filthy and neglected state, screaming abuse at passers-by. The main abnormalities on mental state examination were persecutory ideas, fragmentary talk and auditory hallucinosis. She was found to come from a Huntington family, her husband knew this and had concealed it from the children since he thought that as she had no involuntary movements therefore she would not pass on the disease to the children, and he had disclaimed responsibility for their 'mad mother'.

Sometimes a family member develops movement disorder without dementia or *vice versa*, these are simple variants of the syndrome but the prognosis is no better in either instance since chorea affects muscles that control swallowing and breathing, as well as gait and handling so that progress to death is unchanged. The usual duration of disease is 15 years from the time of diagnosis.

The wider implications of Huntington's chorea gives an interesting view of the interaction between genes and environment in psychiatric illness, family members know they stand a 50% chance of inheriting a progressive fatal disease in middle life and it is for question whether suicide, instability, alcoholism and crime in Huntington families are based on inherited defect or are a reaction to a terrible threat.

Treatment is entirely palliative, medication to control movements, physiotherapy, general care and good nursing in the final stages.

Tay Sach's disease (familial amaurotic idiocy)

This is a rare type of dementia transmitted by a single recessive gene. It is found most commonly in Jewish people but can occur in Gentiles. The clinical picture is of progressive mental deterioration occurring in a previously normal child, though onset in adolescence and later has been described. The child becomes blind, weak and presents a picture of severe mental retardation. Death usually occurs in 2 years.

There is one diagnostic sign namely the 'cherry red spot', a red spot seen at the central foveal area in the optic fundus.

Toxic causes of organic cerebral syndromes

There are many comparatively well known toxic causes of organic brain

F

damage, domestic, industrial and medical, all of which can produce an *acute syndrome or dementia*.

They include drugs; industrial and domestic poisons—particularly the heavy metals; organic chemicals; and carbon monoxide.

Drugs

Many drugs used in medicine and psychiatry act by reducing consciousness, and all such cortical depressants may cause brain damage following coma. It is questionable whether they cause brain damage through chronic abuse. A simple factual statement relevant to this is provided by national expenditure on medication. In 1968 the estimated 'total ingredient cost' of the NHS in England and Wales included £21·6 million spent on drugs acting on the CNS, out of a total drug bill of £108·6 million. If we exclude £5·7 million spent on CNS stimulants and antidepressants, the rest, *i.e.* £15·9 million was spent on analgesics, hypnosedatives and tranquillisers, the last two being the largest group.

In general practice every year there are around 15·5 million prescriptions written for barbiturates and 15 million for tranquillisers. With this in mind any sensible doctor will anticipate at least the possibility of brain damage following the prolonged taking of CNS depressants.

This has been long known and was an important part of medical concern in the days when bromides were the only sedatives available in mental hospitals and when over 60% of mental hospital patients were as ill with chronic bromide intoxication as they were with the psychoses that caused their admission.

Bromide intoxication Bromides are rarely used nowadays, but at one time they were widely used in vast quantities to quieten agitated and excited patients, causing widespread chronic bromide intoxication, often fatal. The severity of chronic bromide intoxication is dose related. In *simple bromide* intoxication the clinical picture is a straightforward *dysmnesic syndrome*: poor retention and recall, apathy and mental inertia. The pupils are usually irregular and unequal, and CNS signs include *tremor and ataxia*. With more severe intoxication patients develop subacute and acute delirium. Other syndromes include hallucinosis in *clear* consciousness but generally chronic bromism causes an organic cerebral syndrome. Withdrawal fits are common. Skin rashes are common in bromide intoxication.

In general psychiatric symptoms appear once the blood bromide level is over 150 mg%.

The list of syndromes caused by bromide intoxication is extensive, the most common picture being delirium though hallucinosis and schizophreniform psychoses *can* occur, plus the associated neurological signs: visual disturbance, ataxia and incoordination. Despite its present rarity there have been recent warnings about its unsuspected incidence in patients who abuse sedatives that contain small amounts of bromide.

Treatment consists of stopping the drug and speeding up its excretion with sodium chloride. There is no justification for the use of bromides, there are far safer anticonvulsants and tranquillisers available and their use is now restricted to *carbromal*, a sedative which has small amounts of bromide. This also can cause symptoms if the dose mounts up. The dangers of bromide are reiterated but occasional cases occur.

In *chronic barbiturate intoxication* the syndrome of ataxia, dysarthria and nystagmus is identical to *chronic alcohol intoxication*, as are the withdrawal syndromes, *i.e.* tremor, fits, delirium, hallucinosis and clouded states. Chronic barbiturate taking can interfere with B_{12} and folate metabolism leading to anaemia and dementia irrespective of the cumulative effects of repeated barbiturate induced coma. Other *anticonvulsant drugs* such as phenytoin and primidone also interfere with B_{12} and folate metabolism and are under suspicion of causing dementia.

Industrial and domestic poisons

Lead poisoning is usually found in industrial workers and produces the characteristic encephalopathy in which the patient is apathetic, weak and dull. Severe lead poisoning can cause delirium and fits. In children chronic lead poisoning frequently occurs if the child is eating paints that contain lead. Nowadays this is relatively uncommon except in old houses where the paintwork is old. This is usually in poorer districts thus chronic lead poisoning is more common. The clinical picture of lead encephalopathy in children includes apathy, failure to thrive and fits.

Mercury poisoning is found in industrial workers and causes tremor, ataxia, dyskinesia and organic impairment.

Manganese poisoning also causes extrapyramidal syndromes, *e.g.* dyskinesia and organic impairment.

Other compounds which cause organic syndromes include anilines, nitrobenzenes, carbon tetrachloride and carbon disulphide. All of these substances can produce chronic intoxication with organic impairment and a clinical picture of subacute delirium and dementia.

Carbon monoxide

Since the introduction of less toxic domestic gas the death rate from carbon monoxide poisoning has fallen. It is difficult to assess what may be the long term effects of chronic carbon monoxide poisoning in heavy smokers and industrial workers. After acute poisoning recovery from coma may be followed by apparent normality for days but is then followed by organic cerebral syndromes ranging from an amnestic syndrome through delirium to dementia. There may be associated Parkinsonian symptoms. Though recovery tends to be complete the extent of permanent damage is related to the depth of intoxication. The late sequelae of carbon monoxide poisoning include apathy, poor concentration, amnesia and irritable depression.

Carcinoma—psychiatric associations

Dementia can occur with cerebral secondary deposits from any primary site, though in practice carcinoma of the bronchus is the commonest cause, hence the importance of chest X-ray in the investigation of any dementia. In addition to this primary carcinomata of lung, ovaries, breast, rectum and prostate may be associated with a syndrome of dementia with symptoms of subacute cerebellar degeneration and peripheral neuropathy (Brain, 1958; McGovern *et al*, 1959).

Epilepsy

Epilepsy and altered mental states

Personality disorders are commonly associated with temporal lobe epilepsy, the association exceeds chance expectation and is presumed to be linked to the epileptic condition. At one time the term 'epileptic' personality was often used to describe personality deterioration in institutionalised epileptics and a variety of traits were named, most of which were rather derogatory. Nowadays the generally accepted view is that this personality type was probably an artefact and more related to excessive medication and institutionalism rather than a specific personality disorder. Immature personalities are said to be associated with epilepsy, the usual features noted include temper tantrums and a tendency to carry on in an irritable unpredictable way. Another feature noted in severe epileptics is 'stickiness', slow and pedantic talk which seems overprecise but somehow never reaches the point.

Taylor (1967) studied 100 epileptic patients in order to find relationships between the mental state and life history and epilepsy. All were temporal lobe epileptics who had undergone temporal lobectomy. Thirteen had been 'normal' before surgery, 48 were 'psychopathic', 30 'neurotic', 16 psychotic and 5 had an 'epileptic personality'. Of the psychopaths 27 were aggressive and 15 immature and 8 of the psychotics had had long term schizophreniform psychoses. Taylor's main general finding was that 'long term personality disorder' is the most frequent finding in patients with temporal lobe epilepsy, although affective changes are often seen'. This study certainly confirms the association between the fits and personality disorder and is another interesting example of the relationship between biologically disordered brain function and psychiatric abnormalities.

The psychiatric aspects of epilepsy go beyond associations with personality disorder, mood disturbance and epilepsy for instance—the general behaviour of the epileptic have been subjects for speculation since medicine first started (Temkin, 1971) Odd behaviour between fits and epileptic psychoses were first described by Falret (1860), later writers have refined and formalised Falret's observations. Most of the observations about behaviour disturbance in epileptics have been made on hospitalised patients. Common and minor disturbances surround the fit, for instance nursing staff can often tell when a patient is 'building up for a fit' despite indications of odd but repeated mood disturbance which may last for days and are relieved by a fit. In the postictal period patients may wander off in a fugue, behave antisocially or become muddled and psychotic for a few days, this is most common after repeated fits.

Epilepsy and violence

Episodic and unexpected violent behaviour is often ascribed to epilepsy, this point was often raised in the days of capital punishment for murder where epilepsy was offered as a mitigating disorder. Falconer reported on

250 temporal lobectomies followed up for 10 years and found no case of a patient charged with a crime committed during or after a fit. Walker (1961) examined the possible relationships between epilepsy and murder describing an inexplicable murder where the accused claimed total amnesia for the event and later had a (L) temporal lobectomy. After death he was found to have a (R) temporal haemangioma. Walker doubted any valid common association between murder and epilepsy and suggested that wherever it is suspected that epilepsy and murder are associated the following six criteria should always be looked for.

1   Presence of true epilepsy
2   Attacks similar to the attack which occurred at the time of the offence
3   Duration of unconsciousness should match the type of fit
4   Degree of altered consciousness should match previous attacks
5   EEG findings should be appropriate
6   Circumstances of the offence should match the person's supposed lack of awareness at the time of the offence

If these criteria are strictly applied the supposed association between violent crime and epilepsy is not proven, the question remains open. There is at least fair clinical support for an association between epilepsy and aggressive behaviour but it seems that this aggression is related to inter-ictal personality disorder rather than to fits.

Epilepsy and psychosis

The occurrence of epilepsy and psychosis has been frequently commented on as an interesting clinical finding. ECT was first used because it was wrongly assumed that there was a negative association between epilepsy and schizophrenia. Many authors however, have commented on schizophreniform psychoses in epilepsy (Hill, 1953; Pond, 1957; Gruhle, 1936) noting onset in middle life when epilepsy has been present for many years. Pond (1957) found these psychoses to be clinically similar to schizophrenia, features such as ideas of influence, paranoid delusions thought disorder and auditory hallucinations being common.

An important problem in explaining any association between epilepsy and psychosis is that these are both common conditions, so that the occurrence of the two together could be accounted for by chance. Slater and Beard (1963) in reviewing epileptic psychoses calculated that epileptics developed 'schizophrenia-like psychoses with a frequency much greater than chance expectation would permit' and concluded that a schizophreniform psychosis *could* be the consequence of epilepsy.

Patients studied were drawn from admissions to the Maudsley Hospital and National Hospital for Nervous Diseases from 1948 to 1959. Criteria for inclusion were

1 Epilepsy
2 Diagnosis of schizophrenia made by experienced clinicians
3 The diagnosis would have been schizophrenia in the absence of epilepsy

A total of 69 patients were studied, 47 of whom had been elsewhere diagnosed as schizophrenic. The mean age of onset of psychosis was 29·8 years after a mean duration of epilepsy of 14·1 years. This suggested that a long history of epilepsy caused psychosis. The psychoses were classified as acute, episodic (20) and subacute/insidious (29). The course of psychosis was classified as improved, fluctuating and chronic (31 patients, *i.e.* most common). Symptomatology was typically schizophrenic except that thought disorder was often organic, though 31 patients had schizophrenic thought disorder. The general conclusion drawn was that these psychoses were *indistinguishable from schizophrenia.*

Further categorisation of patients into a, chronic psychosis and confusional episodes; b, chronic paranoid psychosis; and c, hebephrenia-like, showed that a significant number of groups a and b had suffered brain damage (birth trauma, head injury, encephalitis etc.). There was no evidence that medication, fit control and fit severity determined the onset of psychosis. Temporal lobe disorder was the commonest type (45), diagnosed clinically and confirmed by EEG. All studies confirmed organic damage in 37 out of 56 cases. There was no evidence of increased incidence of schizophrenia in sibs or parents. The authors' final conclusions were that epileptic psychoses may be regarded as symptomatic schizophrenias which arise in consequence of epilepsy.

Temporal lobe epilepsy (psychomotor epilepsy)

The manifestations of temporal lobe epilepsy (TLE) consist of recurrent episodic changes in higher mental function associated with partial alterations in consciousness. This covers the basic features of TLE in which quite frequently the episodic and often bizarre psychological symptoms may lead to diagnostic difficulties.

Consciousness Total loss of consciousness as in grand mal fits, is uncommon in TLE. It is more common to find a partial change in consciousness in which the patient is clouded or confused, sometimes severely. In other cases the patient may appear to be in a trance. Rarely a patient with TLE may develop episodic states of heightened awareness.

Behaviour The original descriptions of TLE emphasised the importance of mouth and tongue movements, *e.g.* chewing lip, smacking and swallowing. These are not essential to the diagnosis though they are frequently part of the aura.

More complicated behaviour such as automatism, repeated acts which appear almost ritual in character, *are* described in TLE as also are fugue states, *i.e.* wandering away after a fit. Epileptic fugues however are brief compared to hysterical and schizophrenic fugues.

Mood Forced thinking is a common experience in TLE as are delay, slowness and interruption of thought. Patients also experience poor concentration and states of bewilderment, incomprehension and perplexity. This may be associated with the repetition of some phrase or question, *e.g.* 'Why am I?'.

Perception The perceptual changes in TLE are probably the best known phenomena in this disorder, these take the form of short lived hallucinatory episodes. It is however, incorrect to suppose that TLE is *always* characterised by olfactory or gustatory hallucinations, these figured largely in early descriptions but it is now recognised although they may be features of the aura they are not diagnostic essentials. Hallucinations occur in any modality but auditory hallucinations are probably the most common. A good diagnostic point to look for is the repetitive content of hallucinosis in TLE. Other and perhaps more frequent perceptual changes include feelings of unreality of the self (depersonalisation) and of the environment (derealisation) and also feeling of familiarity in a situation supposedly previously experienced (*déjà vu*) or feelings of unfamiliarity in a previously experienced situation (*jamais vu*).

8

Affective disorders

INTRODUCTION

Mood change is so common that anyone who says 'I'm depressed' can expect a hearing and may know what he means when he says so. This is true of minor mood disturbance but severe mood disturbance is another matter since it may lead to the unlikely alternatives of being detained in hospital as 'manic' or to the experience of having 100 v AC passed across the head.

The affective disorders are all characterised by a primary disturbance of mood, the polar extremes range from the profound sad dejection of psychotic **depression** to the breezy insightless hilarity of **mania.**

Mood disturbance is recognised as part of an illness only when it is excessive and goes beyond the customary fluctuations of mood that are part of the fabric of ordinary mental life. It is as simple as that—affective disorders are diagnosed mainly on the basis of quantitative mood change; however it has to be said that the division between 'normal' and 'abnormal' mood is largely arbitrary. In affective disorder however mood disturbance is not merely extreme, it is also disproportionate. Another aspect of pathological mood change is that it is unresponsive to outside influence—the depressed patient is not easily reassured nor cheered up any more than is the hypomanic even slightly put off by comments on his exuberant behaviour.

Physiological symptoms are common in affective disorder, *e.g.* weight loss, insomnia, loss of libido and general loss of energy, and they usually follow mood change although sometimes they can be the presenting symptoms. The term depression is used in many ways. 'Depression' is talked about by many and the 'average intelligent person' probably has a vague idea of what he means by it. This vagueness is not confined to laymen, the boundaries between the uses of the word are indistinct.

Endogenous and reactive depression

These terms will be considered later, but an early introduction is necessary: *endogenous* is used to describe severe inexplicable depression and *reactive* to define an 'illness' that is an understandable reaction to an experience. The differences can be summarised thus:

Endogenous	*Reactive*
Severe mood change	Less severe
Diurnal variation	None
Insomnia—early waking	No early waking
Spontaneous onset	Reaction to life experience
Responds to physical treatment	Treated with psychotherapy
Genetic factor	No genetic factor

This classification of depression has caused a persistent even eternal dialogue amongst psychiatrists about the question of relating psychiatric illness to life, a problem that does not trouble the layman; someone experiences loss and is sad and none of his friends are surprised if his sadness is prolonged; they say 'he hasn't got over it'. For the psychiatrist the problem is not so simple, for a start reactive depressions do not necessarily recur given the same precipitant, on the other hand organic psychoses if recurrent do tend to have the same content, usually a garbled version of previous experience. In other words people do not run as true to form in terms of their reactions as they do under the influence of either organic brain damage or genetic inheritance. This latter is seen in families where there is clear history of affective disorder, the incidence and recurrence of depression or mania bears little relationship to experience but an inexorable relationship to inheritance. The problem is made more complicated by the fact that while we take it for granted when unhappy events cause unhappiness we are taken aback when cheery news sometimes triggers off depression!

Making sense

Another important feature of affective disorders in general is that even in the most severe cases it is usually possible to make sense out of them, to feel oneself in the patient's situation in a way which is impossible in schizophrenia. It is easier to empathise with the patient, even if his ideas are exaggerated and delusional, it is still possible to trace *some* connection between feeling and action.

The gloom and pessimism of the depressive is something that we can understand though at the same time we can recognise its disproportionate quality. In the case of the hypomanic, although we are left behind by his restless energy we can see how his behaviour and view of the world are consistent with his elevated mood. In both these disorders there is a recognisable internal consistency which we cannot find in the schizo-phrenic unless we make convoluted mental exercises.

Historical note

Kraepelin was the first to use the term 'manic-depressive' insanity, but Hippocrates made clinical descriptions of affective disorder, Burton wrote extensively of depression in *The Anatomy of Melancholy* and in the mid 19th Century Falret (1854) described 'folie circulaire' and Kahlbaum (1882) distinguished between mild cases of 'cyclothymia' and severe intractable cases 'vesania typica circularis'. After Kraepelin when psychiatrists began to look more closely at manic depressive psychosis they became more aware of morbid depression and realised that depression is more common than typical manic depressive psychosis. Nowadays the term *affective disorder* is preferred as a term to include not only psychoses but also milder types of depression.

AETIOLOGY OF AFFECTIVE DISORDERS

Genetic factors

Early attempts at identifying a genetic factor in affective disorders tended to look for genetic evidence that might support the idea of a polarity between endogenous and neurotic depression. Stenstedt (1959), Winokur and Pitts (1964) and Kay (1959) all found considerable overlap between types of depression in the families studied which makes it in general impossible to justify this idea. However, Leonhard (1959) pointed out that a better dichotomy might be provided by separating affective disorders into bipolar (manic depressive) and unipolar (pure depression) and look for evidence of genetic inheritance in these. Since then there have been a number of reports that suggest a genetic inheritance of this sort quite strongly (Perris, 1966; Angst, 1966; Winokur & Clayton, 1967). In general the findings have been that unipolar psychoses and bipolar psychoses appear to breed true with very little overlap. The percentages of affected family members vary, though not greatly from one series to another. Angst, for instance found the percentage of affected family members in bipolar psychosis as 14·4% (parents) and 21·5% (sibs), and in unipolar psychosis 11·2% (parents) and 12·2% (sibs). Other workers, *e.g.* Hopkinson (1964) and Winokur and Clayton (1967) found also significantly higher incidence of affective disorder in early onset cases.

Twin studies suggest a concordance rate of around 70% in monozygotic and 19% in dizygotic twins of the same sex.

The work so far reported then strongly suggests genetic influence in bipolar and unipolar psychoses which have been shown to breed true in families and which have the great advantage of being relatively easy to identify. The mode of inheritance is not known, clearly it is not simple Mendelian inheritance, the majority view at present is that it is probably a polygenic type of inheritance.

Biochemical factors

Coppen (1967) remarked that some psychiatrists would regard as provocative the linking of biochemistry and affective disorder, a fair comment since many still question the relevance of biochemistry in depression or mania, claiming that any biochemical abnormality found is as likely to be a consequence of the condition as it is to be a causal factor. In fact present evidence does point to an important role of disturbed biochemistry. Simple clinical examples include depression following jaundice and influenza or excitement following steroid or isoniazid therapy.

The success of physical treatment in depression cannot be shrugged aside and as Coppen (1967) commented, antidepressant drugs are now so widely used that it is increasingly hard to find depressives who have not had them.

In depression the first difficulty to be overcome is to find out what types of depression have a biochemical basis. Depressed mood is part of normal life—does this involve biochemical change? Minor mood change is not to be studied in this way though perhaps if we did understand the biochemistry of feeling it might clarify the biochemistry of pathological mood.

But research *has* to be concerned with people *available* for and *willing to be* studied and this has to date been concerned with patients with affective disorders—selected on the basis of severity of illness. Biochemical research tends to follow the patient during and after illness so that the patient is his own control.

There are three main groups of metabolites studied in affective disorders.

1   Cerebral amines
2   Electrolytes
3   Adrenal cortex

Cerebral amines (biogenic amines)

The cerebral amines, adrenaline, noradrenaline and 5-hydroxytryptamine (5HT, serotonin) and dopamine are CNS transmitters stored in free nerve endings and acting on the synapse. When released they are active, when stored, inactive. They are derived from amino acids by decarboxylation and are reduced by deoxidative deamination by the enzyme(s) monoamine oxidase.

The cerebral amine theory of depression is based on the fact that amines are found in higher concentrations in various brain areas in either free or bound form. When bound amines are liberated, the theory is that cerebral stimulation occurs; conversely depression may follow a disproportionate shift from free to bound form. Hence mood change could occur if free amines are released or if release is prevented or oxidation delayed. In effect these mechanisms are thought to explain the actions of various antidepressant drugs, *e.g.* monoamine oxidase inhibitors that prevent destruction of available free amines, and tricyclic antidepressants that interfere with transport across the cell membrane. The storage of monoamines is in neuronal pools whether as 'readily available' monoamines at sympathetic nerve ends, *i.e.* 'available transmitters' to stimulate adrenergic receptors, or as 'deep pool' monoamines stored near neuronal mitochondria, *i.e.* as recently synthesised monoamines.

Some research suggests that tricyclic antidepressants such as imipramine increase amine availability and inhibit 5-HT uptake. Further evidence linking biogenic amines with depression is the severe depression caused by reserpine which depletes serotonin (5-HT) and causes depression in 15% of patients treated with reserpine.

Electrolyte and water disturbance

Any doctor who has looked after dehydrated patients or patients with postoperative electrolyte disturbance will have been impressed by their altered mental states, admittedly such patients may be exhausted and frightened and are more likely to develop odd mental states but the common thread that unites them is electrolyte disturbance. At the CNS basic transmitter level the mechanism is one of polarisation/depolarisation, *i.e.* electron change. Therefore it can be inferred that if CNS transmission is related to mood change then electrolyte diffusion may be relevant.

Early studies on water and electrolyte changes in affective disorder were mainly carried out on patients with cyclic affective psychoses (Klein & Nunn, 1945; Crammer, 1959; Klein, 1950) but in time studies, *e.g.* of sodium and potassium exchange using isotope counting methods (Coppen & Mangoni, 1962) the relevance of ionic change was pointed out. This research showed proportional changes in total body water and in extracellular water after recovery from depression and an increase of 'residual sodium' in depression.

Other electrolyte studies have included sodium changes in mania (Coppen *et al*, 1966) and the possible roles of magnesium and calcium (Cade, 1964; Flach, 1964). The most relevant clinical therapeutic example lies in the use of lithium in affective disorders. Lithium alters sodium transport across cell membranes and is now extensively used in recurrent mania, and in recurrent depression.

Adrenal cortex

Psychiatric symptoms in hyper and hypoadrenalism are well known, the increased adrenal activity in Cushing's syndrome is usually associated with depressed mood, while apathetic depression is a well known accompaniment of Addison's disease. However the relationship of adrenal cortical activity to mood is not clearly understood.

In *summary* we can say that the biochemistry of mood disturbance is at present a mass of biochemical data, most of which suggests a fundamental pathogenic role for amines and electrolyte disturbance.

Aetiology of depression

Age

There is an association between age and depression, certain periods of life are especially vulnerable. Most depressions occur in middle aged and elderly people. This is not to deny that depression does affect youngsters but rather to emphasise the special risk for older people. Ageing brings not merely failure in physical function but also a wide range of psychological and social change. Growing old is not just developing rigid joints and papery skin but also less obvious psychological rigidity, a set attitude and a tendency to be less emotionally flexible and less able to adjust to life change and stress, less able to take strain and uncertainty. Also age brings more stress because of the greater range of responsibilities acquired.

Parents who have met the needs of their children dependent on them for everything find not only that the children are independent but that they are questioning if not deriding authority. So that around the middle years a person faces considerable changes in social role. Earning capacity is at its highest level but with retirement earnings fall away so that the stage is set for uncertainty, particularly in a society which values youth and accords little respect to age. Sexual function is an added area of stress. Fears of loss of sexual potency and notions of missed forbidden pleasures can cause many middle aged men to stray into promiscuity. This produces guilt and self-recrimination. For the middle aged woman the stresses are equally difficult. Mothers may feel less wanted by their children and by their husbands; and the menopause, quite apart from physiological change may present the real threat posed by the loss of childbearing ability. In addition to this people often feel less physically attractive as they grow older and this is something that even the least narcissistic find hard to cope with.

Social class

There is some evidence that depression is more common in middle and upper class people but this may not be absolutely true. What seems more likely is that depression is more often diagnosed in middle class people by middle class doctors, possibly because sharing the same class attitudes etc. the doctor finds it easier to diagnose depression in people who use the right code words, *i.e.* give him the right signals. On the other hand working class people may be less able to indicate their distress to the doctor or may complain about physical symptoms of depression. This is an important area which needs to be investigated. In England social class barriers do exist and are reflected in the form and content of speech and it seems likely that working class people cannot communicate as effectively with their doctor as their middle class colleagues. This is true of their contact with social agencies and courts where working class people frequently lose out on their entitlements because of class barriers and communication problems.

Life events

Many depressions follow on some relatively minor event in every day life. It is often hard to evaluate just how definitely these events can be accepted as causal. But whether or not they are causal it is a fact that they are often quoted by depressed people as being precipitants of their unhappiness. Disappointments in love, personal quarrels in the family and at work, difficult relationships in marriage and such-like. These are constantly quoted by depressives. The point about it is that what people call causes of depression may well be manifestations, *i.e.* the depressed person is more likely to be quarrelsome, more likely to fail in his job and falter in personal decision making and relationships. And when depression really hits home the sufferer naturally looks round for possible causes.

Other life events such as moving house are often quoted as are such things as the death of household pets, especially in lonely and elderly people.

Personality

In the case of manic depressive psychosis the link with personality may be fairly straightforward since the person often has a cyclothymic type of personality but as far as depression goes in general there are no clear links with personality though it may be thought that certain people are more prone to depression if they are over rigid in outlook, mildly obsessional and therefore less able to adapt and take the strains of life. Again immature people may be especially vulnerable to short lived changes in mood particularly in the wake of disappointment and frustration. Another personality type that is linked with depression is the 'depressive personality' usually characterised by a certain quiet gloominess and pessimism of outlook which can be illuminated by flashes of sardonic and wry self-deprecatory humour of a rather attractive sort. Storey (1969) has rightly commented at how little factual knowledge we really have about the role of personality in the aetiology of depression.

Physical illness and surgery

There is a real association here. This must seem like stating the obvious but chronic illness, especially chronic painful illness, is a frequent cause of depression. Also surgery, particularly mutilating surgery, *e.g.* mastectomy or amputation of a limb.

Virus infections such as influenza often cause depression as does infectious hepatitis. Depression is a well known consequence of jaundice.

Depression and aggression

In Freud's paper *Mourning and Melancholia* he pointed out that aggression played a key role in depression in that loss of a love object could result in the person diverting aggressive feelings from the lost object on to himself. One of the consequences of this observation has been at times a tendency for some psychiatrists to try and deal with depression as if it were repressed aggression and nothing else, *i.e.* 'let it all out and you'll feel better'.

Actually it is not as simple as all that. Freud wrote about melancholia, *i.e.* psychosis and never suggested that a quick catharsis would remove depression, and it really is unkind as well as stupid to try and treat a depressed person by telling him that it is all due to his bad feelings etc.

Drugs

A number of drugs can cause depression. They include the sulfonamides, methyldopa and perhaps the most severe of all is caused by reserpine which as we have seen causes depletion of serotonin (5-HT) in the brain. Short lived depressive periods usually follow the withdrawal of amphetamines taken over long periods. Although usually this depression settles quickly this is not always the case and many amphetamine takers complain of chronic depression for long periods after stopping.

Phenobarbitone is another drug that can cause depression if taken over long periods and the same is true of prolonged phenothiazine therapy.

The contraceptive pill, particularly those with a high progesterone content, can cause depression. Also steroids can cause depression, usually during withdrawal.

PRECIPITANTS OF AFFECTIVE DISORDER

Depression

The question of precipitants in depression is an interesting one. Anyone who feels low spirited is bound to ask himself why he should feel like this in the intervals between his family and friends either asking him or telling him why. Also being depressed, tense or even unhappy is a state which leads to preoccupied introspection, often dismissed by others as 'self-pity', no consolation to the person who remains absorbed in a ruminative search for causes of his distress. Nevertheless it is important to discover causes and much psychiatric research has looked at environmental causes and life events in the aetiology of depression. In everyday life people are used to being upset by loss and uncertainty or being cheered and elevated by success, relief of tension and simple events like public holidays.

Bereavement and depression

Grief is a psychological disorder which is usually typified by a change of mood, a loss of function and a picture which is so familiar as hardly to invite comment. Everyone is aware of grief and everyone experiences it. Characteristically it is the predicted response to personal loss, usually it is short lived and on the whole it rarely concerns the psychiatrist because it is self-limiting. It is fair to call it a psychological disorder, despite its universality, for the simple reason that it is associated with symptoms and loss of function. Its transient nature rarely means that outside 'treatment' is needed but as Parkes (1965) has commented 'a bruise or a burn does not cease to be pathological just because it is treated at home', and 'grief is a reaction and is also, because it leads to dysfunction, morbid or pathological'. Engel (1961) compares grief by analogy to a septic wound and refers to the complications of grief.

The relationship of grief to psychiatric disorder becomes of interest if it is possible to demonstrate that bereavement is an important antecedent in the onset of psychiatric disorder; we know that grief is the most typical sequel of bereavement but does bereavement lead to more serious consequences. There have been many attempts to examine this question, some of them will now be reviewed.

In the United States there was a disastrous fire in the Coconut Grove night club in Boston. Lindermann undertook the psychiatric care and investigation of relatives of people killed in the fire and reported (1944) on the psychiatric disturbances encountered. He commented on 101 cases of acute grief and remarked on the presence of a normal syndrome of grief and also on distorted pictures which were like normal grief. However it was not possible to discern from this study what were the main features of normal grief.

A study of widows in the East End of London was reported by Maris (1958). This examined 72 out of 104 unselected widows who were mainly young or middle aged women interviewed about 2 years after bereavement. Maris gave a detailed account of the natural history of grief and distinguished clearly between normal and abnormal grief reactions. Anticipatory grief has been studied by Bozemann, Orbach and Sutherland (1955) in their reports of the reactions of mothers of children with leukaemia when they discovered that there was no hope for their children, and also more recently by Hinton (1960).

Clayton *et al* (1972) examined 109 randomly selected widows and widowers (mean age 61) at one month after the death of the spouse and found that 35% showed typical depressive symptomatology. The depressed group was compared with the non-depressed group on 53 demographic, social and physical variables and there were no significant differences except that fewer of the depressed group tended to have children in the area they considered close. The authors drew the general conclusion that unhappiness and depressive symptoms form an affective syndrome very similar to typical depression but that the relationship between the two remained questionable.

The usual picture of grief following bereavement is determined first of all by the closeness of the lost person, this is a matter of common knowledge. Often the reaction is delayed or the person remains seemingly untouched—the term 'numbed with grief' is well enough known and of course numbing is not peculiar to grief, it can follow any severe traumatic experience, *e.g.* soldiers in wartime, people after disasters etc.

Then, usually in a matter of days the person begins to realise the extent of the loss more fully and becomes more distressed, yearning for the lost one even to the extent of acting as if he were still alive. At this stage periods of anxiety, irritability and even anger often occur, the person feels sad and lonely and is preoccupied with thoughts of the lost one who becomes idealised. Though all would agree on the description of grief there is uncertainty and disagreement about the duration. The figure of 6 months seems to have been selected almost arbitrarily, probably for the simple reason that most bereaved people in general feel rather better after 6 months and are able to return to a normal life. And this is a very important feature of grief namely that grief renders people much less effective in every sense—they cannot cope with their work, have little interest in things or people and feel disinclined for work or pleasure, food, drink or sex.

Some of the most detailed recent studies on the natural history of bereavement and its place in the aetiology of psychiatric illness have been reported by Parkes (1964, 1965). In the earlier of these studies the case records of over 3000 psychiatric admissions were examined. He found that the number of patients whose illness 'had come on within 6 months of the death of a spouse was six times greater than would have been expected had the bereavement not been a causative factor in the illness which followed it.' He found also that 65% of the bereaved psychiatric patients (61 out of 94), had developed affective disorders, a significantly higher percentage than in the non-bereaved clinic population.

In a later study Parkes (1965) studied psychiatric disturbance in the bereaved and examined the natural history of their disturbances. The material for the study included personal interviews with 21 patients who were bereaved and a case note analysis of 94 bereaved patients. All patients studied were included on the basis of psychiatric disturbance which had come on within 6 months of the death of a parent, spouse, sibling or child or during the terminal illness.

The 21 patients interviewed were described in some detail, 17 women and 4 men, mean ages 46·7 and 44·2 respectively. Although the sample was small it was found to resemble the 94 patients in the case note series on most relevant features. A subsample of 14 patients of the 21 was matched for age and sex with the widows studied by Maris and the incidence of the grief features compared, the results are given in Table 8.1.

The object here was to examine the clinical features, the similarities and differences between Maris' randomly selected widows, a non-psychiatric series, and Parkes' strictly psychiatric series. In fact, as may be seen in Table 8.1 most of Maris' features appear in the bereaved psychiatric patients: all subjects were depressed and the majority of both groups were apathetic, slept badly and had a sense that the lost person was still present.

Table 8.1   Grief symptoms in widows

Principal features of grief reported	Unselected widows (Maris) %	Matched subsample (Parkes) %
Depression or anxiety	100	100
Apathy	61	50
Insomnia	79	71
Cultivates ideas of presence	21	21
Sense of presence of deceased	50	50
Performs acts connected with deceased	21	21
Attempts to escape reminders	18	36
Hard to accept loss	23	79*
Blames self	11	79*
Blames others	15	43
	n = 72	n = 14

* $P < 0.001$

There were, however, three features which were more common in the psychiatric group: two of them at a statistically significant level (difficulty in accepting loss and self-blame); the third, hostility towards others associated with the loss (blames others), was more frequent but not at a statistically significant level.

The clinical features of Parkes' interviewed patients were further examined in regard to duration and intensity which were in both instances prolonged and severe. The immediate reaction tended to be characterised by numbness; eight patients described a delayed reaction. Functional bodily symptoms, insomnia, anorexia, and weight loss were common, as were apathy and inertia. The author drew the general conclusion that people who develop psychiatric illnesses after bereavement usually show symptoms which are more intense and prolonged but basically no different from typical grief.

A classification of bereavement reactions proposed by Parkes includes

1   Grief and its variants:
   a   typical grief

b chronic grief, *i.e.* abnormally prolonged and intense usually associated with guilt and self-blame.

c inhibited grief, *i.e.* lasting inhibition of the total picture with the development of other symptoms, apparently common in the very young and the old.

d delayed grief—a chronic reaction which occurs after a delay and may persist for weeks and years.

2 Non-specific and mixed reaction including
  a psychosomatic conditions
  b psychoneurotic reactions including hypochondriacal, phobic and depersonalisation syndromes
  c affective disorders not resembling grief, mania being the most important
  d others including alcoholic episodes

The question of bereavement and grief needs to be considered more fully by psychiatrists, a point well made by Parkes. It may be that it is the universality of grief that has caused psychiatrists to dismiss it as being only of marginal interest when in fact its involvement in the aetiology of psychiatric disorder is at least fairly clear.

Classification of depression

The problems of classifying depression go beyond academic dispute and have become more important since physical treatments, drugs and ECT have been effective in relieving depression and shortening mania. Any classification that can help to choose correct treatment is worth more than a glance. But though classifying depression is difficult and controversial it should be realised that most topics in psychiatry are imprecise and controversial.

In the 1920s in England, when therapeutic optimism in psychiatry was at rock bottom, the question of the reactive/endogenous depression dichotomy was summarised by Mapother (1926) who said that manic depressive psychoses represented a 'merely quantitative deviation from the normal—which could only be recognised as pathological if extensive, excessive or prolonged', 'subdivision' he added 'serves little purpose unless the types discriminated are correlated with differences in the un-known—for example in causation, prognosis and treatment'. This was fair comment at a time when there were no psychiatric treatments beyond general support, sedation and psychoanalysis for a very few neurotics. Aubrey Lewis (1934, 1936) reviewed the symptoms and natural history of depression in papers that remain models of simple clarity and concluded that 'reactive' and 'endogenous' referred to severity and length of illness and that no useful distinction could be made between these categories.

In more recent times Garmany (1958) studied 295 endogenous, 194 reactive and 36 involutional depressives. He looked at constitutional and 'stress' factors, age scatter and treatment methods and could find no significant differences between the three categories.

Kiloh and Garside (1963), Carney, Roth and Garside (1968) who may be called the 'Newcastle' school as opposed to the 'London' school (Mapother, Lewis, Garmany, Kendall *et al*) examined depression by searching for symptom clusters which might differentiate reactive from endogenous types. They prefer the term 'neurotic' to 'reactive' (Kiloh & Garside, 1963) commenting that neurotic and endogenous depression 'have the advantage of being understood by those who profess not to use them' (sic). The 1963 study (Kiloh & Garside) surveyed clinical and social data on patients in a trial of imipramine. Endogenous depressives responded better than neurotic depressives and when the imipramine treated group was examined they showed symptom clusters which correlated positively and negatively with a good response to imipramine, and the clusters of symptoms included items typical of endogenous and neurotic depression.

Factor analysis has been used to clarify the problem. Hamilton and White (1959), Kiloh and Garside (1963), Carney *et al* (1965) have demonstrated a bipolar factor which accounts for an endogenous—neurotic dichotomy, while a recent study Kay *et al* (1969) took factor analysis further by examining 104 depressed patients. The features studied included 18 psychiatric symptoms, 3 physical symptoms, 3 precipitants, 2 personality features, 3 social features and 6 diverse features (age, sex, widowed, duration, ECT, previously ill).

The factor analysis picked out a bipolar factor identified as endogenous (retarded) versus neurotic (complaining). The endogenous factor was associated with ECT and a personality trait 'narrow interests', whilst the neurotic syndrome was associated with psychogenesis and lengthy illness. The important general conclusion was that two-thirds of the patients were diagnosable as 'endogenous' or 'neurotic' depression.

Critics of these studies point out that they tend to find out what they are looking for because the hypothetical typology is based on criteria

already siezed on as identification points in the typology. The last word
in this controversy has not been said—many feel it is hardly worth saying
since in Eysenck's view the controversy is based on an illogical assumption (Eysenck, 1970).

The current state of knowledgeable uncertainty has been summarised
by Kendall (1968) who analysed data on 1080 consecutive depressives
admitted to the Maudsley between 1949–1963. Sixty items were selected
for their possible relevance to a psychotic–neurotic dichotomy. Discriminant function analysis was used since it is a statistical technique that
tests hypotheses rather than sniffing them out, as opposed to factorial
analysis which generates hypotheses by finding them. The results showed
that for every patient a 'diagnostic index' could be derived and that the
index scores had a unimodal distribution. From this Kendall reasoned that
if psychotic and neurotic depressions *are* distinct then a bimodal curve
should have been found. From this and other abstruse statistics Kendall
concluded that depression lay along a continuum, and 'neurotic' depression was another point on the continuum which is determined by reliable
and valid variables.

Kendall's final conclusion was that the continuum model gave good
information about symptoms, treatment and prognosis in a more sophisticated way than by arbitrary assignment to traditional diagnostic categories: '. . . it preserves the traditional stereotypes as the two poles of the
continuum and acknowledges that differences between them are genuine
and not simply questions of severity and chronicity . . . on the other hand
it recognises the impracticability of drawing any clear boundaries between
them.' If we accept the Kendall view and partially accept the Newcastle
view we can say that the continuum hypothesis gives us a linear scale with
identification points, the bimodal view of depression gives us syndromes
whose relationship is nonlinear.

Practical considerations operate to the extent that psychiatrists tend
empirically to use a typology of depression that has at least found official
recognition in the *Glossary of Mental Disorders* (1968), *i.e.*

	Code
Manic depressive psychosis-depressed type	
(including endogenous depression)	296·2
Involutional melancholia	296·0
Depressive neurosis (neurotic depression)	300·4

And this is as good as any!

Clinical features of depression

The commonest early symptom of depression is by definition *mood change* in which a mood of sadness or near sadness is the dominant clinical feature, and the mood change is directly proportional to the severity of the depression. Furthermore all the other clinical features are secondary to mood disturbance, following in its wake in an understandable and predictable way.

Mood disturbance

Mood change is not only prominent but essential to the diagnosis. There can barely be a diagnosis of depression unless there is mood change. Self-descriptions of mood are important and encompass despair, pessimism, solemnity, apathy, grief, fearfulness, gloom, hopeless self-examination and wretchedness, to name only descriptions of a range of altered feeling that is not easy to summarise. So that the common statement 'I'm depressed' may mean a great deal or it may mean nothing at all—it is a statement that must always be examined closely and it should also be realised that the question 'are you depressed?' when unqualified can be equally meaningless.

In *mild cases* the depressed person feels sad and miserable, pessimistic and dejected in a way that seems inexplicable to him when the depression lifts. As *depression worsens* however the relief given by reassurance or change goes, leaving him disconsolate and inconsolable. There are no clear frontiers that divide severe and moderate depression. As depression worsens glumness and discontented irritability dominate the patient's behaviour; his colleagues and friends find him hard, even impossible to please and rally. Family and friends may put it down to 'bloody mindedness' but as he gets worse they realise that the change in him goes beyond this and that maybe he is ill or 'abnormal'. As he gets worse the patient feels overwhelmed by unrelenting pessimism and gloom. Soon his wretchedness is too much to bear, he is surrounded by a feeling of inexorable doom and dread. This feeling may deepen into conviction. Another important aspect of mood change in depression is the lack of feeling, the apathy, loss of feeling which can get so bad that the patient feels 'dead inside'.

Behaviour

The main change in behaviour in depression is a general *lowering of psycho-motor activity*, mental and physical alertness and responses are slowed and become dull. Thinking is slow and laboured, in severe cases to the point where thought is sparse and has no spontaneity, the patient seems so pre-occupied that he cannot attend to what goes on around him. This is reflected in his talk which becomes restricted, slow, ponderous and monotonous. Lack of spontaneity of talk is often noticed early by others, *e.g.* 'he seems to have very little to say—quite unlike how he usually is'. Severely slowed down psychomotor activity is called *retardation*: a slow, halting way of talking and acting that *is* recognisable but which can be mistakenly diagnosed in cases of parkinsonism, myxoedema and myas-thenia gravis. But if these conditions are excluded—depressive retardation is a syndrome of slow talk and action—the patient answers questions after long pauses and with few words, every act seems laboured, and slow. The facial expression and posture reflect this: he becomes stooped and bent, his facial responses are sluggish, his brow is furrowed, mouth turned down, he smiles rarely and wryly. He neglects his appearance and becomes slovenly and scruffy. The ultimate is depressive stupor, rarely seen nowadays, where a severe depressive is inert, inaccessible and unresponsive.

Thinking and concentration often appear to be impaired, but this impair-ment is a reflection of depressive preoccupation, it disappears with improvement of the depressive state.

Delusional ideas: guilt and self-blame

In severe depression the patient may feel so sad and hopeless that the logical outcome is for him to believe that not only is he without hope but that also he is a deplorable blameworthy person, deserving condemnation and punishment. Depression colours a person's view of himself and the world beyond mere self-doubt and minor self-recrimination into delu-sional convictions of guilt and wickedness. This can extend beyond him-self to include family and children whom he can come to believe are damned and beyond hope—this accounts for those depressives who kill wife and children to spare them from the wrath that is to come etc. Depressive delusional ideas of this degree of intensity are rare nowadays but *do* occur and should always be thought about as a concealed possibility when a self-deprecatory depressive smilingly declines treatment or help. Depressive suicide and murder still occur and *always* in a setting of self-blame.

In milder depressions the patient is guilty and blames himself for trivia in an insightless way—guilt feelings are inevitable in depression and may pass unnoticed until a positive statement is made by the patient. This is again always an important sign that needs to be given a proper hearing and never dismissed nor minimised. The doctor should ask the patient how he feels about himself, does he think himself a bad person? etc. Another important consequence of depressive mood is *hypochondriasis, i.e.* fancied ideas or convictions of bodily illness. In mild cases this is little more than fearful concern about the *physiological accompaniments* of depression such as dry mouth, furred tongue, constipation and general lack of energy—any or all of which suggest to the patient that his physical health is bad through some unsuspected malignant illness. *Delusional hypochondriasis* in depression is so severe that the patient believes his bowels or his brain are rotting. In general in depression it is most common to find a hypochrondriacal flavour, the patient just doesn't feel well in an unspecified way.

Perception

Depressed people see the world in a dull light. This goes beyond mere metaphor, depression *does* colour a patient's view of the world. In severe psychotic depression patients often develop auditory hallucinations which reflect the depressive content, *e.g.* the voices condemn him, prophesy doom and damnation etc.

Other symptoms

Most depressed patients complain of physical symptoms which are frequently so prominent as to divert attention from mood change to the extent of totally diverting it. The catalogue of symptoms includes loss of appetite, loss of sexual desire, impotence, a dry mouth, constipation, headache, abdominal discomfort and above all a general feeling of malaise. Anorexia usually causes weight loss though occasionally depressive over-eating occurs as an unhappy depressive tries to compensate for feelings of sadness and loss.

An *admixture of anxiety symptoms* is also common, not confined to apprehension or dread but also the physiological accompaniments such as tremor, sweating and tachycardia. *Elderly depressives* are often agitated with restless semipurposive overactivity such as hand wringing, moaning and body rocking, the total aspect being one of wretched restless despair.

Weeping is common in depression, sometimes it pervades the picture, perhaps more common is episodic weeping related to helpless despair. Other depressives are unable to weep and say 'I'm so depressed, I've gone beyond tears'.

Sleep

All depressives sleep badly, they are wakeful, have nightmares and get up feeling irritable and unrefreshed. Often sleep disturbance is one of the first symptoms and remains persistent and troublesome long after all other symptoms have gone. In severe depression (or endogenous depression) the typical insomnia consists of early waking, the patient wakes up in the early hours and lies awake turning over his problems and worries. This is the traditional description of depressive sleep disturbance but doubt has been cast on this by the findings of Hinton (1966) and Oswald (1965) who found that depressive sleep disturbance tends to be scattered throughout the night. It may be that early waking in depression is an aspect of insomnia that the patient remembers. Oswald and Jouvet (1973) have suggested that depressive insomnia may be the *primary* disturbance since depression may in fact be not a primary mood disorder but a disorder based on alteration of central nervous system arousal. McGhie (1966) has pointed out that there are considerable discrepancies between subjective and objective sleep disturbance while Crisp and Stonehill (1973) noted crucial relationships between insomnia and nutrition in psychiatric patients. The real significance of depressive insomnia is not clear—it may well be that, as is so often the case, patients are right when they say 'I'd be all right if I could get a good night's sleep'.

Suicide and attempted suicide in depression

Suicide and attempted suicide are important complications of depression—depressed patients still kill themselves at a rate that *has hardly been affected by modern treatment methods*. In all cases of depression the doctor should think of suicide as a possible complication, it occurs in a minority that needs recognition. Severe symptoms are an important guide, suicide is rare in mild depression, but there are a number of clinical and social factors which should always alert the doctor.

The first is *retardation* which can precede a suicidal attempt since the *retarded depressive* can become more suicidal as he improves, *i.e.* as retardation lifts and he has enough drive to kill himself. Second is *hypochondriasis* —depressives who believe they have an unrecognised illness often try to kill themselves. In clinical practice it is a sensible move always to be very cautious about any depressive who has one *persistent and dominating symptom* since its failure to improve can lead to self-destruction, the symptoms that are most important include hypochondriasis, insomnia and headache. *Guilt and self-depreciation* are also important predictors of suicide and suicidal attempt. *Social factors* such as being unmarried, widowed or divorced are important, especially in middle aged men. Previous suicidal attempts and family history of suicide are also important. *Associated physical illness* makes the risk of suicide greater.

The most important point to recall is that suicidal talk and suicide go together—old sayings about people who talk about it don't do it are quite wrong.

Diagnosis of depression

Listing the symptoms of depression does not *ensure* that the diagnosis is made—nevertheless it is useful to have a clinical check list.

1 Sleep disturbance, especially early waking and lying awake
2 Loss of energy
3 Loss of appetite
4 Loss of interest
5 Hypochondriasis
6 Impotence, frigidity and loss of libido
7 Irritability, anxiety and tension
8 Indecision and self-doubt
9 Apathy
10 A general feeling of malaise
11 Thinking and talking about suicide
12 Self-neglect
13 Abuse of alcohol and drugs
14 Weight loss
15 Fall off in work record
16 Fall off in interpersonal relationships

However it is possible to make these personal lists more valid and reliable and this has already been done, in fact the number of depression rating scales is extensive. However although rating scales are useful in assessing change in depressive states and to some extent in differentiation in practice diagnosis is a clinical matter which is important because depression is treatable and an important cause of morbidity and mortality.

Severe depression usually presents little diagnostic difficulty since onset is acute and symptoms are prominent. Everything about the severely depressed patient points to the diagnosis: face, posture and bodily movements all contribute to a picture either of inert sluggish misery or agitated despair. Diurnal variation of mood is common and insomnia, particularly early waking, is troublesome and persistent. Bowel symptoms, constipation and bowel hypochondriasis, are also common. They are often near delusional: 'My bowels are blocked with rottenness', this is a general hypochondriacal attitude. Ideas of guilt and self-depreciation which again may be so bad as to be delusional are also common. Above all the severely depressed patient often is sluggish, slow, and retarded and can neither be comforted or cheered up. The clinical picture of *retarded depression* fits well with the traditional description of endogenous depression. At its most severe retardation merges into total apathetic inertia, *i.e. depressive stupor* in which immobility and mutism render the patient totally inaccessible though after recovery he is able fully to recall the attempts that others have made to contact him in his stuporose state.

Mild depression is less easy to spot. A common presentation in mild depression is vague but troublesome physical symptoms which have no structural basis, *e.g.* pains, dyspepsia, flatulence, headache. All of these can be non-specific symptoms. The diagnosis of depression here may be missed because the doctor's attention is diverted by physical symptoms and because mood disturbance may not be striking. In other cases mild depression can present with lack of energy, feelings of exhaustion, general weariness and lassitude. Here the patient rarely mentions mood disturbance until direct questioning reveals that he has been 'just a little down in the dumps lately' but that he has 'put it down to having no energy'.

AFFECTIVE DISORDERS: DIAGNOSIS AND DIFFERENTIAL DIAGNOSIS

Depressive states

The diagnoses of *endogenous* and *neurotic* depression appear largely to be problems of definition: people who *believe* in endogenous and neurotic depression tend to diagnose them and people who are sceptical do not. This may sound like an unverifiable assertion; actually it suggests a testable hypothesis. If there are valid differences between neurotic and endogenous depression then there are, presumably, differences in remission rates and results of treatment. If this is the case then it should be possible to compare the results of *antidepressant* treatment as practised by psychiatrists who believe in a dichotomous concept of depression as opposed to results of *antidepressant* treatment as practised by psychiatrists who do not.

As we have seen the *recognition of depression as a symptom* should not be difficult. What is difficult is to establish its importance. From the clinical point of view *pathological depression* as opposed to normal mood variation, is always diagnosed (1) on the basis of mood change which exceeds in extent and duration the ordinary mood changes that are part of normal experience and (2) on the finding of associated symptoms as already outlined.

Having recognised pathological depression it is important first of all to exclude undetected *physical illnesses* which may simulate 'true' depression. In theory this may encompass a vast array of physical disorders. In practice it means excluding hypothyroidism, Parkinson's syndrome, myasthenia gravis, Addison's disease, megaloblastic anaemia, late onset diabetes and unsuspected renal failure, diagnostic exercises which are, after all, not beyond the range of practice of any competent doctor.

Psychiatric conditions to be excluded are *schizophrenia*, especially in the younger patient, and *organic cerebral syndromes*. In the latter the important diagnostic indices are features which suggest cognitive impairment. *Hypomania* and *mania* present diagnostic difficulties mainly in the differential diagnosis of states of acute excitement. Here the first differentiating point is to decide whether the condition is one of acute organic excitement, *i.e.* delirium or subacute delirium. This diagnosis is made by identifying clouding of consciousness as the cardinal sign. This leaves schizophrenic excitement to be excluded, this is not always straightforward at first, as is mentioned in the differential diagnosis of schizophrenia.

Mania and hypomania

Mania and hypomania are affective disorders in which the primary symptom is *elevation of mood*. The distinction between the two terms is entirely one of severity. *Mania* is a state of high elation and disorganised restless excitement, sometimes coloured by paranoid features and patchy hallucinosis. Grandiose and delusional ideas usually complicate the picture. *Hypomania* is less severe and more common though both conditions are relatively rare.

Hypomania

Hypomania often goes unrecognised, particularly if it occurs in someone whose basic *personality* can be described as hypomanic. These people are always energetic and cheery, they tend to be envied and admired by friends and colleagues because they have such tremendous vitality. They are full of zest, work hard, enjoy life and never seem tired. They are chatty, humorous and optimistic and are rarely put down by happenings that leave most people daunted. Hypomanic personalities seem really to enjoy hard work and diverse leisure interests. Their appetites are kingsized, they can eat, drink and fornicate with great zeal and no guilt. They are cheery people, full of fun—too full for some and too aggressive for others since their restless energy seems to be *their* way of dealing with aggressive feelings and impulses. They enjoy social occasions in an indefatigable fashion, leaving everyone else weary. Often they are touchy and quarrelsome and many find them caustic, unfeeling and rude.

However in hypomania this picture of breezy energy is too much for everyone and exceeds the normal and becomes absurd. Personality traits formerly tolerable if a little irritating now become exaggerated to the point where they become *symptoms of morbid excitement*. The hypomanic personality may be charming but the hypomanic patient is *too charming*—he becomes a wearisome bore—a breezy flow of witty chat is replaced by a relentless flood of talk uttered by a psychotic who can only be interrupted at the risk of harsh rebuttal, irritable anger and noisy swearing. The cheery smile becomes a fixed laugh which lacks mirth or warmth.

In hypomania friendly behaviour becomes exaggerated, overwhelming and embarrassingly intrusive; the hypomanic is familiar and presumptuous, his jokes are no longer witty but noisy, coarse and boring, he lacks tact and utters obscenities in an unthinking way. Ordinary flirtatious behaviour, normally barely tolerable, degenerates into a series of inappropriate propositions to unlikely, though sometimes surprisingly receptive, people. The unbounded energy increases, he eats and drinks too much, stays up all night and will not go when he visits people. Consider the following case.

A hypomanic professional man surprised his friends by unexpected visits accompanied by his mistress. He insisted on describing his elaborate financial plans to develop a neglected country by converting it into a vast sheep farm. Exhausted would-be but disenchanted prospective investors telephoned his doctor for advice about his mental state only to find that his doctor had agreed to give him financial support. This is a good illustration of the way in which the hypomanic can convince the seemingly level headed!

But, inevitably, hypomanic energy becomes self-defeating, the patient is unable to persist with his schemes and flits from one to another. He becomes *distractible*, wanders from the point in conversation and tries to do too much. His optimistic cheeriness is thin, he becomes irritable, impatient and hot tempered. He is overconfident, a boring know-it-all who cannot be restrained, who cannot tolerate interruption let alone disagreement. Nothing can check his flow of talk which embarrasses friends and alarms strangers. If anyone crosses him they are abused, on the other hand he becomes generous and will brook no refusal, he insists on bringing home unexpected and sheepish guests. His talk is extravagant, full of rambling anecdotes but his jollity remains at least *superficially infectious*. At this stage it is usually hard to convince him that he is at all disturbed—in fact any such suggestion can provoke scornful abuse and a telephone call to his solicitor!

Mania

Mania is more severe. Pressure of talk and activity is extreme and disorganised and obviously abnormal. *Pressure of talk* is enormous, the patient cannot be interrupted without an angry and violent reaction. Cheeriness is overbearing and hostile, his unbounded joy and confidence brook no argument. The overconfidence of hypomania is replaced by *delusional ideas*: he is the King of Europe, the inventor of a device to save the world etc.

In mania the *mood disturbance* is often one of exaltation and totally insightless exuberance. *Thought and talk* are uninterrupted and connections

G

between ideas are determined by *casual links* such as rhymes, puns and alliterations, *e.g.* 'What's my name? Well the name of the game is the same. Is my name the same as yours? You put water in ewers. Up yours. Up mine. Don't go down the mine daddy? Baddy, Baddy. Goody. Goody. Who are you calling a prude? The first of the fewd. . . .'

Manic gaiety is noisy and intolerable to everyone except the patient who remains convinced of his absolute rightness about everything. Tactless talk degenerates into a garbled string of puns, rhymes etc., funny for a few minutes but boring after more. His overactivity can be violent if someone tries to interfere, while on the other hand if he is in hospital he is overinterfering—telling doctors and nurses what to do and advising patients to discharge themselves. Manic patients have an unerring knack of picking on some abnormality in nurses or doctors, *e.g.* greeting the doctor as, 'Baldy' etc. Manic patients tend to be unpopular!

The manic patient left untreated becomes exhausted, dishevelled and neglected. A *paranoid colouring* is common in mania, ideas of grandeur, superior ability etc. are part of the *delusional ideas* that may develop. Disagreement with his ideas is interpreted as a plot to deprive the world of his special knowledge, others are conspiring to prevent his good deeds benefitting mankind. These are *paranoid delusional ideas* understandable in the context of the mood disturbance.

Increased energy may lead to sexual promiscuity and real risks of pregnancy and venereal disease. *Wakefulness, weight loss* and *self-neglect* are common, also *abuse* of *alchohol and/or drugs. Hallucinosis* is rare, fleeting and colourful.

In summary mania and hypomania are clinical syndromes where mood is excessively cheerful, all activity is accelerated and where talk and thought become so overactive that the normal flow of ideas degenerates into 'flight of ideas'.

AFFECTIVE DISORDERS: PROGNOSIS AND MANAGEMENT

Prognosis and outcome

The remission rate in affective disorders is high, this has been common knowledge since affective disorders were first distinguished by Kraepelin as 'manic depressive'. The fact that they had a better prognosis than 'dementia praecox' was one of the important differences that Kraepelin commented on.

Physical treatments such as ECT and antidepressants have undoubtedly proved to be excellent methods for shortening illnesses though whether they substantially alter the natural history is open to question, although recent work has indicated for instance that lithium has a definite prophylactic value in recurrent mania.

Therefore we can say that chronic affective disorders of any severity are uncommon; mental hospitals no longer have patients in states of severe depression persisting for months and years. *Chronic mania* is also extremely uncommon. On the other hand *chronic mild depression* is found fairly frequently and is usually related to personality problems and neuroticism.

The important points to be noted in assessing prognosis include:

1   Mode of onset—acute onset favours speedy recovery
2   Clinical features—the more definite the affective nature of the illness the better the prognosis
3   History of previous similar illness—suggests a better prognosis
4   Absence of complicating factors such as associated physical illness or alcoholism suggests a better prognosis
5   Absence of 'atypical' features—suggests a better prognosis

Treatment

The first question to be answered is whether or not the patient needs to be admitted to hospital. This is influenced by severity of symptoms and by the patient's age and social situation. If the patient is suicidally depressed or is an exhausted manic then clearly admission is necessary, otherwise it is always preferable to try and treat the patient at home; as an outpatient; or in a day hospital. Elderly patients, and patients who live alone present another criterion for admission. The object of admission, however, should be quite specific and aimed at as short a stay in hospital as is reasonably possible.

Assuming the patient is in normal physical health the choice of treatment in *depression* includes antidepressant drugs both tricyclic and monoamine oxidase inhibitors, and for the severely depressed, ECT often combined with a tricyclic antidepressant. However, complete management of depression should not stop at medication. Depressed patients need encouragement and support and a chance to discuss their problems and see them in a different light.

In *mania* and *hypomania* lithium is frequently used though its side effects are hazardous. For this reason many psychiatrists prefer to commence treatment with neuroleptics such as the phenothiazines, and use ECT to shorten the manic attack. However, the place of lithium in the treatment of mania and hypomania is now more clearly established and its use should always be considered in cases of affective excitement.

Psychosurgery is sometimes recommended in chronic depressive states where tension and agitation are prevalent, distressing and immobilising symptoms. The problem here is the decision about recommencing psychosurgery. It is no good pretending that it is merely a case of the right operation for the right patient, it is not as simple as that. Psychosurgery is used after other methods have been given a reasonable trial, is never imposed on a patient and is not claimed to be a miraculous form of treatment, but rather a treatment that deserves serious and sensible consideration.

9

The neuroses

INTRODUCTION

Neurosis is a word that is widely used and badly understood. Laymen use the word in a way that encompasses a vague concept of psychiatric disorder that is rarely severe, tiresome to patient and family and in some unspecified way linked to self-indulgence—not so much self-inflicted as self-perpetuated; not so much an illness more a way of life. It signifies an illness from which the sufferer could extract himself if perhaps he was a bit tougher, more independent, less demanding, less egocentric, less importunate and above all less manipulative.

But in psychiatry we need a clearer definition of neurosis. We need to establish the essential clinical features of neurosis and we need to know the value of a term such as 'neuroticism' when applied to people who may be constitutionally more liable to neurotic symptoms, *i.e.* is there such an entity as a 'neurotic' personality? These are difficult questions to answer.

Definition

The first difficulty is that not only is the term *neurosis* used but also the word *psychoneurosis*. In this work the two terms will be taken to be synonymous. Most definitions of neurosis turn out to be descriptions rather than anything else but descriptions that concentrate on the presence or absence of symptoms.

The origins of the term have to do with early ideas of 'weakness' of the nervous system, 'neurosis' as opposed to 'psychosis', *i.e.* severe mental illness or madness. This is an arbitrary distinction no doubt, but one that has some clinical value.

There is no clear unifying element that runs through all neuroses though there is an unstated aspect of neurosis, *i.e.* that neurotic disorders are more likely to have been caused by outside events, by loss, by conflict, in short as sequels of psychological factors rather than by genetic, bio-chemical or physical causes. Psychoses are regarded as more *severe* than neuroses. There are other elements that differentiate these two generic terms, but they are given different weight by different authorities (Table 9.1).

Table 9.1 Definition of neurosis and psychosis by different authors.

Authors	Neurosis	Psychosis
Mayer-Gross Slater & Roth	**a** constitutional liability **b** genetic basis of neurotic disposition **c** comprehensible relation with psychopathic personality **d** symptoms such as tachycardia, sweating, fear, depression, insomnia, faints, fugues **e** no fundamental distinction from psychopathy, *i.e.* personality disorder **f** not defined	**a** severe symptoms such as delusions, thought disorder, personality change **b** organic causes and 'functional' psychoses, *e.g.* schizophrenia and manic/depressive **c** not defined
Freedman & Kaplan (1967)	**a** chronic symptoms **b** role of psychodynamic factors stressed **c** importance of motivation in therapy **d** not defined	**a** thought disorder, hallucinations and delusions are common symptoms **b** physical treatment important **c** not defined
Redlich & Freedman	**a** higher mental functions unimpaired **b** differentiation questionable **c** analogy with water and ice, *i.e.* one is a form of the other **d** not defined	**a** higher mental functions impaired **b** differentiation questionable **c** not defined

Authors	Neurosis	Psychosis
Noyes & Kolb	**a** symptomatic expression of anxiety or the psychological mechanisms unconsciously adopted to control it	**a** personality disorganised
	b no personality disorganisation	**b** break with reality
	c no gross symptoms	**c** capacity for work and relationships impaired
	d defined	**d** defined

From the briefly tabulated comments we may conclude that the differentiation between psychosis and neurosis is something that is implied rather than stated. However from these and other observations we may delineate a general concept of neurosis as being disorders in which there are the following features.

Neurosis

1   Preservation of contact with reality, *i.e.* no symptoms such as hallucinations, delusions, thought disorder or intellectual impairment
2   Symptoms of anxiety common, whether somatic or psychological
3   Minor mood disturbance
4   Symptoms tend to be mild and chronic
5   Insight, *i.e.* awareness of illness is common though the implications of illness in terms of unconscious conflict etc. are not readily available to insight
6   Personality change does not occur

Psychosis

1   Contact with reality is *likely* to be lost, *i.e.* symptoms such as hallucinations, delusions, thought disorder, aggressive and suicidal behaviour are common
2   Anxiety symptoms are absent except in depressive psychosis
3   Mood disturbance likely to be severe
4   Symptoms and syndromes likely to be acute and severe
5   Insight likely to be lost, *i.e.* patient is not aware that he is ill *during* the

psychosis but insight may recur on recovery rather like the insight that occurs on waking from a dream

6 Personality change is common

When we condense these ideas it appears that the differentiating features are:

1 Presence or absence of anxiety
2 Presence or absence of severe symptoms
3 Involvement of the personality

but the overlap between neurosis and psychosis is a fact of life.

THEORIES OF NEUROSIS

Since it is hard to define neurosis it is hardly surprising that it is even harder to account for it. Often the explanations seem to depend on the definitions and for this reason there has been an increasing interest in the concept of 'neuroticism', *i.e.* a constitutional liability to develop 'neurotic' symptoms unrelated to brain damage, possibly related to stress but basically related to an inherited state of emotional instability. The investigation of this started in the 1940s; before then there had been a general suspicion that some people were specially vulnerable to anxiety and ill defined emotional disturbances. Linford Rees and Eysenck were involved in the investigation and treatment of the neurotic casualties of World War II and found firm evidence for a concept of neuroticism as shown by a constellation of attributes and symptoms—a cluster of factors which suggested a factor, 'neuroticism' correlating well with neurosis as diagnosed by psychiatrists.

This led on to a dimensional study of personality—a whole school of experimental psychology founded by Professor H. J. Eysenck whose work has been always related to the scientific principle that gives credibility to a theory only when it is properly tested. His theory of neurosis is essentially one in which neurotic symptoms are the result of maladaptive learning, hierarchically arranged in Pavlovian terms: that is proceeding by generalisation etc. from one conditioned response sequence onwards. Pavlov's theory of neurosis postulated an excessive stimulation of the cortical inhibitory process in conflict with a highly stressed state of cortical excitation leading to overreaction. The Eysenckian school goes further than this and suggests that such a conflict of conditionability leads to defective, *i.e.* maladaptive learning, manifest as a persistent maladaptive response.

Behaviourist theories of neurosis have influenced treatment in the development of behaviour therapy—a treatment of neurosis in which the aim is to remove the distressing symptom since the basic philosophy is that the neurotic disorder is a representation of a learned maladaptive response, and once the response is *unlearned* then the patient is better. This theory of neurosis is quite opposite to the psychodynamic theory of neurosis which has been most influential in psychiatry in Western society at least, since Freud's first tentative proposals for a dynamic model of neurosis based on his observations on cases of hysteria. Freud's basic statement, later modified by the psychoanalytic school, was that neuroses develop given a defined set of criteria namely:

1   A state in which a person is immobilised by conflict between fear and drive and that basically the drives are sexual
2   The resulting conflict is unresolved—so that the person neither recognises the significance of the conflict nor does he have available the emotional apparatus to come to terms with the conflict, *i.e.* to 'work through it'
3   The offending drives are dissipated or at least rendered *less recognisable* through mechanisms such as repression or displacement.
4   The repressed drives are however not made impotent by being out of sight and have a tiresome tendency to show up as neurotic symptoms
5   The conflict is likely to have started in childhood

Theories of neurosis then are, at present, unsatisfactory—in many instances the theory and the description of neurosis overlap considerably. This is true of the clinical psychiatric concept of neurosis in which it is regarded as an *illness* where anxiety is prominent and where certain symptoms are *absent*, *e.g.* delusions, hallucinations, thought disorder and personality change. All this is tied in with the notion that neurotic anxiety develops in the face of unspecified threat to the psychological integrity of the sufferer. However there is more to *neurosis* than its existence as an individual disorder. Sociologists have pointed out that neurosis can not only be coloured by sociocultural factors but that the incidence of neurosis may well be a largely culture bound phenomenon.

In both instances a good example is provided by the falling incidence of conversion hysteria in Western society. In the days when hysteria was the favourite topic of neurologists and psychiatrists, when Charcot's clinics in Paris had become a pantomime of histrionic collapses and pseudopsychosis, it was likely that the only way in which a neurotic patient could get medical attention was by developing a 'physical' symptom. Also many areas of personal experience were just not regarded as topics that could be discussed with anyone so that the distressed person with problems and conflicts could only obtain medical/psychiatric help if he or she presented with a 'physical' disability. Counselling about problems of living was handled by the clergy within the context of established religion and infrequently by doctors in terms of moral exhortation, whilst the poor relied on charity seasoned with sermons.

But Freud and the psychoanalytic school put an end to this situation by forcefully suggesting the role of the emotions in neurosis thus liberating people from certain cultural influences of the time and making it *acceptable* for patients to present with emotional disturbance. At this point it is interesting to reflect on the fact that diagnosis and treatment of patients is influenced by doctors' attitudes. At all events it has become easier to be neurotic in the 20th Century.

An ironic example of this is in the ways in which 'cowardice' was dealt with by the British Army in two World Wars. In World War I many private soldiers were shot for cowardice. By any standards most were exhausted men who had broken down under stress. The incidence of 'cowardice' in officers seems to have been lower. Closer examination suggests that breakdown in officers was more likely to be diagnosed as an illness and called 'shell shock'. In World War II however the Army recognised that *soldiers*, whatever their social class, can be overwhelmed by fear, exhaustion etc. and developed facilities to treat patients many of whom would no doubt have been shot in World War I.

In more recent times the work of Hollingshead and Redlich (1958) has shown up the ways in which the diagnosis of neurosis or psychosis can be directly related to the patients' social class and to the psychiatrists' professional attitudes. In the United Kingdom an increasing number of studies have revealed that neurotic disorders are common (Logan & Cushion, 1958; Kessel, 1960; Goldberg & Blackwell, 1970). They form a high proportion, up to 24%, of doctors' patients. And yet despite their common occurrence the neuroses provide doctors with constant difficulties in management mainly accounted for no doubt by their persistent symptomatology and unpredictable response to treatment.

ANXIETY

Clinicians are usually impressed by the prevalence of anxiety as a symptom. A distinction is usually made between *normal* and *morbid* anxiety: normal anxiety being a familiar emotional response to frightening and stressed situations, morbid anxiety being an exaggerated response which tends to become chronic or be unrelated to stress or else triggered off by specific signals. The word has been derived by mistranslation from the German *Angst, i.e.* fear, used freely by Freud who drew no distinction between fear and anxiety.

In psychiatry however anxiety and fear are regarded as different. The features of anxiety as summarised by Lewis (1967) are as follows:

1 An emotional state with the subjective experience of fear or something like fear (*o.g.* terror, horror, alarm, fright, panic, trepidation, dread, scare)
2 The emotion is unpleasant
3 It is directed to the future
4 There is no recognisable threat, or the threat is out of proportion to the emotion it evokes
5 There are subjective bodily discomforts and manifest bodily disturbances

In common clinical experience the feelings of dread, panic and physical symptoms of adrenergic overactivity are well known enough, it may be thought, for anxiety to be easily recognised but this is not always so. Often the physical symptoms lead the patient to various specialists—to the physician for palpitations and chest pain, to the gastroenterologist for abdominal pain, churning or diarrhoea etc., or the neurologist with numbness and tingling in the limbs, or headache.

Often anxiety is an important feature in depressive states and may be found in organic cerebral disease. In adolescence and old age anxiety is usually found to be related to the patient's special situation. In the adolescent it is a well recognised part of the turbulence and self-doubt of maturing into adulthood and in response to the real stresses of adolescent life. In old age it is usually a reaction to loneliness, general falling off in the quality of life and the fear of death. In the middle years anxiety may be part of a reaction to uncertainty, unfulfilled ambition and changing status and role. All this then should suggest the universal nature of anxiety and indicate the difficulties encountered in discovering its aetiology.

It would be simple to describe anxiety in terms of specific syndromes, *e.g.* in affective disorder; in pure culture—phobic anxiety; and deal with clinical syndromes alone but doing this overlooks the wider implications of anxiety as studied by psychologists and physiologists.

We can start by acknowledging that anxiety is such a widespread symptom that it overlaps a good deal of psychiatric diagnosis. This also suggests that it must be a fundamental response to a variety of stresses. At the experimental level *anxiety* is regarded as *biological entity* in its own right and not a mere symptom. This has led to a growing body of knowledge about anxiety in *psychophysiological terms*. This brings out an important difference between the clinical and experimental approach, the former relating it to syndromes and the latter seeing it as a response as universal as hunger and as open to study.

Psychodynamic formulations of anxiety have tended to dominate the field for many years. They are diverse but have come mainly from the psycho-analytic schools. Freud (1936) for instance, regarded anxiety as the basic trigger of repression, thus repression was a way of dealing with the anxiety caused by the reverberations and conflicts set up by instinctual drives. And the instinctual drives described by Freud in this instance were the fear of castration and the fear of the loss of love. Later psychoanalytic writers stressed different aetiologies of anxiety. Otto Rank (1952) popular-ised the concept of 'separation anxiety', *i.e.* anxiety set off by the un-conscious mind being disturbed by the separation from the mother. Adler (1938) on the other hand thought anxiety was an expression of recognised threats to the life style. Other dynamic formulations have been concerned with the concept of existential anxiety where anxiety is seen as a response to the fear of ultimate dissolution, of non-being.

A more specific dynamic formulation of anxiety places anxiety in the parent/child relationship, here anxiety is a response to stress in the relation-ship following normal dependence on parents which has shifted into a pathological dependence. Even the most independent and mature adult often feels a bit helpless when faced with hard tasks and problems and this may contain echoes of childhood anxiety. Anxiety too may become inter-woven with a sense of right and wrong and associated ideas of guilt and punishment.

The symptoms and manifestations

Subjective emotional symptoms

Anxious patients describe how they feel in many ways. They may say that they feel 'strung up' or nowadays 'strung out' or 'uptight', tense, panicky, fearful or 'in a sweat'. They may use a wide range of words to describe the feeling like terror, apprehension, dread etc. that is for them the central pervading type of distress that has overtaken them. This feeling often goes with tension and depression. Depressed mood is easy to comprehend, tension is not quite so clear. It is often not just a strung up, taut feeling but is also a feeling of *muscular* tension. Limbs and muscles feel heavy and tight and the patient may find himself clenching his jaw, gripping things hard and be seen to tap things, clench and unclench his fist. His talk may be quick, he seems irritable and jumpy.

A list of presenting complaints of anxiety given by patients includes statements as follows: 'feel anxious; feel tensed up; can't relax; feel afraid; as if something nasty will happen; tight feeling in my chest; feel strung up; feel uptight; feel strung out; limbs achy and heavy; can't keep still, can't sit still; can't swallow; can't breathe; tummy churns over; feel sweaty; heart keeps missing a beat; got a choky feeling; feel as if I'm fainting; tight feeling in the neck; numb in my arms and legs; butterflies in my tummy' etc.—in a sense the list is endless in its universal recapitulation of uneasy distress of all sorts.

Physical symptoms and manifestations

The physical symptoms of anxiety are entirely those of autonomic disturbance: sympathetic overactivity, tachycardia, palpitations and chest discomfort are probably as common as any, as are a dry mouth, tremors, sweating and restlessness. Loose bowels and frequent micturition, nausea, abdominal discomfort and vomiting also occur. Anxious patients sleep fitfully, have no appetite and lose weight. The physical symptoms interweave with the emotional disturbance as previously described and often are overshadowed by indecisiveness, lack of energy and a general difficulty in concentration—'I can't think, can't remember things, can't cope somehow'.

Recognising anxiety and appreciating its significance

Many of the problems that have arisen in recognising and understanding anxiety may have been reinforced by the tendency to regard this complex phenomenon as a straightforward clinical syndrome. Lader (1972) suggested that anxiety is 'best regarded as an emotional response syndrome' and postulates a model of anxiety based on psychophysiological research findings.

The semantics of anxiety need to be clarified—although the word is used in a number of ways it should be used in psychiatry in a more limited way to signify the emotional response and its subjective qualities and associated physiological disorders. Actual examples of the flabby use of the term are numerous, too many psychiatric discussions are still punctuated by arguments where one psychiatrist asks another why the point in question is making his opponent anxious? Another more absurd example may follow an antisocial and disruptive outburst by a sociopath. A discussion of the event may provoke a lofty enquiry as to why this has made a junior doctor 'anxious'? These are only two examples of the way in which the meaning of the word is debased by the unthinking. Similarly it is absurd to talk of 'unconscious anxiety' since anxiety is by definition a subjective experience and terms such as 'unconscious anxiety' are catch all phrases used to conceal ignorance.

It appears that an important component of anxiety relates to uncertainty and ambiguity. Rollo May (1950) for instance sees anxiety as being linked to emotional impotence in the face of uncertainty, a theme which recurs in existential writings. And why not? Learning to cope with ambiguity whether of information, of feeling or of meaning is very much unhappily part of the experience of maturation.

Physiology

Physiology has been extensively reviewed by Lader *et al* (1969, 1970, 1971, 1972). The biochemical and physiological changes are most marked in both anger and anxiety—'white with anger; pale with terror; wide-eyed with terror; trembling with rage; choked with fury' etc.

The measurement of the physiological substrate of anxiety covers cardiovascular investigations: muscle blood flow, skin blood flow, pulse and blood flow while brain activity has included EEG studies showing increased alertness, characterised by increased beta and diminished alpha activity.

The consensus of physiological findings points to *increased CNS arousal* which is regarded as a non-specific response since physiology measures levels of arousal and not discrete emotions. Anger, sex and anxiety all produce similar physiological changes.

Lader's model of anxiety (1972) incorporates 'trait' anxiety as a personality attribute 'I tend to get anxious' as opposed to 'state' anxiety; 'I am anxious now'. He regards conflict determined anxiety as an interaction between internal and external stimuli.

Finally Lader suggests that anxious people are physiologically overactive and that this is reinforced by their impaired adaptability which leads to a vicious circle situation which prolongs and reinforces rigid pattern of response.

Phobic anxiety—phobic states

Though anxiety is recognised as both a symptom and as a syndrome there is one special variety of anxiety that has been more extensively studied in recent years and this is included in the generic term 'phobic anxiety' which covers phobias, single and multiple, simple and complicated. The topic has been definitively reviewed by Marks (1969). The term *phobia* (from the Greek *Phobos* meaning flight, fear or terror) is used in psychiatry to describe a variety of fear which is distinctive in that it is disproportionate, irrational and involuntary and tends to lead to avoidance of the stimulus that provokes it. This distinguishes it from *normal* fear which is a biological response to alarming situations. The difference between the two states lies in the irrationality and disproportionate quality of phobias which may so affect a person that he changes his whole life in attempts to avoid the phobic stimulus. Also phobias tend to be concealed since patients find others unsympathetic or frankly disbelieving of their symptoms.

The aetiology of phobias is linked to the aetiology of fear itself, an instinctual biological drive found in more highly developed animals. Genetic inheritance is important as exemplified in timid as opposed to aggressive animals, in man genetic inheritance is *less* obvious. Types of fears and phobias are related to the type of stimulus, heights, open spaces, darkness, unknown situations etc., and are also related to early childhood experiences. Fear is expressed via the autonomic nervous system, the subjectively unpleasant experience of fear is obvious but the mechanisms of fear are not fully accounted for though contemporary theory favours the importance of learning theory, *i.e.* conditioning, without assigning it total causality.

Phobic states tend to be more common in women than men (Marks &

Gelder, 1960) but general prevalence rates are hard to estimate. Studies in the UK and USA suggest that although up to 20% of psychiatric patients have phobic symptoms, phobic disorders account for less than 3% of cases seen (Marks, 1969). Personality studies are inconclusive but suggest at least the importance of a dependent type of personality. Psychophysiological studies suggest higher levels of arousal as opposed to the average person, psychoanalytic studies stress the importance of the symbolic meanings of phobias. Neither theory accounts for phobias entirely and the theories are not mutually exclusive.

Phobias may be classified according to special stimuli, *e.g.* aquaphobia (fear of water), agoraphobia (fear of open spaces) etc., but in general it is found more useful to divide them into *phobias* which are *secondary* to depression, obsessional disorders etc., *i.e.* to another psychiatric syndrome; and those *which exist on their own, i.e. phobic states.*

Marks (1969) recommends that they are divided into phobias of external stimuli (Class I) and internal stimuli (Class II). Typical examples of Class I phobias include the most common, *e.g.* fears of heights, open spaces, animals etc. as opposed to phobias of illness or phobias of harming others.

Agoraphobia

The most important phobic state is *agoraphobia*—the 'classic' phobic anxiety state. This is a clinical syndrome in which the patient has a recurrent fear of going into open places, a fear which characteristically quite rapidly moves from a fear of open places to *a fear of going anywhere at all outside the home* leading to the 'housebound' syndrome. The majority of such patients are middle aged women. The syndrome is clear cut, widespread and not heavily limited by culture. The syndrome tends to start in the early thirties, the family backgrounds are unremarkable (Marks & Gelder, 1965) and the personality equally so although some describe them as 'passive, shy, dependent etc.'

The syndrome may come on suddenly, however, usually the history is of episodes of unease and fear in open spaces. Panic, palpitations and fear of collapse inevitably complicate the picture and gradually ensure that the patient's activity becomes progressively more limited, *i.e.* to a housebound state, or else leads to a state of uneasy compromise where the patient learns how to avoid symptoms and has available islands of safety. Sudden onset after witnessing an accident or some public spectacle is often quoted as relevant but it is suggested that such examples merely represent intensification of phobias already present.

Agoraphobia is frequently complicated by mood change, depersonalisation and other anxiety symptoms—the most unpleasant of which are *panic attacks*, autonomic storms of palpitation, sweating, tremor and tachycardia against a setting of intense dread. Roth (1959) described a phobic anxiety syndrome associated with *depersonalisation* and noted a high incidence of associated temporal lobe disturbance. At this point it is worth noting that depersonalisation is generally a symptom which patients find extremely distressing.

The management of agoraphobia This is something on which there is one specific area of agreement; namely that it is difficult to treat. This is true of phobias in general though in more recent times results may have improved as clinicians have taken more interest in phobic patients and have had their interest reinforced by the successes of behaviour therapy particularly *desensitisation*. Desensitisation is by now the most widely practised type of behaviour therapy.

Fears are common, phobias are not so common but where they do occur they can cause great hardship to the patient even though he or she may find all sorts of ways of altering life to make it more liveable. But inevitably the severe phobic disorder leads to a state where the patient has to seek help. And this raises an important point since the patients who come for treatment are inevitably the most handicapped. This leaves one to speculate about how much might be achieved in the sphere of *prevention*. Marks (1969) points out that the patient who seeks treatment is part of a highly selected group since he has exhausted simple measures, attempts at self-control, friendly and not so friendly advice. Therefore prevention offers itself as a way of avoiding phobic states, but the most that may be said about this is that children should be brought up in a way that encourages them to face frightening situations with the essential back up provided by stable sensible parents.

On the other hand it should also be said that *education* and *training* are important. Good practical examples of this are found in the ways in which people are *taught* to swim or to do parachute jumps. In each case the instructors inspire confidence by their own calmness and experience and desensitise the learner from any fears he may have by gradually permitting the learner to become totally familiar with the skill, all the time encouraging him and rewarding success in acquiring the skill with approval and praise.

After traumatic experiences, *e.g.* motor accidents etc. people may easily become phobic, this has been known for a long time and commonsense advice has always been to drive again as soon as possible before a phobic reaction develops. This is sound advice and has been borne out by clinical experience. But the psychiatrist needs guide lines for the management of phobias that have already become established. These will be considered under the following headings:

1 General measures
2 Medication
3 Desensitisation
4 Psychotherapy

General measures

As in most psychiatric disorders no treatment is of any use until the patient's complaints have been systematically examined by taking a full and detailed history. This is not in itself therapeutic but provides the only basis for the sensible planning of therapy. A clinically important and useful tactic here is to set out a careful analysis of how the patient spends a typical day since this will soon reveal the extent of the handicaps imposed by the phobia.

Time is an important factor—the longer the phobia has been present the more difficult it is to eradicate it. Phobias present for more than 2 years need the most intensive treatment (Marks, 1969). The psychiatrist should adopt a positive and encouraging attitude. Most phobic patients feel totally defeated by the time they consult a psychiatrist and the last person they need is someone who conceals therapeutic pessimism behind unsympathetic detachment. The patient needs to be advised about the usefulness of islands of safety and advised about the various ways in which the impact of phobias can be reduced by simple measures such as the sensible use of medication and by ensuring that public occasions are more easily encountered if there is a supportive person present. The agoraphobic patient should be encouraged towards self-help via organisations such as the 'Open Door' where he will find solace in sharing the problem and learning from the experience of others. One of the most useful practical advices given by the 'Open Door' is to have a telephone! Neighbourly help in going out shopping etc. are simple things to provide for the agoraphobe, simple help for a friendly person to give and invaluable to the patient.

A good example of the success of simple methods in phobic states was a 42 year old executive who had severe phobias of public speaking, something that was in fact one of his main tasks as director of training in industry. For about 2 years he had managed to conceal it and avoid any public collapse etc. by altering educational programmes, and making excuses but when he asked for help he had exhausted these stratagems and his employers were beginning to notice. The nature of his work, fear of loss of earnings and status made desensitisation impractical so he was given diazepam 10 mg tds to qds. The medication controlled his anxiety symptoms sufficiently to enable him to start with small conferences (up to 20 people) then gradually he became able to address larger and larger meetings (up to 500) though 2 years later he still took diazepam at least before a meeting. However, 3 and 5 years later he was untroubled by his phobia but always carried diazepam 'as a standby', but rarely took it!

Medication

In the past, sedatives such as barbiturates, *e.g.* amylobarbitone, were often prescribed and gave good subjective relief. Nowadays they are less popular mostly because of the dangers of dependence and chronic intoxication. The *tranquillisers* especially the benzodiazepines are the most popular, chlordiazepoxide and diazepam are probably the front runners. They are excellent for short term symptom relief in the person who has to face particular ordeals but it is doubtful if they are any more effective in the long term.

Antidepressants are useful if the patient *is* depressed and has secondary phobic symptoms though in primary phobic states it is now suggested that the monoamine oxidase inhibitor phenelzine, and the tricyclic antidepressant, clomipramine (anafranil) are effective, not only in suppressing symptoms but as a treatment for the phobic disorder.

Occasionally the psychiatrist may see a patient with alcoholism or sedative dependence and find that this has developed as a result of casual self-medication by a phobic patient.

Desensitisation

Of all the techniques of behaviour therapy desensitisation is to date the most useful and the most widely employed, especially in phobic states (Wolpe, 1958; Rachman, 1959; Eysenck, 1960).

Desensitisation consists in teaching the patient not to experience anxiety when faced with a frightening stimulus. Its origins lie in the commonsense observation that people can progressively learn to experience such a stimulus and lose the phobic response but has become formalised in terms of learning theory, in which the phobia is regarded as a learned maladaptive response which is lost by graduated exposure to a series of stimuli akin to the most feared. Wolpe suggested the term *reciprocal inhibition* to encompass a process in which an unpleasant stimulus and a pleasant one are linked and the latter gradually replaces the former. In practice the pleasant stimulus is provided by a state of subjective relaxation. This is taught by a variety of techniques, all involving an end point of relaxed calm.

The patient is then asked to make out a list of frightening stimuli and to rank them in order of severity. Thereafter though there are differences in technique the principles of treatment are the same. After the patient has learnt and successfully experienced a technique of relaxation the next step is to encourage the patient to imagine the least frightening stimulus of all whilst in a state of relaxation. The patient is instructed to indicate feelings of anxiety by raising one hand, feelings of relaxation by raising the other. The process is repeated until the patient can imagine a frightening stimulus without feeling anxious and is then encouraged to move stepwise up the hierarchy. Obviously it is not in practice quite as simple as that but that is basically how it is done, usually backed up by instructing the patient to practise the technique when alone. For more detailed examinations of behaviour therapy and in particular desensitisation it is advisable to consult what are now standard references and texts (Wolpe, 1958; Rachman, 1959; Eysenck, 1960; Marks, 1969; Marks & Gelder, 1965).

Psychotherapy

It may seem surprising that psychotherapy is listed last since the traditional view has been that psychotherapy is the first choice treatment. This is no longer acceptable. The claims for the effectiveness of psychotherapy were never established in contrast to desensitisation which, despite its acknowledged shortcomings has, at least, been well tested and it could be added more stringently tested than any other psychological type of treatment. However it is not merely a question of claiming simply that desensitisation is 'better' than psychotherapy (Gelder *et al*, 1967; Gelder & Marks, 1968). Phobic symptoms disappear quickly with desensitisation but the inter-personal aspects of therapy are never overlooked in behaviour therapy that is sensibly carried out.

However psychotherapy *is* used and when it is the aim is to find out the symbolic meaning of the phobia in the hope that this insight will help the patient to improve.

This leads to perhaps the most contentious area in psychiatry, namely whether or not psychotherapy is useful in the treatment of the neuroses. This question is examined more fully under psychotherapy, suffice it to say that at least as far as phobic disorders are concerned there are no controlled studies of psychotherapy but that desensitisation *has* been subject to controlled studies and at present is regarded as the first line of treatment. However this is mainly true of uncomplicated phobic disorders and is not true where phobias are part of larger scale personality problems. In these cases psychotherapy is still thought to be most useful.

Prognosis

A simple rule is that the more acute the phobia the more treatable it is and the better the prognosis. Single phobias are more treatable than multiple phobias. The *agoraphobic syndrome* is the core problem of the treatment of phobic disorders since it renders patients incapable of leading an ordinary existence. Secondary depressive features should always be treated and when treated the syndrome may improve. On the other hand it seems likely that the majority of agoraphobic patients endure a phasic illness with periods of remission hastened and intensified by positive and en-thusiastic therapy.

HYPOCHONDRIASIS

Persistent concern over fancied illness, *hypochondriasis*, is part of the differential diagnosis of a large number of main symptoms ranging through every system. The hypochondriac, the person who imagines he is ill, fears he is ill or even knows he is ill in some way that doctors cannot seemingly clarify, is well known in fiction and well known in real life. But hypochondriacal concern is a serious symptom which needs to be sensibly investigated and which should not be dismissed impatiently even though the most hypochondriacal patients can test a doctor's patience very sorely.

The psychiatric view of hypochondriasis is conflicting: some maintain that *all* hypochondriasis is secondary to some psychiatric disorder be it anxiety, depression or hysteria; others maintain that even after these conditions have been excluded there remains a hard core of patients who are 'essential hypochondriacs', *i.e.* they are hypochondriacal people and that is that.

From the *clinical point of view* it is certainly easier to consider hypochondriasis as a symptom and examine the differential diagnosis since in practice a large number of patients are referred to the psychiatrist for the investigation of hypochondriacal complaints. At this stage it is important to try and clarify what exactly is a hypochondriacal complaint. In general doctors seem to apply an arbitrary scale to the recognition of a patient's subjective awareness of bodily discomfort. This has practical value in that some patients bear pain more readily than others and this observation is useful in deciding how to use analgesics in a rule of thumb sort of way.

However it does seem likely that doctors and nurses tend to play down a patient's complaints of pain and discomfort except when the patient has malignant disease. On the other hand chronic painful disorders may not receive sufficient attention, in fact it is highly likely that despite the range of pain relieving drugs the medical profession is on the whole rather bad at relieving pain except in dire circumstances. This observation must weigh heavily in any discussion of hypochondriasis since the topic is concerned with not only fancied illness but with exaggerated concern over illness and discomfort, and the latter is something that it is too easy for doctors to judge too harshly.

Pain is a badly understood phenomenon, in fact the most that can be said about it with absolute certainty is that it is unpleasant. This basic attitude should be borne in mind when considering *hypochondriasis* since quite frequently the patient's mode of stating his complaint may somehow offend the doctor's expectations and incorrectly suggest hypochondriasis. Having made this reservation we can acknowledge that there *are* patients who complain of symptoms, sometimes vague, sometimes specific, who are found on examination to have no physical disability but who remain convinced of physical illness despite *explanation and reassurance*, and these patients we regard as hypochondriacal.

Explanation and reassurance are terms that need to be amplified. It is remarkable to find how many patients find the doctor's explanation inadequate. Explanation of symptoms and their causes takes *time*. It is no good expecting a patient to accept a 'there's nothing wrong with you' type of explanation.

This may seem an oversimplification to the doctor but when it comes to explaining to patients, the medical profession still lags very badly, even to the extent of warning about drug side effects or even advising how to take prescribed medication. Part of this comes from the ancient tradition of the omniscient physician, part comes from the doctor's fear of creating hypochondriasis and part from the doctor's experiences of giving explanations and finding them badly misunderstood. However there is increasing evidence that on the whole it is better to explain as much as possible and that people in general benefit from it.

However it is possible to exclude misinformation and ignorance as causes of apparent hypochondriasis since it disappears when proper explanation of the symptom is given. But this leaves those patients in whom this does not occur and this is what hypochondriasis is about. The first task is to clarify the patient's subjective complaint in simple terms so that one knows exactly what the patient is complaining about. This is important, *e.g.* sometimes patient's complaint is described as 'headache' when in fact he is complaining of numbness or tingling on the scalp.

Next the psychiatrist should exclude the following psychiatric syndromes: 1, schizophrenia; 2, affective disorder; 3, anxiety; 4, organic syndromes; 5, personality disorder; 6, obsessional neurosis; 7, phobic state; 8, hysteria; and 9, malingering.

Schizophrenia   Here hypochondriasis tends to be bizarre and delusional in florid illnesses although many early schizophrenics complain of vague bodily symptoms that seem to have no meaning in physical terms.

Affective disorder   Hypochondriasis is a common clinical feature in depressive illness and probably accounts for the majority of persistent hypochondriasis in middle aged and elderly patients.

Anxious patients often present with hypochondriacal concern focused on a somatic expression of anxiety, *e.g.* palpitation, chest discomfort, nausea, muscle tension.

Organic syndromes   Here hypochondriasis is more likely to be an important complaint in an elderly patient with dementia.

Personality disorder   Hypochondriasis can be a cause of persistent visits to the doctor especially by patients with inadequate personalities.

Obsessional states   Here the hypochondriacal complaint is usually recurrent, and has a strongly compulsive quality often related to other obsessional symptoms, which when examined emerges as compulsive fears of illness rather than of conviction.

Phobic state   Phobic states may overlap with obsessional states in that the patients basic problem is actually *fear* of illness rather than belief that he has it.

Hysteria   In conversion hysteria, hypochondriasis is usually closely allied to functional loss and a situation that involves gain.

Malingering   Malingering means feigning illness. It is uncommon but should always be included in the differential diagnosis of hypochondriasis.

HYSTERIA

The term hysteria is generally applied to disorders in which there is a loss of bodily function without any evidence of structural disorders: but to get a correct understanding of the use of the term it is necessary to know something of its historical background since the concept of hysteria has given rise to confusion and uncertainty particularly since the term is used in a number of ways.

The word hysteria derives from the Greek *hystera* (uterus) and is an indication of the fact that the Ancient Greeks and Romans recognised certain types of psychological disorder but believed that they occurred only in women and that they were caused by abnormal uterine movements. During the Middle Ages, as we have seen, many states which would now be recognised as psychiatric disorders were thought to be caused by demonic possession, and books such as the *Malleus Maleficarum* contained descriptions of clearly recognisable case histories of psychiatric syndromes including hysteria.

In the 19th Century there was a revival of interest in hysteria in an attempt to explain strange neurological syndromes involving sensory loss, paralysis, trances and odd behaviour. The French physician Charcot described 'classic' signs of hysteria but these were mainly bizarre manifestations which were the response to suggestion on the part of histrionic patients.

The general principles underlying the concept of hysteria, *i.e.* of lost function plus no structural damage were advanced to a theoretical level by Pierre Janet and by Sigmund Freud, at a time when hysteria was a topic hotly disputed by doctors.

Janet suggested that the hysteric underwent a splitting or dissociation of consciousness so that the alteration of function became almost autonomous leaving the patient genuinely unaware of what had happened. Freud took this idea further and suggested that hysterical disorders were the sequels of traumatic experience in which the person had failed to go through an appropriate emotional response, had repressed the response below consciousness but that the response became converted into a symptom. This led to the term *conversion hysteria* which is central to psychoanalytic theory since it relates symptom formation to the dynamic influences of sexual conflict and led Freud to speculate further about the dynamics of human behaviour since his intellectual curiosity and clinical interest were stimulated first of all by a puzzling syndrome.

So there is general agreement that in hysteria a patient can suffer a loss or impairment of function in almost any part of the central nervous system that is ordinarily subject to voluntary control but that this loss occurs at an unconscious level, *i.e.* the person does not knowingly fabricate the illness. Confusion arises and seemingly always must arise from the fact that it is hard to think of such a disorder as being distinct from malingering or simulated illness. It appears possible that there is a continuum that extends from hysteria to the malingerer, the latter is said to be comparatively rare and occurs in special situations where malingering may serve a fairly obvious purpose, *e.g.* in prison etc. This tends to be the majority view amongst psychiatrists, however some suspect that psychiatrists may be unduly diffident in acknowledging the true extent of malingering.

A general theory of hysteria postulates functional loss in the central nervous system at a level beyond consciousness which is a reaction to stress in a person either constitutionally vulnerable or in a normal person in conditions of intolerable stress. Severe ordeals such as in war, exhaustion and exposure to bombardment etc. may cause almost anyone to break down in this way if pushed to the limits of endurance. Cultural influences must also be taken into account. In primitive unsophisticated societies psychiatric illness may not be a recognised or accepted concept so that a person is only permitted to break down in a 'physical' way. Epidemics of hysterical disorder are also recognised—the disturbed 'bewitched' children of Salem Mass, the Nuns of Louvain—both of these are good examples of epidemic hysteria in relatively closed societies involving young women. These populations are especially at risk as pointed out by McEvedy (1970) in his observations on a 'virus illness' that caused fainting amongst school-girls in Derbyshire on the occasion of a Royal visit.

Further confusion has arisen over the use of the term since it is used in a number of ways—to describe conversion hysteria, as a label for a personality type (hysterical personality), to describe exaggeration of existing disease (hysterical overlay) and by laymen (and some doctors) to describe disordered 'out of control' behaviour ('she's hysterical').

Conversion hysteria

This may be regarded as the 'true' hysterical disorder. It can present in a wide number of ways in the nervous system affecting motor and sensory function and with disordered mental states. Hysterical disorders are usually dramatic—loss of vision, loss of speech (hysterical aphasia), difficulty in swallowing (globus hystericus), loss of sensation (hysterical anaesthesia), inability to move a limb or limbs (hysterical paralysis), can arise. This makes the careful investigation of all neurological symptoms of the utmost importance since hysteria will be included in the differential diagnosis of many neurological disorders.

Disordered mental states may be caused by hysteria, in severe forms psychosis may be mimicked (hysterical pseudopsychosis).

In conversion hysteria the patient develops a loss of function which conforms to his own notion of what an illness is like. On examination there are no signs of structural damage to the central nervous system. Sensory loss is haphazard and paralysis is unaccompanied by changes in muscle tone or reflexes.

The diagnosis of hysteria therefore is not easy and is very much the province of the expert since some structurally based diseases can present with what at first sight appear to be hysterical signs. Also the liability to conversion hysteria may be increased by brain damage, in childhood and in senility.

Some of the most dramatic varieties of hysteria include somnambulism and hysterical fits. In the former the person walks around in a trance-like sleep, and in the latter develops fits which may be mistaken for epilepsy. In hysterical amnesia there is total memory loss quite unlike that found in brain damage usually following a traumatic event.

Hysterical personality (histrionic personality)

This term is used to describe people whose personalities show persistent signs of emotional immaturity into adult life. The level of emotional maturity is infantile and the hysteric may on the one hand show many of the attractive features of childhood but carry into adult life many of the less attractive aspects of infantile behaviour. Tendencies towards being unduly egocentric, importunate, manipulative and demanding are hall marks as are undue vulnerability and inability to sustain mature interpersonal relationships.

Histrionic behaviour is the rule, to be the centre of interest and attraction a byword. All needs require immediate gratification—failure to meet them causes histrionic reactions—literally 'creating a scene'. Rather like a small child in fact.

The quality of the hysteric's behaviour is dramatic and urgent, problems are stated in louder voices and in more vivid colours. And they tend to take the centre of the situation very speedily, progressing from one emotional crisis to another leaving behind a trail of bewildered observers. Instability or lability of mood is common, depression is described in colourful terms but the mood changes quickly. Emotional responses are shallow and superficial.

It is said that people with hysterical personalities are more likely to develop conversion hysteria and though this may be the case it has not clearly been shown to be true. Perhaps it is more important to emphasise that conversion hysteria is not the exclusive province of people with hysterical personalities. Given enough stress almost anyone can break down in a hysterical way.

Difficulties in maintaining interpersonal relationships extend in to all aspects of behaviour. In the sexual sphere the hysteric is flirtatious and shallow, so that marriage may prove disastrous for them for they lack the ability to weather the emotional demands of forming a stable union. In the past it has often been said that the hysteric is frigid but this is not necessarily true; what is more likely is that the hysteric's sexual encounters may be less than fulfilling because of his or her genuine emotional shallowness. Many of the qualities of the hysteric's behaviour can be put to profitable use particularly in the entertainment business where their vivacity and capacity to manipulate may be put to shrewd use and their histrionic ability used to the full. The superficial charm of many hysterics itself may lead them into a series of disturbed relationships since they speedily tire of new friends and lovers.

It is important that the term is not used as a pejorative label. This is quite improper but unfortunately often seems to be the case. The possession of various character traits and modes of behaviour should not lead to a moral value judgement by the observer. People are what they are not from choice but as a result of the complex interaction of genetic inheritance, environmental learning and life experience.

Hysterical exaggeration or overlay

In all sorts of illnesses a patient's symptoms and signs may seem to be more colourful than expected. Unconscious exaggeration on the part of the patient is common and often dictated by fear and uncertainty. If there is an element of gain in the sick role then the patient may exploit this in a hysterical way, particularly if he or she is receiving attention previously denied.

'She's hysterical'

The term is frequently loosely used to describe behaviour that is exaggerated and out of control. This is not in any sense a valid way of using the term since uncontrolled behaviour may arise from a much wider series of psychological and social causes.

A general theory of hysteria and its causation

The role of the hysterical personality has been mentioned. It is likely that a genetic factor operates here but early childhood experience has to be taken into account. A child who shows early signs of hysterical character tendencies may frequently have its behaviour reinforced in to a hysterical pattern by the unwise indulgence of an unstable or doting parent who accedes to all its whims thus confirming the child's expectations that this is a reasonable way of going on and that relationships with others are to be gained by manipulating them and obtaining speedy gratification of urgent needs under the threat of tantrums and noisy displays of frustrated resentment.

Brain damage may release hysterical manifestations since it causes a lowering of control of higher central nervous system activity. A person of late middle age or an elderly person may develop a hysterical reaction because control of higher mental activity is impaired by the beginnings of dementia. Again in mental subnormality hysterical reactions can occur on a similar basis since the subnormal person is lacking in the basic equipment to direct his or her behaviour in a stable and well adjusted fashion and may react to minor frustrations by developing hysterical signs, usually of such an unsophisticated sort that they are near to frank malingering.

Perhaps the most important thing to be said about the appearance of a hysterical symptom is that in most cases it is a danger signal, a call for help. It has been likened to the tip of an iceberg in this context. It may overlie genuine organic disease, it may herald the onset of a more serious psychiatric disorder or it may overlie a series of deep seated problems of which the patient has at the best only partial awareness. And for this reason all hysterical manifestations need thorough investigation.

The psychodynamic explanation of hysteria related it to conflict, where unconscious wishes and desires are repressed by the patient and channelled into loss of physical function. This loss of physical function is the only route perhaps by which the patient may preserve his or her psychological integrity against the overwhelming and anxiety provoking threats posed by intolerable conflict arising from the pressures of totally unacceptable wishes and desires forced into the deceptive calm oblivion of unconscious mental life.

Loss of function in hysteria may ultimately be regarded as being a sign of impending loss of control, and that loss of control may relate to the inherent instability of a genetically inherited personality disorder, to overwhelming stress or to damage to the brain. It is almost as if the sufferer switches out circuits and isolates the stressful experience and anxiety into a pool of lost function.

The possible role of hysterical personality may be traced to the histrionic and exhibitionistic behaviour of patients at the Saltpetriere and was reinforced by Freud's clinical description of cases with hysterical syndromes. From these descriptions there rose the idea of a specific personality type, the 'hysteric' who was presumably more liable to hysterical syndromes, otherwise the eponym is meaningless. To date there is no published series of patients diagnosed as suffering from hysteria who have been shown to have a significantly high incidence of a hysterical personality. The literature on hysteria does not suggest that it is a unitary syndrome any more than does the epithet 'hysterical personality' suggest anything more than that a psychiatrist has observed that certain patients are consistently histrionic, flirtatious and manipulative, and display a degree of non-cooperativeness with doctors which tends to induce doctors to interpret their refusal to cooperate as indicating the presence of a personality disorder. Undoubtedly some people remain tiresomely and manipulatively overdemanding throughout life. They are not easy to deal with whether they are ill or not and when they are ill they are certainly worse. It is probably safe to call them *histrionic* or *immature* and leave it at that, for the label hysterical too often causes doctors to prejudge the outcome of a plethora of symptoms which are always problematic and which may overlie some very serious disease. People with too many symptoms get called hysterical too easily.

Any discussion of the aetiology of hysteria is a good example of the uncertainty of the whole concept of hysteria and the difficulty that persistently impedes any useful discussion of hysteria in operational terms is that hysterical illness is a concept that tends to be approached by doctors in a way that may be regarded as a variety of double think. On the one hand the medical profession makes public statements that hysteria is an illness, yet privately many honest doctors would concede that their internal statement of hysterical disorders includes a series of illnesses in which conscious simulation is more forceful than functional loss caused by internal conflict. And yet the bulk of published works on conversion hysteria have increasingly stressed the importance of internal conflict as an important aetiological agent.

The logic of this all is relatively simple and whether the theory is stated in Freudian, neo-Freudian or eclectic terms in essence it amounts to this. First, everyone is assumed to have limits of tolerable internal conflict and limits of individual reaction to forces acting on them from outside whether these forces are obvious as in the case of battle, or less obvious as in the case of personal struggle in interpersonal relationships. Secondly, it is assumed that the basic response of a person to any such influence is to become anxious. Thirdly, it is postulated that people have varieties of ways in which they can cope with anxiety. For many people anxiety is a threat to their psychological integrity and the hysterical response can be regarded as one in which intolerable anxiety or unspecified conflict is so intolerable to the person that the nervous system shuts off the threat by switching off a series of functions in the central nervous system. In this way the symptom complex of lost function as represented by paralysis makes the person 'ill' and recognised as such. It also provides the person with a mode of living which permits him to avoid any type of decision making in the face of conflict and, more than that prevents him from having even to consider areas of internal conflict let alone doing anything about them.

Now this type of explanation has some value since it is a way of constructing an aetiological model. But we can take it further in considering hysteria and consider the relevance of brain damage or poor brain function acting as a trigger where integration of central nervous system is less controlled, so that switching out the central nervous system circuitry becomes more likely through plain lack of control. Some support for this idea is found in the finding that hysterical symptoms can occur more easily in the brain damaged.

The basic problem of hysteria remains unresolved; namely is there such a thing as a hysterical illness? To be sure under conditions of extreme terror, exhaustion and so on people do break down in a way where they lose function, but in fact the basic concept of hysteria is not relevant to this sort of breakdown since anyone may develop it under sufficient stress in much the same way that anyone may break a leg. This leaves us with the uncertainty of hysteria as a useful diagnosis since its neat summary by Slater (1965): 'No evidence has yet geen offered that the patients diagnosed from hysteria are in medically significant terms anything more than a random selection. . . . The only thing that hysterical patients can be shown to have in common is that they are all patients.'

And there still the matter rests. Some people become ill in a way that conforms to clinical expectation and others become ill in a way that has a stagey peculiar quality to it.

It looks as if hysteria is:

1 Protean in manifestation
2 Impossible to diagnose positively
3 Too often diagnosed in the absence of positive findings
4 Often overlies organic illness

This view has been clarified by Slater (1965) who comes down uncompromisingly on the side of rejecting its value and emphasising its dangers. His study of 112 cases diagnosed as hysteria of whom 85 were followed up, revealed that after 9 years 12 were dead, 14 were totally disabled and 16 were partially disabled, and only 19 symptom free. This prompted his comment that patients diagnosed as suffering from hysteria are nothing more than a random selection. The lack of consistency in the medical condition of 'hysterics' suggests that there are other qualities that cause someone to be labelled hysteric and Slater suggests the following:

1 Absence of positive physical findings

2 A multitude of symptoms
3 Evidence of psychogenesis offset by the comment that trouble, discord, anxiety and frustration are so universal in life that their temporal association with illness does not imply causation
4 The presence of suspect symptoms such as aphonia and amnesia
5 The presence of certain personality traits which tend to provoke hostility from doctors.

Management

In managing a patient with conversion hysteria attention is first of all directed towards the lost function whether it be loss of vision, paralysis, loss of sensation or whatever. The psychiatrist aims to restore lost function gradually rather than suddenly since sudden dramatic relief such as has been produced by hypnosis may be followed by development of others.

In the case of acute conversion hysteria the technique of abreaction is sometimes used. In this the patient is given an injection of a sedative, usually intravenously, and then in a state of drowsy altered consciousness the patient is allowed or encouraged to ventilate pent up feelings. This is frequently associated with restoration of function, usually suggested to the patient by the doctor.

Long-standing conversion hysterical symptoms are much less easy to treat, it should be commented that many cases of chronic conversion hysterical paralyses have ended in permanent contractures of the limbs and even amputation.

The avoidance of chronicity is therefore of great importance and much was learned about this from experience in World War I where soldiers with hysterical paralyses often remained untreated. In World War II cases of acute conversion hysteria were treated with heavy sedation, continuous sleep in fact, and then given vigorous rehabilitation and physiotherapy thus avoiding chronic loss of function. In a sense the treatment of conversion hysteria aims at avoiding chronicity and this can be achieved by positive and confident management. Doubt and uncertainty feed hysteria and suggest prolonged disability to the patient.

Psychological understanding of the dynamics of the illness is a necessary part of the investigation of the patient but it is hard to claim that it necessarily means radical cure for the patient. Encouragement and confident rehabilitation are fundamental. Psychotherapy in depth is very much the province of the expert. It has been said that hysteria is the most psychogenic of disorders yet the results of prolonged psychotherapy are far from satisfactory. In many instances prolonged therapy may take on the character of persuasion and be effective.

In the case of hysterical personality disorders there is always the hope that the patient will mature with time, and this probably happens more frequently than is given credit. Prolonged intensive psychotherapy of an analytic type is again an expert undertaking and full of difficulties since the hysteric tends to become overdependent on the therapist to a degree which becomes a handicap in itself.

Treatment of depression when it occurs is usually along conventional psychiatric lines using antidepressant medication where necessary. Perhaps the most useful treatment remains the most undramatic namely, gentle support in the long term. The hysteric will need to be supported through crises and through good and bad spells of his or her life. This treatment though unspectacular is probably as good as any. In the past marriage was often recommended as a 'cure' and undoubtedly caused great unhappiness to patient and spouse.

OBSESSIONAL DISORDER (OBSESSIONAL NEUROSIS)

Obsessions are contents of consciousness which are unpleasant, recurrent against a sense of inner resistance and which are usually regarded by the sufferer as silly, absurd or mad. Obsessional neurosis is rare, tends to be concealed and is usually chronic though the epidemiology of the disorder is uncertain. This may be because it is generally rare or because it does not come readily to light since obsessional neurotics often conceal it and do not recognise it as illness as it is so close to normality in mild cases. The prevalence rate is not known, most psychiatrists agree that it *is* uncommon and that patients often have severe and crippling symptoms.

In severe cases concealment is aided by the fact that patients often go to incredible lengths to hide obsessional symptoms from others as they are sure that others would deride their absurd behaviour since their compulsive rituals may be bizarre, and are only offset by the patient's distress at his own apparent folly.

Very good accounts of the sufferings of the obsessional are found in John Bunyan's *Pilgrim's Progress* and in the writings of Dr. Samuel Johnson.

H

Obsessions and normality

Many obsessions have a magical quality about them so that the person feels safer if he either performs a ritual or repeats a phrase. This is part of normal experience in childhood, there must be few people who have not known this in childhood and adult life, particularly in times of danger and stress, fancied or trifling. At school, it is common for children to discover some act that has to be performed which makes them feel safe from trouble or failure. This can extend into university life. Many medical students have personal rituals that they carry out at examination. The same quality applies to good luck charms and mascots and to common superstitions. We tend to smile at them but may feel vaguely uncomfortable if we don't carry them out.

Kraupl Taylor (1966) has commented on a familiar example of this in medical practice where hand washing and scrubbing in such minor procedures as injections confer nothing on the outcome of the injection, any more than does cleaning the skin with cotton wool and spirit yet this always is religiously carried out.

Stafford-Clark (1970) observed the use of compulsive checking by flight engineers in Bomber Command in the Royal Air Force in World War II. Instrument checks would be carried out as many times as possible, this was associated with the idea that this would ensure a safe return. Often this was recognised by the fact that the engines failed to start due to overheating associated with delay in ignition while checks were prolonged.

Magic and the superstition of primitive peoples again are very similar phenomena and they play a more forceful role in the culture of primitive societies than in developed countries.

The psychiatric significance of obsessions is exemplified in obsessional disorders, in the obsessional personality and in the presence of obsessional features colouring other psychiatric disorders.

Obsessional disorders

The term obsessional disorder is synonymous with terms such as obsessional neurosis, obsessional state, obsessive compulsive disorder and obsessive-compulsive neurosis. The term obsessional disorder is preferred since it is comprehensive. In fact the basic definable characteristics of obsessional and compulsive symptoms which are primary in this disorder relate simply to the definition of obsession and always includes these characteristics:

1   Obsessions are always experienced against a feeling of inner resistance

2   They are always obtrusive in the mental life of the patient

3   They always induce fear, apprehension, anxiety, even dread in the patient

4   They seem absurd to the point of unbelievable idiocy as far as the patient is concerned whose retention of insight is fragmented. On the one hand he knows he is ill, on the other he is forced to act as if he didn't.

5   The obsession is experienced by the patient as something alien to him.

Clinical aspects

Varieties of obsessional disorder are described but it is hard to know just how useful this is. Perhaps the crux of it is that certain obsessional syndromes stand out because of their particular symptomatology, *e.g.* some patients are crippled by the need to carry out complicated and extensive rituals involved with basic activities such as eating, washing, dressing or defaecation. Consider this following case.

A 44 year old woman of eccentric personality and genteel upbridging was tortured by compulsive eating rituals. In these she had to search through every meal for any solid particle exceeding about 0·5 cm in diameter. This reduced her daily life eventually to a chronic preprandial search which took hours and ended up with her failing to eat ice cold inedible meals. When admitted to hospital she was suffering from severe malnutrition and vitamin deficiency that caused an organic psychosis.

Other patients are troubled with insistently persistent obsessional thoughts which at times render them incapable of sustained action and may be complicated by depressive mood. Others are afflicted by obses-sessional uncertainty and doubt about everything to the extent that they can accept nothing as certain and indulge in no activity because they doubt the rightness or wrongness of every action—in the words of Descartes 'To doubt everything that is not clear, to avoid precipitancy and to divide up every difficulty into as many parts as are possible, and neces-sary for its better solution: also to proceed from the simplest and plainest facts.' This type of obsessional disorder is usually called *folie de doute*. Others are troubled by the urge to utter blasphemies in Church, or in any place of worship, so-called 'contrast ideas'. A 40 year old professional man was troubled by an intolerable urge to shout out obscenities every time he took Communion. This made him so guilty that he tried to kill himself.

Such a case was described by the monks Kramer and Sprenger in the

Malleus Maleficarum in their account of a man who brought his son to them supposedly possessing a devil. He was impelled by his obsessions to stick out his tongue when he genuflected in church or passed a statue of the Virgin. In other cases obsessions are complicated by phobias (irrational fears) which assume bizarre dimensions and complicate life to an intolerable degree. Consider the following case.

A 30 year old married woman had obsessional fears of impregnation which started as fears of intercourse and pregnancy and then extended so far that every time she touched things such as door knobs, cutlery, kitchen utensils, indeed anything, she was beset by obsessive fears of picking up semen on her fingers. This led her to endless genital washing which reached its worst when she habitually scrubbed her vulva with a nylon dish scourer covered with cleaning powder.

The obsessional personality

Some people are from their earliest years conscientious and methodical to an excessive degree. They tend to be meticulous and scrupulous in a way which makes them honest and dependable but always tortured by guilt and fear of giving offence. This shows itself in behaviour and talk loaded with apologies, qualifying clauses and self-deprecatory statements which recur in a predictable and often irritating way—'I'm afraid that. . . . Of course I wouldn't wish to disagree but. . . . Pardon me if I appear to be disagreeing . . .' etc. Often these statements may be their only way of dealing with internal aggressive feelings which no doubt give rise to anxiety which can only be dispersed by endless apology and qualification.

Otherwise talk is precise, pedantic and systematic to the point of boredom and their outlook is moralising, even self-righteous and rigid to the extent that friends and colleagues temper their regard for their probity with mild amusement at the rectitude of one, say, who cannot see anything even mildly funny in the trifling dishonesties that often make social life more bearable for the average person. Often the sense of moral rectitude is tiresome and superior, extanding to the point where they are incapable of seeing anyone else's point of view so convinced are they of their correctness and so fearful are they of change. 'I can't help feeling that you haven't really understood me or you would agree with me.' Indecision, vacillation and a hypochondriacal attitude go with this personality and indeed their rigid systematic behaviour makes them valued colleagues, particularly as subordinates. They do not make good leaders, so hidebound are they by detail and formalism, probably the most disastrous example of such was Lord Haig in World War I. He was rigid, conscientious, indecisive and totally without imagination. Often their correctness and regard for detail dissociates them from any feeling at all, for instance Adolf Eichmann, the Nazi exterminator and Himmler. Their humour when present is arid and donnish, palely coloured by old maidish archness at supposed impropriety. People with this personality possess many traits which rightly are valued: honesty, sobriety, punctuality, neatness, systematic thought and ordered lives but they possess them to an excessive degree.

Obsessional features colouring other psychiatric disorders

In primary affective disorders it is sometimes the case that the patient is troubled by obsessional thoughts, compulsive acts etc. This tends to happen when the obsessional personality develops depression in late life, a recognised complication of the obsessional personality.

Schizophrenia may be coloured by obsessional features. In the early stages this may lead to diagnostic difficulties since it may be hard to distinguish whether ruminations or preoccupation with overvalued ideas is based on delusion or is an obsession. In fact schizophrenics can develop obsessional symptoms. Usually these features tend to be more bizarre than customary obsessions and tend to conceal underlying delusions that can only be elicited by prolonged and patient interview.

Obsessional symptoms in organic brain disease

It has long been recognised that obsessional symptoms and in particular compulsive acts and utterances may be a complication of postencephalitic states. Actually this is not a very common occurrence and hardly presents a real diagnostic problem in recognising the significance of obsessional symptoms.

In dementia the condition of 'organic orderliness' has already been commented on. This represents a person's attempt to preserve order in the face of recognised disorganisation in brain function.

The natural history of obsessional disorder

This has been reviewed by Pollitt (1960, 1969) Grimshaw (1965) and Kringlen (1965). On the whole obsessional disorder is rare constituting about 0·25 to 3·1% of psychiatric in-patients and a similar percentage of out-patients. The onset tends to be early in life, before 25 and rarely after 45 (Pollitt, 1969) and usually the illness starts with phobias and rituals (Kringlen, 1965). Often obsessional disorders start quite suddenly and as has been remarked earlier the patient conceals the symptoms which cause him such shame.

The outcome of obsessional illness apparently is less grim than formerly has been taught, in fact there is good evidence of variability of symptoms and the possibility of spontaneous remission. One of the difficult clinical problems presented by these patients is the fact that their symptoms are bothersome, often handicapping and always preoccupying to a degree that wearies the doctor long before the patient.

Treatment

The cornerstone of treatment is the recognition by the doctor that the illness may be episodic but always long drawn out, and that the patient will never yield to his worst fears and that simple support and reassurance are always very helpful. It is particularly important for the obsessional patient to know that he is neither mad nor unique. Tranquillisers may be used to relieve tension, and antidepressants to relieve depression. In severe cases psychosurgery is sometimes used (Bridges, 1973).

I0

Schizophrenia

The term schizophrenia is well known and poorly understood. In psychiatry it is used to describe syndromes in which severe personality change occurs in the absence of organic cerebral damage. These syndromes usually come on relatively early in life and have a poor prognosis. The trouble about the word schizophrenia comes from the fact that psychiatrists disagree about its meaning. This is related partly to the history of psychiatry and the beginnings of psychiatric classification, and in all respects epitomises the real problems that surround the use of the medical model of psychiatric disorders amongst which schizophrenia is conventionally regarded as a serious mental disorder, a psychosis that leads to total disorganisation of the personality. Kraepelin was the first clinician to describe the symptoms and natural history, calling it dementia praecox; Bleuler called it schizophrenia.

In modern clinical psychiatry there is disagreement about the essence of schizophrenia but general agreement that there is a recognisable and discernible population that develops this syndrome. Some regard it as a genetically determined illness, others regard it as a syndrome that can be explained in terms of a person's life experience, others regard it as a mysterious syndrome of severe psychological breakdown which, until proven otherwise, probably is based on multifactorial aetiology. All are agreed that once the diagnosis is made the outlook for the patient is dubious, at best he may emerge as a mildly damaged person, at worst a lost disintegrated person living in a world of inner directed fantasy, delusion, hallucinosis and muddled thinking. The original descriptions stressed the importance of special clinical types, *e.g.* simple, hebeprenic, catatonic and paranoid schizophrenia. Nowadays though it is conceded that these types may occur, the real clinical importance lies in the recognition of a syndrome that can be recognised as something we call schizophrenia.

Kraepelin regarded dementia praecox as a psychosis which started in adolescence and led to dementia. He thought that the symptoms indicated a lowered integration of volition, emotion and behaviour and emphasised the likelihood of a genetic factor which transmitted the disease and he suspected that brain damage or metabolic disturbance would turn out to be the cause of the disorder. He used the word 'dementia' as he believed that the end of the illness was intellectual defect. Nowadays it is realised that organic dementia does not occur in schizophrenia.

Bleuler re-examined the whole concept of dementia praecox and pointed out that dementia did not occur and that any resemblance to dementia was superficial. His observations emphasised not so much the *deterioration* of the schizophrenic but rather the *fragmentation* of psychological processes. He looked for links between the psychopathology of the schizophrenic and his previous experience, in many ways a novel idea since hitherto the content of 'insanity' had been supposed to bear no relationship to previous life experience. Bleuler commented on the relative importance of schizophrenic symptoms—thought disorder was given prime importance as he suspected that it probably followed a brain physiological disturbance whilst other symptoms were 'psychological'. He believed that the *schizophrenic process* could be altered by psychotherapy and stressed the importance of the doctor–patient relationship.

After Bleuler had re-defined the syndrome, its status remained more or less unchanged as psychiatrists tacitly assumed that it was a reaction to life experience in a genetically predisposed person. This meant bending the observed facts since 50% of schizophrenics are people with a stable premorbid personality and no family history.

During the past 40 years there has developed a general concept of schizophrenia as a disorder that is related to fairly specific family disturbance but also there has been increasing interest in the possibility of disordered brain biochemistry in schizophrenia. Many lines have seemed promising but have been discarded usually on the grounds of faulty methodology. Genetic studies have been contradictory; some will be reviewed.

Diagnosis

The biggest obstacle in understanding schizophrenia is the lack of agreement about its status as a disease, something that was first defined in 1896. Before then the situation was confusing, there was a general idea that there was a condition called 'insanity' but classification was imprecise although earlier writers had been impressed by abnormal mental states which started in adolescence and progressed relentlessly to apathy and personality change in adult life. The physician Arateus of Cappadocia wrote of patients who 'enter into such a degradation, that, plunged into an absolute fatuousness, they forget themselves, pass the remainder of their lives as brute beasts, and the habits of their bodies lose all human dignity'. The significance of this ancient observation was lost for over a thousand years before the human race re-discovered the notion of humane care for the mentally ill.

In the 19th Century there were many descriptions of abnormal mental states, *e.g.* John Connolly, the reforming physician of Hanwell Asylum who advocated the release of patients from restraint wrote 'Young persons not infrequently fall into a state somewhat resembling melancholia without any discoverable cause of sorrow and certainly without any specific grief; they become indolent or pursue their usual occupations or recreations mechanically and without interest; the intellect, the affections, the passions all seem inactive or deadened and the patients become utterly apathetic'. In the mid 19th Century, despite such accurate descriptions as this the interest in psychiatric classification reached a state of comic uncertainty: Heinroth described 48 mental illnesses while in 1860 Neumann rejected all mental disease categories in favour of 'insanity'.

In 1868 Kahlbaum described 'catatonia' and later Kraepelin used the term 'dementia praecox' originally coined by Morel, to summarise early onset of mental illness leading to deterioration but distinct from manic-depressive psychosis and in so doing achieved a breakthrough in classification and started the diagnostic scheme which remains the basis of clinical psychiatry. Kraepelin always rejected a purely psychological aetiology believing dementia praecox to be a constitutionally determined brain disorder.

Bleuler redefined dementia praecox as *schizophrenia* and viewed it as an illness midway between organic brain illness and a dynamic reaction. The symptoms were primary and secondary, the former included thought disorder, incongruity of affect and ambivalence and autism. Bleuler's words carried authority and still do but, as has been pointed out by Kendell (1972), psychiatry has been marked by authoritative statements based on assertion rather than on accurate data collection.

Bleuler's most important observation, apart from proposing the term schizophrenia, was to refer to 'the schizophrenias' thus implying that schizophrenia is a syndrome rather than a single cause disorder, thus schizophrenia may be as general a term as fever or hemiplegia.

Present clinical uncertainty has been reviewed by Kendell (1972) who in acknowledging the confusion commented on the diagnostic differences between various countries. This is shown by Cooper *et al* (1972) who found that when truly comparable patient populations were examined that the diagnosis of schizophrenia was made 'nearly twice as frequently in New York as in London' and that many patients diagnosed as schizophrenic in New York would be in London regarded as depressed, neurotic or as having personality disorders. In New York State Malzberg (1959) found that the rise in schizophrenic admission rate over 20 years was inversely related to the affective disorder admission rate, while in 1972 the World Health Organisation Study on the diagnostic criteria for schizophrenia used in nine countries (Colombia, Czechoslovakia, Denmark, India, Nigeria, Taiwan, UK, USA and USSR) showed that in all of the countries save the USA and USSR the diagnostic criteria were *fairly* uniform.

American texts frequently define schizophrenia in a way that would be quite unacceptable in Europe, a typical recent example where the author acknowledged its unacceptability in Europe was provided by Kohn (1973) —'Those severe functional disorders marked by disturbances in reality relationships and concept formation': a definition that is broad, but as Kohn remarked, he used it 'not because I think it superior, but because it is the usage that has been employed in much of the relevant research'.

Diagnostic problems resolved or unsolved?

Schneider was definite about the diagnosis of schizophrenia since he said that there are symptoms of *first rank importance* (Schneider, 1959; Breakey & Goodell, 1972)—such symptoms are said to be diagnostic of schizophrenia 'in the absence of coarse brain disease' (Fish, 1967). They include:

1 Hallucinatory voices which repeat aloud the patients' thoughts: German, *Gedankenlautenwerden*; French, *echo de la pensée*

2 Thought withdrawal and thought insertion

3 Hallucinatory voices discussing or commenting on the patient's acts or thoughts

4 The feeling of having lost possession of thought—that they are being broadcast or shared by others

5 Feelings of bodily influence

6 Feelings of being controlled from outside

7 Delusional perception

Actually it appears that clinicians tend to regard these symptoms as diagnostic in the same way that they regard delusions and thought disorder as key symptoms of schizophrenia. A questionnaire study of diagnostic practice of British psychiatrists reported by Willis and Bannister (1965) found that thought disorder and affective incongruity were rated as the most important symptoms. A similar study carried out in America (Edwards, 1972) reported virtually the same findings, which is surprising in view of the known diagnostic differences.

This suggests that Bleuler's symptom list is credible but untested though some credibility is lost when Bleuler's symptoms such as autism and ambivalence are found to be hard to define, unreliable and may occur in the normal.

The clinical subdivisions of schizophrenia and special varieties such as residual and latent schizophrenia etc., have been described but provide little help in resolving the diagnostic impasse; clinical subtypes are either obvious or else useless.

Up to 30% of people diagnosed as schizophrenic have none of Schneider's first rank symptoms. This lack of clinical reliability is familiar and has led to a search for *an operational definition of schizophrenia*. Feghner *et al* (1972) have put forward the following based on American experience and thus subject to the diagnostic differences between the USA and the UK.

A Both of the following are *necessary*:

1 A chronic illness with 6 months symptoms before first evaluation without return to previous psychosocial adjustment

2 Absence of affective symptoms that would be sufficient to make a diagnosis of affective disorder or *probable* affective disorder

B The patient must have at least *one* of the following:

1 Delusions or hallucinations without significant perplexity or disorientation

2   Speech that makes communication difficult because it is illogical or hard to understand

C   At least *three* of the following must be present for a diagnosis of *definite schizophrenia*, and *two* for a diagnosis of probable *schizophrenia*.

1   Single status
2   Poor social adjustment or work history before onset
3   Family history of schizophrenia
4   No alcoholism or drug abuse within 1 year of diagnosis
5   Onset before age 40

Aetiology of schizophrenia

Since there is disagreement about the definition of schizophrenia it is hardly surprising that there is an equal amount of uncertainty about aetiology. For many years there has been a general air of conflict about whatever might be 'the cause' of schizophrenia, on the supposition that there might be one discoverable cause, which when revealed, would explain everything. But at present there must be few who take this idea seriously and there is general acceptance that schizophrenia is likely to have a multifactorial aetiology; that the illness/syndrome arises from an interplay of factors, personal and psychological, genetic, biochemical and social. However, the concept of multifactorial aetiology does not exclude the crucial intervention of one set of factors in a given case, thus in some instances it is likely that disturbed family relationships trigger off the attack, while in another a genetic factor is the most important.

In truth we do not really know how much weight to attach to any particular factor though many would argue that genetic inheritance is the best understood and most definite aspect of aetiology, though this view has been shaken in recent years by disparate genetic findings. And it is this uncertainty that prompts further diverse enquiry. At present we may say that the strands of the aetiology of schizophrenia are tantalising and elusive ranging from high quality genetic studies through conflicting biochemical theories to well thought out psychosocial theories of family interaction which have an immediacy and conviction that reflect one's own clinical experience. But at the end of it all there is no general consensus of aetiological theory. Physical treatments such as ECT and neuroleptic drugs point to the role of disordered biochemistry in the acute illness, on the other hand these methods are less useful in the chronic illness where social rehabilitation has been given great impetus by the work of Wing which has shown how careful re-education and training can fit someone previously thought untreatable into a more productive and enjoyable mode of life.

Since knowledge is slender the best we can do is review aetiology under the factors that have been most carefully studied.

All discussions about the aetiology of schizophrenia are handicapped, some might say mentally handicapped, from the start by disagreements about definition though these problems have been clarified by such researches as the WHO Pilot Study and the USA–UK diagnostic study (Cooper *et al*, 1972). As if this were not enough, the problems of definition are, for many, reduced to near absurdity by disagreements as to whether or not 'schizophrenia' as a concept is to be regarded as a type of illness, a way of labelling the socially intolerable or a way of labelling family outcasts driven into eccentricity by tangled family relationships. This is a knotty academic point which should not be allowed to obscure the fact that a remarkably constant proportion of any population studied so far does develop a syndrome with fairly constant abnormalities of feeling, conduct and thought that we may usefully regard as an illness since it leads to a general fall off in a person's life style, efficiency and happiness often to the point of suicide or to an end point of bewildered incoherent disorganised lost behaviour that leaves him as a long term patient in hospital, totally unable to enjoy the mainstream of human existence. If this is not an illness then it is something very like one!

Epidemiology, incidence and prevalence

The incidence of schizophrenia has usually been worked out by psychiatrists who have surveyed populations, interviewed people and made the diagnosis using their own criteria (Wing, 1972). Despite the varying populations studied the estimated rate of incidence between ages 15 and 40 is between 0·5 and 1·0% (Book, 1961) though Eaton and Weil (1955) and Book (1953) had found rates very different in special communities such as the Hutterites of North America who seemed to have a much lower incidence (Eaton & Weil, 1955). Also a much higher incidence rate was found in North Sweden (Book, 1953). These differences can however be practically explained in terms of case finding and criteria. Certain other races have been shown to have higher rates of incidence of schizophrenia

—the Tamils of South India and Ceylon (Murphy, 1959; 1965) the people of North West Croatia (Crocetti *et al*, 1964) and Irish Catholics (Spilzka, 1880; Pollock, 1913; Malzberg, 1940) and more recently by O'Doherty (1965) who found that both the Irish admission rate and bed occupancy rate were double that in England. Hospital admission rates for schizophrenia are very different in the USA and UK, in 1960 24·7 per 100 000 as opposed to 17·4 but here the difference is to some extent accountable for by differing diagnostic criteria, however, this difference does not exist between England and Ireland.

Other epidemiological aspects of schizophrenia touch on class and social mobility. Many writers for instance have noted a higher incidence in those who emigrate to another country as opposed to those who stay behind (Odegaard, 1932; Murphy, 1965; Mezey, 1960) whilst others have noted a higher incidence in the centres of towns, probably related to social isolation (Hare, 1956; Sainsbury, 1955). Others have noted a tendency for schizophrenics to drift downwards in the social scale, not only through limited earning capacity but also possibly to a preschizophrenic drift into inertia before the condition was recognised.

Personality

Many writers have stressed the importance of the premorbid personality structure of the schizophrenic. As ever, one is confronted with the difficulty of assessing personality but a 'schizoid personality' has been described. This is a personality type which can be seen to contain the seeds of schizophrenia. Schizoid individuals display behavioural traits such as seclusiveness, abnormal shyness, hypochondriasis, emotional coolness and indifference, fanaticism and eccentricity. However, there is some difference found by various workers in the incidence of these abnormal personalities before the onset of schizophrenia. Bleuler found a 34% incidence of schizoid personality in a series of schizophrenics. Other workers have found a higher incidence but it has to be admitted that up to 50% of schizophrenics show no evidence of previous personality disorder. Nevertheless the finding of personality disorder in an individual suspected of the slow development of schizophrenia may be a useful pointer towards the diagnosis. Further evidence of the possible role played by personality abnormality in the aetiology of schizophrenia is demonstrated by the increased incidence of deviant individuals in the families of schizophrenics.

Physical illness

Physical happenings such as illnesses, operations or accidents can commonly precipitate an acute schizophrenic psychosis or bring about remission in an established one.

Life changes

Recent research suggests that schizophrenic onset and relapse are significantly preceded by life changes such as moving house, loss of a job, bereavement, etc. The implications of this may be that the schizophrenic has a low tolerance for change or overstimulation.

Psychological factors

The role of psychological factors in the aetiology of schizophrenia is far from clear. Common clinical experience teaches us that schizophrenia may be triggered off by any variety of psychological stress.

A comprehensive theory of the aetiology of schizophrenia would postulate that the schizophrenic process is mediated biochemically, *i.e.* follows a biochemical final common path, that the illness occurs in a genetically predisposed individual, and that this disturbance may be triggered off by a variety of physical or psychological stresses or both. It would certainly seem at the present time that this theory of multiple aetiology is the most profitable one to follow in research.

Schizophrenia appears to be a complex disturbance occurring at many levels in which hereditary, psychological, neurophysiological, sociological and biochemical factors may all play relevant parts.

Theories of aetiology in schizophrenia

Family interaction studies

Anyone who speculates about psychiatric aetiology may form at least a theoretical model in which the family may be thought of as exerting a potent influence in psychiatric illness in general and schizophrenia in particular. In recent years theories of family interaction have been put forward with greater force and more convincing evidence. The theories centre on communication within the family and postulate ways in which communication disorders might predispose to psychiatric breakdown.

It remains a matter for debate as to how powerful these factors may be despite rather emphatic statements that have been made by writers such as Lidz *et al* (1966), Wynne and Singer (1963) and Bateson (1900), in the USA and Laing (1960) and Laing and Esterson (1960) in the UK. The debate is intense, even heated in the case of schizophrenia, between those who visualise it as a genetically determined biochemical disorder leading to psychological malfunction and those who see it as an understandable, predictable reaction to conflict and ambiguity within the network of family relationships. The idea of the family's role in the aetiology of psychiatric disorder is not new: Pinel, Griesinger and Kraepelin all alluded to it in more than casual fashion.

But current interest in the family tends to view it as an emotional time bomb where ambiguity, hidden meaning and veiled hostility are the explosive ingredients. This interest may well be an outgrowth of the cultural climate of an age when communication is keenly studied and when communication has become so prolific as to saturate. There is an excess of communication in society via the press, television, the media, experts and self-appointed experts. In science and technology the flood of information overwhelms to the stage where no one person can keep abreast of the developments in his own specialty. Hence the need for information retrieval systems. Our society exists against an immense background noise of words: a flood that too easily engulfs the individual who can become in computer language, the subject of 'information overload'. Current sociological and psychiatric interest in family communication failure as an aetiological factor in psychiatric disorder started in America—a country where the concept of the family has been romanticised as if the family was a present from a deity unfamiliar with the communal life style of the People's Republic of China.

This interest in the family started with Adolf Meyer who was impatient with 19th Century descriptive psychiatry which must have seemed to him to be rigid, sterile and unsympathetic to the point of being unconcerned by the possibility that family life could mould personality development or cause illness. So Adolf Meyer took a novel step since he regarded psychiatric disorders not as syndromes which might eventually be explained in terms of brain malfunction but rather as disorders that could be explained as the individual's own personal, even idiosyncratic adaptation—the outcome of a series of forces to which he had been subjected. Meyer laid great stress on family influences as a general series of factors but was unexpectedly vague about details. This view of psychiatric aetiology was not shared by many of Meyer's contemporaries who had become absorbed in psychoanalytic theory. Freud himself was uncommitted about the role of the family since he stressed the importance of the individual's unconscious drive, conflict and childish fantasy, giving the parents a secondary role as individuals rather than as a group of abnormal communicators.

These theoretical misgivings were not shared by enthusiastic psychiatrists and social workers who recognised the family as a cauldron of strong brew. This was intensified by the Child Guidance Clinics of the 1920s where planned counselling and therapy of parents and children were regarded as a way of preventing neurosis, psychosis and delinquency—high-sounding aims which were never achieved.

At present there is soundly based interest in the role of the family in the aetiology of psychosis. Whether it is by tangling communications with the sick family member, giving ambiguous instructions, misinterpreting what he is saying or manoeuvring him into a position where parental messages are so inconsistent that he is forced to opt for psychosis as a refuge from an immediate world that is incomprehensible and uncertain. Thus 'withdrawal' becomes an adaptive manoeuvre. These hypotheses need careful examination and certain studies will be described. Before this we need to look at the 'normal' family, since though there are an increasing number of family studies they are selective in that they concern families that have been studied because they have at least one member defined as abnormal. The 'normal' family, *i.e.* the family that does not include an obviously sick person, is taken almost for granted, it seems to be assumed that families which do not produce deviant people are probably functioning normally. This assumption is accepted as fair but at the same time it should be realised that there are no hard and fast rules governing behaviour within the family though there are enormous differences between cultures; each of which imposes on its members general family structures.

In Western society the family hierarchy has altered considerably in the past 100 years and it is no longer easy to make predictions about the behaviour of a 'normal' family. A reasonable supposition is that 'normal' family members would be affectionate, supportive, honest and consistent in their relationships with one another. This supposition assumes an ideal state of perfection similar to the way in which people tend to regard themselves as stable, correct, mature and well informed. We have learnt much about communication within 'abnormal' families but we are ignorant about modes of communication in 'normal families'. The works of novelists such as Thomas Mann, James Joyce, Nancy Mitford and Ivy Compton-Burnett give vivid pictures of tangled and hidden meaning that may seem overdrawn but which leave the suspicion that even in 'normal' families communication is not necessarily as clear and unambiguous as we might expect. Most families have family jokes and special use of language which might easily bamboozle well intentioned and often naive researchers. These speculations are introduced only to suggest a proper note of caution in evaluating family interaction models.

Family interaction studies have been *heavily concentrated on schizophrenia* and the most important examples include the works of Lidz and associates, Bateson and Wynne and Singer, some examples of which will briefly be reviewed.

Spiegel and Bell (1959) reviewing parent/child studies in psychiatric aetiology pointed out many inconsistencies in these areas and set out a list of supposed parental pathological traits that had been quoted in the literature since 1930. The list includes parents who have been classified as: *abusive; cold; controlling; covertly rejecting; dependent; domineering; emotionally unstable; fearful; hypochondriacal; inadequate; masochistic; neurotic; over- achieving; overprotective; overtly rejecting; passive; poor self-adjustment; poor social adjustment; punitive; sadistic; successful; submissive; uncritical; underachieving; unhappy;* and *wavering.*

A glance at this list leaves an impression of inconsistency and lack of meaning. Recent work however has been more sophisticated and has moved away from epithets in a search for abnormal types of communication within the family. Mishler and Waxler (1969) have stated the four questions that family studies in schizophrenia set out to answer:

1 What are the patterns of family interaction that are related to the development of schizophrenia?

2 What is schizophrenia and what are the psychological mechanisms through which family patterns of interaction enter in to the development of the schizophrenic process?

3 How do these interaction patterns persist over time, that is, what individual and family junctions are served that help to maintain the schizophrenic forms of interaction?

4 What are the preconditions for these patterns of interaction, *i.e.* what are the personal and social attributes of family members that are associated with the development of the processes.

Lidz

Lidz and associates have been particularly interested in family interactions in schizophrenia. Their basic hypothesis is that muddled relationships, ambiguous communication and uncertainty between parents and child can lead to schizophrenia: a hypothesis which is in general backed up by their studies (providing allowance is made for the diagnosis of schizophrenia).

The Lidz approach began in the course of orthodox psychoanalytic study of families but latterly Lidz and associates have examined the family as a whole and its possible influence in producing schizophrenia in one member. Lidz regards the family role structure as critical and has moved from psychoanalytic theory to sociological theory to explain abnormal family relationships. He even went as far as defining an ideal marital relationship which would be most beneficial to the children—'What appears to be essential can be stated simply. . . . The spouses need to form a coalition as members of the parental generation maintaining their respective gender roles and be capable of transmitting instrumentally useful ways of adaptation suited to the society in which they live.' Roughly translated this presumably means that parents should be stable and consistent if they hope to bring up stable children.

However Lidz and associates found in their studies of schizophrenic families that there was a definite incidence of abnormal marital relationships which apparently contributed to schizophrenia in the children. Two types of marital disturbance are described: marital *schism* and marital *skew*. Skew is defined as a state of superficial harmony which barely conceals the pathological domination of one partner by another, marital schism is marked by discord and dissent, the parents communicate in a way that is either coercive or full of mutual defiance. In either case the child is given a distorted image of the parent by the other, both of whom compete for the child's affection in a devious and mutually denigrating fashion. Thus a 'schizophrenogenic' family is thought to be wholly pathological—a group in which one member is selected to be schizophrenic, *i.e.* to fulfil a particular role. There is an excellent fictional account of such a situation in the novel *The Elected Member* by Bernice Rubens.

It is suggested that schizophrenic girls are more likely to come from 'schismatic' backgrounds and schizophrenic boys are more likely to come from 'skewed' backgrounds where a disturbed mother dominates a passive husband. In either instance the child is drawn into conflict between parents and opts for or is driven into psychosis out of self-protection. To prove such a hypothesis controlled family studies are needed, also studies that employ careful methodology. A good example of the latter is the study of Waring and Ricks (1965) who examined 50 schizophrenics seen previously at Child Guidance Clinics. They split the patients into 'chronic' and 'recovered' and compared them with controls. They found that 55% of the mothers of the chronic patients were borderline or actually psychotic as opposed to 16% in the recovered group and 22% in the normal group. The relationship between parents were classified as follows:

1 Emotional divorce (ED), *i.e.* cold hostility
2 Pseudo mutual masking (PMM), *i.e.* a facade
3 Extreme marital skew (EMS), *i.e.* one submissive spouse
4 Schismatic conflict (SC), *i.e.* violent discord

The schizophrenic's and normal's parental backgrounds were rated as in Table 10.1.

Table 10.1 Parental relationship and schizophrenia.

Type of parental relationship	Chronic schizophrenic %	Recovered schizophrenic %	Normal %
Emotional divorce	35	17	4
Pseudo mutual masking	12	12	4
Extreme marital skew	7	2	0
Schismatic conflict	20	10	24

The general conclusions drawn were as follows:

1 Chronic schizophrenics tend to come from families where one or both parents are psychotic or borderline psychotic
2 The relationship between parent and child tends to be mutually dependent
3 The parental relationship is most likely to be either severely skewed or emotionally divorced
4 Recovered schizophrenics tend to come from depressed families
5 Normal families do not produce schizophrenics

Such a study is superficially convincing but is questionable on at least two counts: firstly the small sample size and secondly the criteria for the diagnosis.

The best we can say is that odd and eccentric people are more likely to produce schizophrenic children than are 'average' parents but this hardly accounts for the fact that 50% of diagnosed schizophrenics have no family history. This does not imply rejection of Lidz's work but rather qualified acceptance.

Another approach is provided by Wynne and Singer (1963, 1964) who have examined the modes of communication in the families of schizophrenics and found that it tends to be vague and meaningless. (Have they ever examined the proceedings of certain parliamentary debates?)

For Wynne and Singer the family milieu and its communication network are the basis for a child's learning how to live, an almost naive assertion with which few would quarrel. The child learns in the family how to act, feel and think in an acceptable way and becomes aware of the relative importance of family members, again self-evident. From this early experience the child carries over what he has learnt into adult life. But if the child grows up in a family where communication is vague and ambiguous he is likely to become someone who thinks vaguely and cannot easily relate with others. Wynne and Singer have identified the thinking disturbances and communication modes of the parents of schizophrenics. They categorise one type of disorganised and fragmented thinking as *amorphous*. In the families of schizophrenics whose thinking was found to be amorphous the whole family atmosphere seemed misty and undefined, conversation was patchy, desultory and disconnected from feeling. Also the parents were detached from each other *and* the child.

They described another form of thinking called *fragmented*—it was reasonably coherent but lacked consistency and meaning. These families were quarrelsome and acrimonious and always inconsistent in relationships, switching almost at random from blame or disapproval to half hearted encouragement that bewildered the children. Family language was idiosyncratic and full of private codes that served further to confuse the child.

Wynne and Singer's findings may be summarised thus: A person's ways of dealing with what he sees around him and interprets it is a biologically directed and integrated function which is based on perception, zoning in on relevant areas, maintaining attention at a congruous and appropriate level thus providing a data base of perception, intuition etc. about the environment in a coherent way that is appropriate and also means something to the 'average' person, *i.e.* it is not overloaded with personal jargon or symbolism. These abilities depend in part on genetic inheritance and in part on how a person learns to communicate with early key figures in life, *e.g.* parents. If he is perplexed, bewildered or stunned by his parents' communications and how they relate with him then it is hardly surprising if he develops into a person whose communication and emotional apparatus is in a state of permanent malfunction, and this goes beyond being merely someone who is 'hard to get on with'—it is a state in which a person's communication and relationships and rapport are always idiosyncratic and often psychotic.

The most intriguing finding was that styles and forms of thinking in Wynne and Singer's families were stable in adult and fluid in children, and finally that a preponderance of children who became schizophrenic had been pathologically compliant and subservient. One is left to speculate about the prescience of such children.

Bateson

Bateson is a social anthropologist who has explored the ways in which a family communication system could become so abnormal as to edge someone into psychosis. He proposed the 'double bind' theory of schizophrenia which suggests that the parent imposes on the child a special type of ambiguity which is binding, threatening and internally inconsistent. The basis of Bateson's approach is that communication consists not merely of words but that non-verbal cues can signal feeling and instruction, so that non-spoken communication may be in direct contrast to the words spoken. We may assume that in schizophrenic families there is often total communication failure, common clinical experience confirms this. The garbled *verbigerations* of the chronic schizophrenic are pure noise with little or no information content, whilst in less severe cases communication is at least impaired. Bateson's contention is that someone who is later diagnosed as schizophrenic has acquired family communication methods in childhood from his parents. He says that in childhood the preschizophrenic is bombarded with 'double bind' signals, an experience in ambiguity which leads to psychosis, since the child becomes bewildered by parents who give out inappropriate requests, entreaties and commands which contain implied negative injunctions. In effect he is advised to disobey the commands he receives and can only expect rejection, disapproval or punishment whatever he does. The result is that the child learns to avoid rejection or punishment by speaking and behaving in an ambiguous or meaningless way which might deter punishment. Thus his speech and behaviour become so idiosyncratic as to defeat common understanding and eventually ensure his recognition as schizophrenic.

Laing

R. D. Laing and A. Esterson have gone further than Bateson in their observations on communication in the families of schizophrenics. Laing tends to regard schizophrenics not so much as ill people but rather as people who have been judged to be eccentric or unacceptable in behaviour by a society which defines 'normality' and 'deviancy' in an arbitrary and often politically directed way. Thus Laing questions very seriously the medical model of psychiatric disorder.

The essence of Laing's model of psychosis lies in his sensitivity to ambiguity and also in his trenchant criticisms of the many absurdities that Society permits itself in its seeking out and persecution of those who deviate from its expectations. Inappropriate behaviour may be judged as sick, psychotic, psychopathic, deviant or 'abnormal', even criminal by society in a way that is never consistent, often expedient and frequently malign. Judgements of social behaviour may thus be used to identify, as deviant and in need of 'treatment' or punishment, all sorts of people who are inconvenient, tiresome, etc.

Laing's position clearly sees the psychiatrist as someone who is used in political persecution not confined to authoritarian regimes but also in countries who preach liberalism and lock up various types of dissidents in the name of 'treatment'.

The psychiatry of Laing has aroused enthusiasm and opposition of equal intensity. Its most widely read statements are in the *Politics of Experience* (1967) where Laing totally rejects a medical model of psychiatry and substitutes an alternative model which many have found confusing. Laing's views are controversial and no psychiatrist of any sense should enter the controversy without reading what Laing has to say rather than relying on clever rehashes such as that provided by Siegler *et al* (1969). They open their analysis of Laing's psychiatry with the somewhat ominous if not relevant observation that they are members of the 'square' older generation who know what is best and that '*The Politics of Experience* is not good for bright young schizophrenics'.

Laing's basic statements about schizophrenia seem to encompass a political–social theory of schizophrenia, *i.e.* as a role which a person is obliged to adopt because he cannot live in an intolerable world—psychiatrists have been excessively preoccupied with a patient's behaviour and paid no attention to his experience. Diagnosis is a label given to people in certain social situations and in effect the patient becomes the victim of a special sector of the social system. Doctors, nurses, social workers deny the patient his individuality and 'treat' him in hospitals where the treatment process can only serve to make everything worse for him. Hospital admission procedures etc. are a form of ritual social degradation. At the same time Laing offers the view that schizophrenia is 'itself a natural way of bearing our own appalling state of alienation called normality . . . madness need not be all breakdown. . . . It may also be breakthrough. It is potentially liberation and renewal as well as enslavement and existential death.' It is not an illness to be treated but 'a voyage'.

Now this is confusing stuff for the doctor brought up on a strictly medical model of psychiatric illness but just because Laing's statements are worded in a challenging way and are unscientific this does not discredit them in the way that many have suggested.

He argues that we cannot look at madness without looking at society and its corporate behaviour, a point that cannot be shrugged aside conveniently, human society has behaved and continues to behave in a grotesquely violent and destructive way. Genocide and the threat of nuclear war are taken almost for granted by a society that becomes enraged at the antics of adolescent drug takers and ignores the massive neglect of the elderly and chronic sick. As to the treatment of schizophrenia Laing is again on strong ground, there is as yet no convincing evidence that treatment has altered its natural history, the main advances have been in improving disturbed behaviour and hallucinosis and in caring for patients in a more humane fashion.

These are sensible points and Laing has reminded doctors not to dismiss as nonsense everything that a schizophrenic says. The weak points in Laing's views seem to be that he overvalues psychosis as an illuminating enriching experience and also that he hardly appears to offer a better alternative to conventional humane psychiatric treatment.

The controversy remains and Laing remains an uncompromising original man whose writings have already affected a whole generation of young people who are less ready to accept a conventional distinction between sanity and madness. They may be right.

General comments on family interaction theories

Neither Bateson nor Wynne regard family interaction factors as *causes* of schizophrenia but rather as elements in a family relationship that is so tangled and disturbed as to make him act in an odd way and be regarded as ill. The main criticism of the studies is that the definition of schizophrenia is unacceptable as it is too broad. The theories are stated in an imprecise way and there seems to be a tacit assumption running through all of them that we know exactly how 'normal families' communicate. This assumption is less than fair. People who live close to each other often use slang and condensed language which might seem odd, eccentric, even psychotic to an outside observer. Some of the writings on the topic are hardly notable for their clarity either. The great merit of family interaction studies is that they have shown up how easily ambiguity can pass unrecognised by the incurious and unaware. The lack of controls in family interaction studies is an important flaw but it does not devalue their interesting content and speculative atmosphere. Speculation is unpopular nowadays but not as yet forbidden.

Another interesting aspect of Bateson's work is that schizophrenia is viewed less as a continuous process in one person and more as an intermittent state affecting only one member of a group that shares a crazy communication network. The selected family member is thus in an impossible situation, since he can only keep the morbid interaction going in an attempt to defend himself against it. Taken further, this means that the family needs only one obvious schizophrenic since his continued psychotic existence preserves some stability in the family, *i.e.* 'We're all right because he's mad isn't he?'

Genetics of schizophrenia

The present state of knowledge of the genetics of schizophrenia is not so definite as had been supposed. Penrose (1971) reviewed the topic covering symptomatology, onset, family incidence, relationship to affective disorder, twin studies and biochemical genetics. His conclusions are not easy to dispute. First he emphasises that the term schizophrenia is as general as epilepsy or mental subnormality, and that since the diagnosis is based on mental symptoms it does not identify one specific disease, thus, in his view effective genetic studies are hardly possible. He regards twin studies as inconclusive while conceding that heredity and environment are involved in aetiology, leaving genetic studies at best providing limited conclusions since strict Mendelian inheritance is excluded: although in some cases a single recessive gene may operate, in others multifactorial inheritance, whilst sex linked genes may operate as major or minor influences. He suggests that in certain cases inborn biochemical error may eventually be identified and comments on the association between known sex chromosome abnormalities such as Turner's and Klinefelter's syndromes with schizophreniform psychoses.

Slater (1970) takes a more optimistic view since he concedes the difficulty of operational definition of schizophrenia but points out that for the purposes of genetic study it may be satisfactorily defined thus 'An illness affecting the mind and the personality of the patient in a way which is seldom completely resolved. After an attack of illness there is nearly always some degree of permanent change of personality. . . . We conceive this personality change as basically organic in nature so that we cannot expect to define it completely in solely psychological terms. Its main effect is to erode the capacity for functioning at the highest conceptual level . . . illnesses of this kind may be imperceptible in onset . . . more usually they occur in one or more acute attacks of relatively severe illness. Symptoms may include focal disturbances of central nervous function occurring in a setting of general lucidity; hallucinations (especially in the auditory field), passivity feelings, primary delusional experiences and rather typical forms of thought disorder.'

Slater's many observations on the genetics of schizophrenia are based therefore on careful definition and long term follow up and lend weight to the authority of his statements on the central importance of a genetic factor in schizophrenia. The question of genetic inheritance is not a 'once off' one but, despite Penrose's misgivings most psychiatrists accept its relevance.

Until recently it seemed fairly certain that the genetic basis of schizophrenia had been proved since the work of Slater and Kallman showed a clear association between schizophrenia and the closeness of relationship to a schizophrenic family member, especially high in monozygotic twins who showed a concordance rate of up to 80%. Then in 1963 Tienari and Kringlen separately reported much lower concordance rates, Tienari 10% Kringlen 27%. However, more recent twin studies such as that of Gottesman and Shields (1966) report a concordance rate of 40% in monozygotic twins.

Sources of error in genetic studies have been reviewed by Rosenthal (1961), these include sampling and diagnostic errors apart from the basic objections to twin studies inherent in factors such as their having been reared together and that they may be a deviant sample through premature birth.

The present state of knowledge suggests that genetic factors do operate in schizophrenia and that inheritance is probably polygenic.

Table 10.2 Concordance for schizophrenia in monozygotic *twins* variously reported.

Luxenberger (Germany)	1928	67%
Luxenberger (Germany)	1934	33%
Luxenberger (Germany)	1936	52%
Essen Moller (Sweden)	1941	0–71%
Kallman (USA)	1953	69%
Slater (England)	1953	65%
Tienari (Finland)	1963	10%

Odegard (1963) examined the prevalence of psychiatric disorders in the relatives of 202 consecutive admissions observed in the long term (minimum 12 years) and found a higher prevalence of psychopathy, criminality and alcoholism in the schizophrenics and manic/depressives families. Furthermore families tended to breed true in that schizophrenia was more common in schizophrenic families, likewise manic depressive psychosis but near relatives of manic depressives rarely developed schizophrenia. Near relatives of patients with 'other psychoses, mostly paranoid' showed random prevalence of psychosis/psychiatric disorder. Heston (1966) studied the prevalence of psychiatric disorders in the children of schizophrenic mothers who had been separated from their mothers in the first week of life and reared in foster homes compared with children of non-schizophrenic mothers similarly reared. This study is an important one in that it supports the likelihood of a genetic factor in schizophrenia.

The 47 experimental subjects were all children of schizophrenic mothers in an Oregon State Hospital, the 50 control subjects were a carefully matched sample of institutionally reared children. The subjects were all thoroughly evaluated and the main finding was that psychiatric pathology was more prevalent in the children of schizophrenic mothers and also that the only cases of schizophrenia occurred in the children of schizophrenic mothers. Some of the findings are shown in Table 10.3.

Table 10.3 Prevalence of psychiatric disorders in children of schizophrenic mothers

	Control	Experimental
Number	50	47
Mean age	36·3	35·8
Schizophrenia	0	5
Mental subnormality	0	4
Sociopathic personality	2	9
Neurotic personality disorder	7	13
No. spending over 1 year in institution	2	11
Total years institutionalised	15	112

Almost half of the schizophrenic mothers' children developed psychiatric disorders. Heston noted also that the remaining half showed a high incidence of artistic and creative ability.

From these examples it is possible to draw at least a firm conclusion that genetic inheritance in schizophrenia is important but that it does not account for all cases since at least 40 to 50% of schizophrenics have no family history of the disorder.

Zerbin–Rudin (1967) tabulated the expectation of schizophrenia for relatives of schizophrenics based on 25 different investigations (Table 10.4).

Table 10.4 Expectation of schizophrenia for relatives of schizophrenics

	Expectation %
Parents	4·38
Siblings	8·15
Children	12·31
Grandchildren	2·81
First cousins	2·91
General population risk	0·85

Biochemical theories

The biochemistry of schizophrenic patients has been exhaustively studied. Early work concentrated on searching for abnormal sera, foci of infection, endocrine malfunctions etc. but in practice one may discount virtually all of the work done until 1952 when Hoffer, Osmond and Smythies put forward a tentative hypothesis of schizophrenia as a brain located biochemical disorder. After 20 years these early writings (1952, 1954) have a simplicity and certainty about them that has now been lost as the real experimental difficulties have been fully appreciated.

The original idea was that there might be a substance; 'M' substance which would be somewhere between mescaline and adrenaline, be a hallucinogen and be produced in the brain. They pointed out for instance the hallucinatory effects of 'pink adrenalin', *i.e.* adrenaline that goes pink and causes hallucinosis, and speculated that schizophrenia could be caused by adrenochrome in the brain or by some abnormal brain metabolite. It turned out to be not so simple, adrenochrome does not exist in the brain and brain biochemistry is harder to study than was thought in 1952.

At present the status of disordered brain biochemistry in the aetiology of schizophrenia can be summarised under three headings (Smythies 1968):

1 The aberrant catecholamine hypothesis
2 The faulty transmethylation hypothesis
3 The melatonin–harmine hypothesis

The aberrant catecholamine hypothesis is based on the known similarity between noradrenaline, dopamine and 5-hydroxytryptamine (5-HT or serotonin), all known central transmitters and hallucinogens such as psilocybin, psilocyn and dimethyl tryptamine (DMT).

The hypothesis postulates an abnormal metabolite in the biological stress mechanism causing the metabolite to be produced and leading to a positive feed back mechanism that would perpetuate the psychosis. Initial support to this was given by the findings of Friedhoff and Van Winkle (1962) who reported DMPE in the urine of 60% of schizophrenic patients —the so called 'pinkspot'. It remained unproved however, since studies were uncontrolled as to diet, drugs and stress.

The faulty transmethylation hypothesis was given some support by Kety's finding that feeding methionine to chronic schizophrenics caused worsening of symptoms, suggesting a crucial role for methionine as a source of methyl groups.

The melatonin–harmine hypothesis is based on the chemical similarity of the pineal hormone melatonin to the hallucinogen harmine. In 1965 Greiner and Nicholson noted excess melanin in schizophrenic's body cells, particularly in patients who had *not* received phenothiazines which cause pigmentation. The hypothesis postulates a congenital enzyme deficiency causing a metabolic block leading to excess production of a harmine-like hallucinogen instead of melatonin (itself a serotonin derivative).

Perhaps the best summary of the dangers inherent in studying the biology of schizophrenia is that of Kety (1969):

'Those interested in exploring the biologic aspects of schizophrenic disorders cannot with impunity ignore the psychologic, social and other environmental factors which operate significantly at various stages of their development. Leaving aside aetiologic considerations, it is clear that exogenous factors may precipitate, intensify or ameliorate the symptoms and confound the biologic features of chronic schizophrenia are created by prolonged isolation and hospitalisation will become apparent with the increasing adoption of community-oriented treatment. Examples are readily found in which uncontrolled nutritional, infectious or pharamcologic variables may have accounted for specific biochemical abnormalities in populations of chronic schizophrenics.'

Mednick and McNeil (1968), on a purely psychological approach, summarise thus:

'It may be difficult . . . to isolate aetiological factors through studies carried out with individuals who have lived through the process of becoming and being schizophrenic. The behaviour of these individuals may be markedly altered in response to correlates of the illness, such as educational, economic and social failure, prehospital, hospital and posthospital drug regimens, bachelorhood, long-term institutionalisation, chronic illness and sheer misery.'

In other words, it is all very difficult.

CLINICAL TYPES OF SCHIZOPHRENIA

Hebephrenic schizophrenia

This type usually starts insidiously in adolescence. Personality change is extensive and malignant. Sometimes a bout of depression comes before obvious schizophrenic change—a good reason to be wary of 'depression' in adolescence, particularly if it comes on out of the blue and is unrelated to customary adolescent stress. The chief symptom in hebephrenia is *thought disorder* which is usually severe when the illness peaks, at this stage talk becomes incoherent and neologisms become common. Volition falls away, the patient becomes aimless and purposeless, although sometimes a false impression of mental activity is suggested by an interest in philosophy or metaphysics which the patient may take up in an attempt to order his disconnected thinking. The patient is usually dreamy and vague because he cannot think clearly, this may lend him an air of spurious profundity that can mislead the uninformed. Thought disorder, often obvious, is not always so and may be hard to detect or demonstrate. Often people will go to great lengths to explain the non-understandable, it is almost as if they find it impossible to accept the idea that someone's mental state could be so disorganised.

Delusions are usually odd and bizarre rather than sinister. In the early stages the patient may be vaguely but persistently hypochondriacal and visit the doctor frequently to seek reassurance about fancied illness. *Emotional changes* are characteristic and are neatly summarised by the word 'silly'. Affect is shallow, the patient smiles and giggles frequently in an empty inappropriate way. *Auditory hallucinosis* is an inevitable symptom. Regressive infantile behaviour, *e.g.* incontinence and gorging are also common in chronic hebephrenia. Sexual promiscuity in the early stages may be a troublesome social problem and is usually casual and detached. In the later stages of the illness withdrawal and total inaccessibility are common, the end point is affective incongruity, buffoonery, mannerisms, and fragmentation of thought and talk. This is a type of schizophrenia where the personality is truly destroyed.

Paranoid schizophrenia

This type of schizophrenia is particularly interesting, first because in many ways it is less like an illness than other schizophrenias and secondly because it tends to run true to form. It is less like an illness because it is nearly understandable. Though deluded, the paranoid schizophrenic's ideas often have a distorted relationship to past experience, also the process is less destructive of the personality: this is probably related to relatively late onset when the personality is fixed.

The clinical picture is dominated by paranoid delusions either of persecution or grandeur. There is often a baffling interplay of real experience with paranoid misinterpretation in the early stages and this may lead to the diagnosis being overlooked or postponed since a *paranoid state*, so called, *could* be a transient reaction to justice, unfair sacking, romantic disappointment, missed promotion, etc. But sooner or later a true paranoid schizophrenic picture emerges when delusions are expressed with force and absolute conviction. Auditory hallucinations are common and bring to the patient added proof of the conspiracies that enmesh him. A generally negativistic attitude is usual: the emotional state is cool and detached.

Often the patient's premorbid personality has been odd. He has been a man who never could fit in easily with his colleagues: people felt uncomfortable and strained in his distant presence. He may be described as always having been morose or sullen: 'keeps himself to himself'. He gave a general impression of coolness and aloof unfriendliness. His conversation was usually sparse; he took offence easily, was touchy and over-sensitive. His colleagues have found him hard to get on with, often too the personality contains elements of humourlessness and strained pompous solemnity. Others may notice that he is offhand, truculent or impatient and prone to complain about fancied insults. This may have led to his having become more cut off from his immediate circle who over the years have found his brusqueness and ready sarcasm hard to take. At the end of it all the detachment from him by his colleagues reinforces his own preferred alienation from a world that he finds hostile and frightening.

The onset may be either acute or insidious, in the latter instance it is hard to pinpoint as to *when* the patient became recognisably psychotic, at the same time neighbours etc. express little surprise. Whether the onset is quick or slow it is easy to be wise after the event. There is often a *strong affective colouring* to the illness. This is especially true when the paranoid schizophrenic becomes ecstatic, has ideas of cosmic revelation or becomes enraged by feelings of persecution. This is a dangerous state which may lead to assault or murder. He may develop into the sort of person who barricades himself in his home and has to be removed by armed police. But usually the onset is slow, so that over a period of months or years a lonely oversensitive person ends up with an elaborate system of delusions which may be very skilfully concealed. In fact of all schizophrenics the paranoid is most likely to go virtually unrecognised as such for years, whilst being regarded by his friends as, at best, an odd seclusive chap.

Paranoid schizophrenia *can* lead to severe personality disorganisation but this is much less likely than in other schizophrenias. This is probably because of the later age of onset: also many seem to 'burn out' so that although the patient remains bound to his delusions they are less forcefully expressed, can be concealed and he achieves a compromise with them and carries on a relatively normal social existence. Other paranoid schizophrenics are unable to cope in the world, their delusions lead them into quarrelsome conflict and they may find a refuge in mental hospitals where their delusions are tolerated more readily than outside.

Catatonic schizophrenia

Motor disturbances are common in catatonic schizophrenia leading to excitement or decreased activity causing stupor. In excited catatonia the patient may explode into a flurry of overactivity, punctuated by a torrent of disorganised talk shouted incessantly. The emotional state is angry and enraged—excited catatonics can be dangerous people—though fortunately nowadays it is a rare condition.

In the past excited catatonia often led to death from exhaustion 'fatal catatonia' as it was called, where a patient remained highly excited, untouched by sedatives, refused food and drink and eventually died. This was before the discovery of ECT and neuroleptic drugs. In stuporous catatonia, psychomotor activity is slowed, even halted. At first the patient is slow and clumsy and says little except monosyllables. Detachment from reality is total and as activity runs down the patient becomes inaccessible to the point of stupor, drooling, incontinent and needing to be tube fed, at least this is how it was before ECT. Catatonics may take up strange fixed postures, or lie in bed with the head a few inches above the pillow, or may show echo reactions, mechanically repeating the examiner's words and gestures (echolalia and echopraxia). Passive movements of the limbs shows them to be stiff—a state compared with wax 'flexebilitas cerea'. Facial mannerisms are common, *e.g.* pouting of the lips ('schnauz krampf'). Usually onset is acute and the illness quickly ended by ECT but in the past stuporous patients needed feeding and total nursing care. Catatonic defects are usually incoherent speech, neologisms, mannerisms and stereotyped behaviour.

Simple schizophrenia

Simple schizophrenia fits least well with the general run of schizophrenic symptomatology since diagnosis seems to be made by exclusion. Simple

I

schizophrenics say little or nothing, so this makes it difficult to find thought disorder or delusions, either or both of which tend to be surmised. The real malignant features of simple schizophrenia lie in the severe deterioration of behaviour and total disorganisation of the personality that occurs. The onset is always early and insidious. The main symptoms are emotional and behavioural. In both spheres there is a general falling off. Emotional responses are diminished, feeling becomes shallow—the patient is abrupt, rude and unconcerned by other people's feelings. This indifference moves to callousness, even unthinking cruelty to animals and people. It is not easy to be exact about this emotional change, it is a gradual loss of appropriate emotional response. The lack of feeling exasperates and bewilders family and friends alike but their reactions leave the patient untouched. Delusions and thought disorder are presumed but rarely proved since the patient's talk is always monosyllabic and evasive.

The clue to the underlying process lies in the patient's incongruous responses to his own diminished state, his lack of concern for himself or for the worry and distress that his behaviour has caused to other people. His detachment is totally crude and uncompromising. At the same time *changes in behaviour* occur; these include lowered energy, drive, volition and ambition, leading to a state of inert apathy and the picture of a human being who is empty, colourless and without insight. Gradually he becomes more asocial and drifts downwards as he is neither interested in anything, nor able to earn and support himself. So he can end up as a vagrant or a petty recidivist criminal, albeit an ineffectual one. Some simple schizophrenic girls end up as prostitutes or indulge in empty helpless promiscuity. Sexual drive is usually low though affectless sexuality can lead to pregnancy and venereal disease. Occasionally there are outbursts of ill directed impulsive activity. Some simple schizophrenics end up as rather boring eccentrics who tag themselves to cults, etc. whose activities they barely comprehend, but the bulk of simple schizophrenics end up as ineffectual unemployable people. Delinquency is trivial and repetitive: incompetent pilfering, indecent exposure or bestiality in the local farmyard are typical.

Often it is hard to decide whether the patient is a simple schizophrenic or has a personality disorder. Simple schizophrenia has a bad prognosis, and treatment is probably least successful for the true simple schizophrenic.

Schizophrenia—other and less certain clinical types

Other types of schizophrenia which are described include: *latent schizophrenia; residual schizophrenia; late onset schizophrenia; oneirophrenia; pseudoneurotic schizophrenia;* and *schizoaffective disorder.*

Latent schizophrenia This is a confusing term, familiar though to the puzzled clinician confronted with a patient who seems as it were on the brink of schizophrenia but not quite over the edge. This suggests that the term is unsatisfactory, most honest psychiatrists would agree with this. It is generally used, as might be suspected to describe *borderline* states, where frank signs of psychosis are absent but where the patient's general life style is aloof, detached, cool, remote and eccentric. In practice it *probably* means schizoid personality disorder.

Residual schizophrenia This is a term that sounds unsatisfactory yet is not. It is used to describe the impairment of personality left after a schizophrenic attack is over. The personality defect in such cases may be summarised in the words 'diminished' and or 'blunted'. The patient is less responsive to others, he seems less warm, less able to relate with others than formerly. His thinking is not grossly distorted as in schizophrenic thought disorder yet there remains an air of peculiarity and oddness about it. He is limited in his general responses and personal and social effectiveness as compared with his former state. Although the term is not so widely used as formerly there may be merit in further investigation of a clinical entity that has been neglected, since its presence or absence could well be a valuable testing ground for the effectiveness of current physical treatments, *i.e.* are residual schizophrenic states less common than formerly?

Late onset schizophrenia This is another important term since there has been disagreement about the age related aspects of schizophrenia. In general it has been said that schizophrenia rarely starts after age 40 yet numerous clinical reports suggest otherwise. Roth (1961) in particular has emphasised the fact that patients in the 50 to 70 age group develop psychoses, clinically indistinguishable from schizophrenia which may be regarded as late onset schizophrenia or late paraphrenia. The difficulty in classification has arisen from Kraepelin's use of the term paraphrenia which for practical purposes is best taken to mean late onset schizophrenia.

Oneirophrenia In the 1930s Mayer Gross (1930) described schizophrenic psychoses in which the patient was in a state of *clouded consciousness* and had panoramic dream-like hallucinosis usually vivid and highly coloured. At the time when Mayer Gross described them the clinical importance of these psychoses was that they were acute and recoverable, at a period when physical treatments were not available. Nowadays they are probably rarely diagnosed since anyone who is 'schizophrenic' is likely to receive physical treatment that shortens the illness. The importance of recognising these oneiroid (dream-like) states is that the prognosis is good since acute onset and anomalous clinical features such as clouding *are* good prognostic features.

Pseudoneurotic schizophrenia   Hoch and Polatin (1949) described a variety of schizophrenia characterised by 'pan-anxiety', *i.e.* pervasive anxiety symptoms, sexual problems and failure to respond to psychotherapy. The rationale of their hypothesis being that any neurosis which failed to respond to prolonged psychotherapy was not in fact a neurosis but an unrecognised type of schizophrenia. The mental state of such patients as described was typified by words such as amorphous and diffuse. The existence of pseudoneurotic schizophrenia is extremely doubtful, in fact many have suggested that a better name would be 'pseudoschizophrenic neurosis', since the condition fulfils none of the basic criteria for the diagnosis of schizophrenia. This position is shared by the author who finds the term positively misleading. It is included only for the sake of completeness.

Schizoaffective disorder   Another confusing term, yet one which has a certain clinical honesty about it since it implies diagnostic doubt, in itself not a bad thing since the diagnosis of schizophrenia once made can effectively ruin someone's life.

   The term is applied to psychoses in which there is a mixture of schizophrenic and affective features. In general the prognosis is better than in 'pure' schizophrenia, another example of the way in which 'atypical' features improve the prognosis in schizophrenia.

Late onset schizophrenia

This topic has been more extensively studied now that people are living longer. Bleuler (1943) was the first to describe a good sized series: 130 cases with onset of schizophrenia between ages 40 and 49, including less than five over 60. But nowadays late onset means onset between 40 and 65 and more authors have described these syndromes, excluding patients who began to be ill before age 50 (Lechler, 1950; Funding, 1961; Fish, 1960; Kay & Roth, 1961; Kay, 1963).

Post (1967) commented that some 10% of first admissions over the age of 60 have schizophrenic symptoms. The clinical picture is usually paranoid in type. Hallucinosis may be present but not always and extreme schizophrenic symptoms such as catatonia, speech disorganisation and affective flatness are rare in elderly patients.

Post described 100 patients examined over 10 years. The criteria for inclusion were the development of a paranoid syndrome not organic in type, which was persistent or which persisted after affective symptoms had been removed. 'Schizoaffective' syndromes were also excluded. Of the series, 24 were identified before phenothiazines had been discovered. Of the 69 patients treated with phenothiazines 61 did well and the general conclusion was that good results were clearly related to drug treatment.

Post concluded that these patients were not a clear cut group of schizophrenics but included three main groups: *'schizophrenia-like psychoses'* (37); *paranoid hallucinosis* (22); and *schizophrenia* (34). From this Post inferred that the three diagnostic categories might be a continuum.

In this way the three syndromes are viewed as manifestations of schizophrenia of varying strength. Genetic factors did not seem relevant. Perhaps the most relevant comment is that most of the patients were people with long histories of poor personal relationships. Also factors such as deafness, single or widowed state and social isolation seemed to be relevant. One group, those suffering from paranoid hallucinosis was very clearly seen to be made up of people with long-standing, often severe paranoid personality disorders.

Symptoms of schizophrenia

The early symptoms are sometimes as diffuse and as vague as the early experience of being schizophrenic. The writings of former schizophrenics such as Schrieber and S. Faudenmaier suggest that it must be a strange nightmarish experience where the bizarre becomes normal and the normal is bizarre. It must resemble a dream where one is full of inexplicable fear and apprehension: a state in which other people seem to be unexpectedly familiar with one's thoughts and actions, where smiles and nods assume a fearful significance and where chance remarks seem full of unintended meaning. We cannot accurately set out the subjective experience of being schizophrenic except to compare it to bad dreams and also the terrible uncertainty that must be provoked by reality previously taken for granted.

To the outside observer often the early symptoms of schizophrenia are marked by a diffuse change in feeling and perception which troubles the patient but leaves him unable to describe it and also a gradual drift away from commonly accepted reality into a personal and symbolic view of the world where the boundaries of the self become obscured and reality is less concrete. If we add to this difficulty in thinking clearly, a tendency to draw wrong conclusions from innocent events and an unsettled incongrous emotional state we have all the ingredients of continuing personality disorganisation.

The symptoms of schizophrenia may be considered as follows:

1 Delusions
2 Thought disorder
3 Perceptual disorder
4 Emotional disorder
5 Motor and behaviour disorder

Delusions

In schizophrenia delusions are important manifestations: they are inexplicable and come out of the blue and have no tangible relationship to previous experience nor the understandable quality of a delusional idea as in severe depression. The schizophrenic delusion is always a primary failure of judgement—an idea comes into the mind—it is alien and weird and not related to the patient's personal and cultural background and value system. The delusion is the most psychotic aspect of schizophrenia. Sometimes there is a disguised tangled symbolism in delusion but it is usually hard to see any real practical importance in this. Delusions in schizophrenia are internally consistent and serve a purpose by reinforcing the eccentric position of the schizophrenic so that he is able to explain everything that happens to him in terms of his delusions. Ideas of reference are common in schizophrenia, here the patient refers commonplace happenings to himself in a way that has a special meaning for him. Delusions may be fantastic, even grandiose, a patient may believe that he is Jesus Christ or that he has strange supernatural powers etc. At the same time delusional conviction is offset by muddled thinking and abnormal perceptions, the patient feels uncertain of what is going on around him so he is likely to misinterpret trivial happenings and believe them to be sinister. So it is hardly surprising that ideas and delusions of persecution are common, so common that persecutory content often dominates a schizophrenic illness to such an extent that the word paranoid has become condensed to mean 'persecutory'.

The mental content in schizophrenia is paranoid: and whether this is persecutory, grandiose or whatever, the point is that it is beyond reality, inexplicable and strange.

Schizophrenic delusions have variously been classified, *e.g.* as primary and secondary (Bleuler); the primary delusion comes out of the blue and is inexplicable, while the secondary delusion is explicable. Others have classified schizophrenic delusions on the basis of content, *e.g.* grandeur, diminished status, persecution, hypochondriacal, erotic and religious (Jaspers) but there seems little point in doing this.

Delusions of reference are particularly common in early schizophrenia and require special mention. Outside trivia are observed as having some special meaning which may be pleasant but is usually frightening, *e.g.* a patient said 'When I came out of my home the other day and walked to the station I noticed a funny thing. That there was a van outside the shop on the corner and the driver said "Where is —— street?" in a funny way and he wanted me to say something. After that in the station people were nodding and pointing to things in their papers about me. It was worse at work where everyone seemed to know about something and kept on smiling and made signs to me, and they wanted me to do sexual acts which I know and can prove.'

Jaspers stressed the importance of *delusional perception* and *delusional awareness*. These terms are confusing but are used and their meaning should be clarified. *Delusional perception* describes the schizophrenic experience of seeing everyday objects and perceiving that they have a different meaning, *i.e.* the perception is normal but the meaning is misinterpreted. *Delusional awareness* is used to describe feeling of imminent cosmic revelation, profound insight and brilliant understanding that is common in the onset of schizophrenia. The important thing always to bear in mind is that true delusions are inexplicable, alien experiences, where false judgements are made and where the whole environment takes on an entirely different meaning.

Thought and language disorder in schizophrenia

Bleuler was the first to emphasise the importance of disordered thinking in schizophrenia, his view, no doubt influenced by the Associationist School of Psychology, was that the abnormality was a *loosening of associations*. Mental processes were, according to this school, linked in a predictable series where like was linked to like so that the 'mind' was a card index of information stored in some incomprehensible way. This school of psychology flourished at a time when the brain was regarded not only as the organ of the mind but an organ in which each region had its special function, so that each area was autonomous rather like Germany itself before 1870. This followed the work of Gall and Spurzheim, the early 19th Century German anatomists who examined the brain and mapped it out scientifically and then went beyond available knowledge by claiming that there were parts of the brain that were responsible for virtue, truth, love, honesty etc., and created the bogus but always entertaining subject of phrenology. We may laugh at phrenology—a 'science' based on the belief that bumps on the skull reflected brain structure and function—but it is only just over a hundred years ago that new born Royal Princes of England had their heads examined by doctors who informed the public that the new Royal Prince had a 'good share of honesty and understanding'. So Bleuler was in tune with his time although before him Moreau de Tours had compared psychotic thinking to the vague drifting thoughts that people experience as they fall asleep.

In schizophrenia there is often a *basic disturbance* in the thought process, schizophrenic thinking is often highly abnormal beyond the limits of idiosyncrasy to the extent of being a process that cannot be shared or understood.

Not *all* schizophrenics have thought disorder, *i.e.* it is not a sufficient or necessary feature which could make it 'pathognomonic'. The nearest we can go is to say is that when schizophrenic thought disorder is present in someone who has no organic brain disease then the diagnosis of schizophrenia is nearly certain. On the other hand there *are* non-thought disordered schizophrenics.

What then *is* meant by schizophrenic thought disorder? There are ways of identifying it and defining it but its real meaning and significance eludes us.

From the *clinical* point of view thought disorder is recognised by the particular way in which the patient talks, expresses ideas and handles concepts. The starting point is that the thought disordered person does not use ordinary logical sequences, deductions and inferences, in severe cases cause and effect may be interchanged, these symptoms are not hard to spot because the person talks nonsense. But in less than severe cases it is different. Talk is hard to follow, it is vague and 'woolly' drifting into irrelevancy and straying from the point. The person draws half relevant conclusions from inferences that are nearly but not quite right. The links in language and thinking are unclear, ideas follow each other in a casual and drifting way while the patient is trying to explain some seemingly abstruse ideas that concern him.

Language often is enriched by symbolism that arrests by its quirkish, paradoxical and somehow half right nature. But the enrichment is spurious because one ends up liking the language but unable to understand a word of it. The meaning is lost in elliptical references, condensation of meaning, special language etc. often producing a vivid effect, this is important. Schizophrenic language is not to be shrugged aside because it seems nonsensical, this is wrong and bad psychiatry. Every patient deserves to be heard and listened to. But often schizophrenic communication has an almost random quality which leaves the interviewer fairly baffled! Many have looked for a specific disturbance common to all thought disordered thinking. This is an attractive line of enquiry but has turned out to be less helpful than expected. The following put forward various ideas.

1 *Von Domarus* noted that many schizophrenics would regard A and B as identical if they both had one identical property, *e.g.* 'Jim Smith is a blacksmith. I am a blacksmith. Therefore I am Jim Smith'.

2 *Goldstein* pointed out that schizophrenic thinking is concrete so that the patient can neither abstract from the concrete nor generalise from the particular. For this reason tests for thought disorder have been used which require the patient to find an abstract generality from a concrete statement, in practice this means asking to interpret the meaning of a proverb. To be of any use this assumes that the patient is of at least average intelligence and that the proverb used is familiar to him—it is no good producing an obscure Chinese proverb that he has never heard of! The patient should be asked whether he knows what a proverb is and the proverb should be read out clearly to him, he should be asked to repeat it and asked to explain it.

A typical schizophrenic interpretation is as follows—'People who live in glass houses shouldn't throw stones', 'Well, if they did they might break the windows.' This sort of test is limited since such a concrete interpretation is only given by a schizophrenic who has thought disorder that can usually be detected in ordinary conversation. Also concrete thinking is not specific to schizophrenia, it occurs in organic cerebral disease.

3 *Cameron* (1942) commented on overinclusion as a specific thought abnormality in schizophrenia. Overinclusive thinking is a type of thinking in which irrelevant and casual topics become absorbed in to one concept-meaning and logical distinction is obscured and fuzzy.

4 *Bannister* (1968), the English psychologist, has to date provided the most illuminating observations on thought disorder. Bannister has been influenced by personal construct theory as described by Kelly (1955). This is a psychological theory in which *events* are accorded less importance than the ways in which they are *construed*. Bannister (1968) exemplifies this neatly as follows 'Thus if we contemplate a young lady crossing a bridge (lay construing), then we may equally construe her as a 'series of moments of force about a point' (engineer's construing), 'poor credit risk' (banker's construing), or as 'a mass of whirling electrons about nuclei (physicists construing), as a 'soul in peril of mortal sin' (theological construing), or as a 'likely dish' (young man's construing). Bannister's point is that constructions of what goes on have explanatory and predictive value irrespective of who is doing the construing.

As applied to schizophrenic thinking Bannister's work (1968) is particularly of interest since he has shown that the differences between thought disordered and non-thought disordered people lie in their conceptual view of the world.

At the end of it all the clinician has to shift as best he can in the knowledge that many schizophrenics think in an odd idiosyncratic way, using their own rules of logic and influenced by irrelevant and random associations.

The subjective experience of thinking   As described by schizophrenics this is usually that they find it hard to think clearly. Many describe how they cannot concentrate, cannot control their thoughts, find it hard to work out problems or understand things. Unable to think clearly the patient is forced to look for ways of explaining what is happening to him. This *may* account for severe thinking disturbances described by many schizophrenics where they say that their thoughts are not their own, that thoughts are inserted into or withdrawn from their heads or that their thoughts are being broadcast aloud (Gedankenlauten werden).

These subjective experiences of thought disturbance are probably peculiar to schizophrenics—thought withdrawal and broadcasting are amongst Schneider's symptoms of first rank importance. We may regard them as verbal expressions of the schizophrenic's attempts to make sense of what seems to be going on around him. Though these thinking disturbances are important schizophrenic symptoms. The term *schizophrenic thought disorder* is properly restricted to the *special disturbance of conceptual thinking found in many schizophrenics*. Other abnormalities experienced by schizophrenics include *thought block* where the mind goes blank. This is not peculiar to schizophrenia but occurs also in *anxiety* and *depression* and in normal people *under stress, e.g.* interviews and examinations. Another experience is *pressure of thought* where thoughts seem to crowd through the head with bewildering intensity. Often the schizophrenic's muddled thinking leads him to search for meaning in mysticism and metaphysics and obscure philosophy which he can link with his own difficulties in handling concepts and seemingly find solutions—inevitably illusory.

Schizophrenic language This is often strange. Where thought disorder is severe, talk becomes incoherent and incomprehensible, in these cases the term 'word salad' is used—a psychiatric reminder of Boyd's comments on terms such as 'hardbake spleen' and 'bread and butter pericardium' where he remarked 'this has been so likened by those who see in every pathological condition a resemblance to an article of diet'. Anyone interested in linguistics will be fascinated by schizophrenic use of slang, jargon, alliteration, metonymy and condensation and also by the way in which words are emphasised sometimes with inappropriate gesture and facial expression, and by the way in which ordinary words and neologisms assume special significance and symbolism. Chronic schizophrenic language is often stilted and peculiar, neologisms are common, as in verbigeration, *i.e.* repeating the same phase again and again, and the use of meaningless and limited phraseology, stereotyped speech.

The diagnosis of thought disorder The diagnosis rests very much on clinical experience. In severe cases it is easy to spot—fragmented speech, thought withdrawal and incomprehensible relationships between ideas are not hard to recognise, but in less severe and early cases it can be difficult. There are no simple diagnostic rules; the things to look for are vagueness and lack of clarity, difficulty in concentration, talk that is hard to follow, uncertain in direction and baffling in outcome. These things are inter-woven with peculiar and symbolic irrelevancies. Often schizophrenic talk may seem normal if the patient chooses to make brusque and perfunctory answers. This situation puzzles the student, undergraduate and post-graduate alike. There seems to be little wrong with the patient who gives terse, even vaguely humorous answers in a laconic, non-committal way—he seems to be 'holding his cards close to his chest', He may answer questions with knowing smiles, nods and non-specific remarks such as 'it could be', 'well, possibly', 'that is conceivable' etc. This means that inter-view should always be long and careful where thought disorder is sus-pected.

Motor and behavioural symptoms

Schizophrenic motor and behavioural symptoms range from violent excitement (catatonic excitement) to stupor. There is no disagreement about these symptoms as being part of the psychotic process. On the other hand, it is hard to know how much importance to attach to some of the 'classical' motor disturbances of schizophrenia, *e.g. automatic obedience,* where a patient repeats movements suggested to him by the examiner or *echo reactions* where the patient repeats the examiner's words (echolalia) or actions (echopraxia). These odd behaviours, usually said to be schizo-phrenic symptoms, may in fact be features imposed by prolonged stay in an institution. Long term inmates of any sort lose initiative and drive, and may behave in a dull mechanical repetitive way.

The most common change in behaviour in schizophrenia is a general falling away in activity, loss of energy, initiative, drive and interest. This is often something that leads to the family seeking help—'He just sits around doing nothing; not interested in anything; will not go out; says nothing; just looks into space.' Other schizophrenic change in behaviour may be a change of interest from work towards some obscure eccentric hobby or pastime. The most disabling inactivity is catatonic stupor where the patient is inaccessible to speech or human contact though in a state of clear consciousness. The stuporous patient does not reply to questions and lies absolutely still neither asking for nor accepting food nor drink. Regressive symptoms such as incontinence occur and in prephysical treat-ment days such patients needed total nursing care and feeding. After recovery stuporous patients report everything that has gone on around them, they describe how they felt unable to move or respond but cannot say why. This is true of schizophrenic inactivity in general: just because a schizophrenic is inert and slow this does not mean that he is unaware. Other motor abnormalities noted include awkward, stilted movements and the inappropriate use of gesture, odd grimacing and smiling. Schizophrenics are often said to be 'negativistic', *i.e.* inexplicably uncooperative. This uncooperative resistance to do what is asked is striking, but is unrelated either to resentment or depression and may be really an expression of schizophrenic indecision and inability to pick out the relevant from the irrelevant.

Habitual expressive movements or *mannerisms* are part of normal communication, in schizophrenia pathological mannerisms may be quite striking: the patient makes faces, uses gestures in a stilted and incongruous way. In chronic schizophrenia mannerisms often degenerate into *stereotyped* movements which are always repetitive and without meaning, though originally linked to a mannerism that holds symbolic meaning. Words, phrases, gestures, walking around, elaborate movements of the arms etc. all become incorporated into stereotypy. Other disturbances include *echo reactions* as previously described. Echo reactions and automatic obedience are rarely seen nowadays and were probably institutional artefacts, symbols of anergia and neglect. Eliciting echo reactions and automatic obedience carry an air of clinical pantomime and solemn absurdity, they are deplorable quasi assaults on the integrity of the unprotected, disadvantaged sick.

Perceptual disorder in schizophrenia

Ordinarily people take reality for granted since on the whole their perception of the environment remains relatively unchanged; the surroundings are recognisable and 'feel' real. Although new surroundings often seem strange they are explored with interest. Sounds and sights have an intensity that is predictable like most bodily sensations. In every day experience the quality of perception is hardly altered much except in fatigue and intoxication with alcohol or drugs. But in schizophrenia severe changes in perception are common, it is likely that schizophrenics are overloaded with sensory information. The normal flow of sense data is too much for the schizophrenic and this leads to misperceptions and misinterpretations of sensory data. It may be that the schizophrenic is unable to identify what it is relevant and important from the mass of information that normally is sorted out by the central nervous system.

Whatever the mechanisms may be the clinical fact is that *perceptual disorder is common in schizophrenia*. Some regard such perceptual disorder as a primary disorder, others as secondary and uncertain. The former idea is true of classical 19th Century German psychiatry and mainstream contemporary psychiatry. The commonest perceptual disorders are *hallucinations* usually auditory. These include sounds, clicks, whistles, whisperings and voices which may be loud or soft, single or multiple. Hallucinatory voices (phonemes) may mock, insult, instruct, comment on the patient or repeat his thoughts aloud. The range of hallucinatory content is wide and should always be carefully asked about. True visual *hallucinations* do not occur, visual images described by schizophrenics turn out to be *misperceptions of reality* or *delusional perceptions* where objects are seen in altered strange ways.

Though *auditory hallucinations* are rightly stressed as the most important perceptual disorder in schizophrenia the range of disturbance is much wider especially in the early stages. For instance the patient may say that his awareness of reality is heightened or lowered or that the experience of reality is changed in an ineffable way. Objects around him seem altered, strange or familiar in a way that is akin to the *déjà vu* phenomenon. In short there is a wide range of perceptual change.

Emotional symptoms

Emotional incongruity is the classical *emotional* disturbance in schizophrenia, referred to by Bleuler who thought it very important. He regarded emotional ambivalence as a typical example of the fragmented responses and disintegration that are the essence of schizophrenia. In its most severe form *emotional incongruity* is shown by complete dissociation of emotional responses from events, bad news provokes little or no reaction or in severe cases a totally inappropriate one. In chronic schizophrenia loss of feeling is so striking that it is often referred to as *flattening or blunting of affect*. In this state the person has no emotional display or feeling.

In early schizophrenia on the other hand, emotional changes are often less specific, and may mask the diagnosis. There are no special clinical symptoms here but it is important to know that early schizophrenics often develop severe anxiety—states of fear and apprehension with little associated content. This can lead to panic where the patient rushes blindly around attacking fancied enemies. In other cases a depressive state precedes acute schizophrenic symptoms. However many schizophrenics have premorbid personalities in which emotional responses were limited. They were cool, detached, remote people who remained unmoved by outside events, and were brusque, rude and bitter. A cool detached emotional tone as part of the personality structure is often an important premorbid feature but this applies at most to 50% of schizophrenics, the rest are people with apparently normal personalities. In early schizophrenia patients often complain of loss of feeling, or of the feeling of having lost feeling (Jaspers). They notice their diminished response to outside stimuli, they feel detached from others and feel separated from them as if by a 'pane of glass'. This change is noticed by others who find it hard, even impossible to relate or empathise with them. Personal contact and relationships deteriorate, the patient loses contact with friends and family who find his increasingly dreamy, remote detachment progressively harder to bear.

SCHIZOPHRENIA: DIAGNOSIS AND DIFFERENTIAL DIAGNOSIS

Diagnosis

Throughout standard texts there is general agreement on the difficulties of precise diagnosis since objective criteria are few and agreements on definitions are tenuous (Mayer Gross *et al*, 1969; Freedman & Kaplan, 1969; Noyes & Kolb, 1969). Nevertheless psychiatrists are in general agreed on the existence of schizophrenic patients and their needs for management. Proper management starts off with rational diagnosis, always providing that diagnosis is recognised as a presumptive statement rather than as a label which, once attached to a person, can never be removed.

The diagnosis then is not made on the recognition of one or two symptoms such as delusions and hallucinations but is properly made having given proper consideration to factors in the history and mental state which may be summarised thus:

1   History:
    Age of onset of symptoms
    Mode of onset of symptoms
    Family history of schizophrenia
    Personality change
    'Endogenous' quality to symptoms, *i.e.* unrelated in form or content to previous life experience

Absence of temporal lobe epilepsy, amphetamine or hallucinogen abuse

2 Mental state:
   Thought disorder (highly specific)
   Primary delusions (highly specific)
   Feelings of bodily influence (highly specific)
   Motor disorders (highly specific)
   Emotional incongruity (less specific)
   Hallucinosis (less specific)

Some authors have emphasised the usefulness of the 'praecox feeling' in diagnosis, *i.e.* an intuitive suspicion based on the patient seeming to be odd and eccentric. This is a hard sign to justify, though clinical experience encourages *wariness* about patients whose coolness and detachment precludes empathy. In practice it can be said that while diagnosis may be relatively easy in florid cases and in cases that conform to a clinical type such as *catatonia* or *hebephrenia* the main diagnostic problems are presented by *young patients with a first illness* and indefinite symptoms. Here it is wise not to rush to the diagnosis of schizophrenia, better to take time fully to evaluate the patient and this may take weeks or more.

Differential diagnosis

The differential diagnosis includes:

1 All causes of personality change, *e.g. organic mental states* of whatever type, acute psychoses triggered off by LSD or amphetamines, and TLE. Organic cases will be excluded by proper recognition of clouded consciousness and the fact that delusional content is much less formulated than in schizophrenia. Drug induced psychoses will be excluded by careful history taking and recognition of other signs of drug misuse. TLE will be recognised by the presence of episodic disturbance backed up by EEG studies.

2 *Affective disorders* lead to diagnostic problems mainly in the case of states of acute excitement. At first it may be impossible to make an accurate diagnosis because of the extent of the patient's disturbed mental state. However, the *hypomanic* and *manic* patient will usually show *flight of ideas, punning* and *elation*; all of which have more *congruity* than schizophrenia which tends to be far more disorganised. The depressed *patient who is paranoid* may appear schizophrenic; but again the paranoid or

delusional content is an outgrowth of the depressed mood and is to that extent understandable. *Mental subnormality* may enter the differential diagnosis of simple schizophrenia, especially if the patient has always been someone with limited attainments. *Hysterical disorders* should also be considered; here the patient is likely to be histrionic and gives a strong suspicion of 'acting mad'. Also the presence of obvious precipitant happenings gives a good lead.

Management, outcome and prognosis in schizophrenia

The general consensus now is that 40% or more of patients diagnosed as schizophrenic return home free from symptoms in under 3 months. Of the remaining 60% about one-third will remit sufficiently well to live in the community and the remainder will be split into two groups: one remaining chronic but non-progressive, the other tending to get progressively worse and in need of prolonged hospital care.

Outcome studies in schizophrenia have not as yet *clearly* demonstrated that *physical treatment* with *phenothiazines* has altered the natural history of the disorder but they have shown that these medications improve symptoms effectively, ensure a quick return to the community and a better chance of a more independent existence (Hirsch *et al*, 1973). In other words they give a preferable quality of life as opposed to prolonged hospital stay and institutionalism. And for this reason *early treatment* with phenothiazines is the method of choice. Other physical treatments such as ECT are much less useful, in fact it is doubtful if ECT does more than calm the agitated schizophrenic and get the catatonic out of stupor. When used in this way it should be given on an 'ad hoc' basis. *Neuroleptics* then are the mainstay of management with the special advantages of once monthly injections of *fluphenazine decanoate* for patients who refuse or neglect medication. Otherwise the choice lies between aliphatic phenothiazines for the more agitated patients and piperazine types for the inert schizophrenics.

It is always difficult to give an accurate prognosis in schizophrenia but there are some important prognostic indices. Favourable points include:

1   *Acute onset*—illnesses that come on quickly tend to subside quickly
2   *Onset following psychological or physical precipitants, e.g.* following surgery, or in the puerperium

3 A stable premorbid personality and a stable social background
4 Affective or atypical clinical features
5 Superior intelligence

Bad prognostic indices include:

1 Insidious onset
2 Severe thought disorder and affective flattening
3 An asthenic body build
4 Subnormal intelligence

Despite the more intensive care that is now available for schizophrenic patients, the relapse rate remains high and its occurrence unpredictable though changes in the social environment are significantly associated with the return of florid symptoms (Brown & Birley, 1968; Birley & Brown, 1970). These observations have led to closer examination of hypotheses such as those of Wynne (1968) in which close but distorted family relationships and communications were held to be significant aetiological factors in schizophrenia. Hirsch and Leff (1971), for instance were unable to replicate Wynne and Singer's findings. The difference is no doubt accounted for by the real diagnostic differences that exist in the UK and USA as examined in detail by Kendell *et al* (1972).

Brown *et al* (1972) examined the possible influences of family life on the natural history of schizophrenia and found that relapse was not so much related to sophisticated factors in intrafamilial relationships but much more to failure to take medication, insufficient support for relatives and the level of change in the patient's environment. These, perhaps more simple findings suggest that the schizophrenic patient is highly vulnerable to change and minor emotional involvements and challenges, something that many clinicians may have suspected without being able to prove.

Community care of the schizophrenic patient

It has long been recognised that chronic schizophrenic patients can easily learn bad habits, at its worst this is seen in mental hospitals in backward countries where schizophrenics are allowed to stand naked, smearing themselves with faeces in cheerless rooms. This sort of behaviour in schizophrenics has nothing to do with illness and everything to do with neglect. The best types of institutional care were able to help many schizophrenics to live a reasonably independent existence but the whole process has been made much easier by the use of neuroleptic drugs and by a therapeutic atmosphere of sensible and liberal encouragement. When psychiatrists found that neuroleptic drugs restored patients to a better contact with reality they started discharging them from hospital and the average duration of hospital stay for schizophrenics in English mental hospitals fell from 2 years to 6 to 8 weeks. However, merely sending the patient home is not good enough. And it is from this that the idea of *community care* began. Now in fact there is really nothing very spectacular about the idea of community care for the mentally ill despite the reverential tones in which the concept has been discussed. But although the idea is pretty simple it seems that it is hard to put into practice; there are reasons for this and they will be reviewed.

The first reason is *historical*. For many years 'mental illness' was an idea that doctors acknowledged in a vague sort of way but everyone knew that such people would never get better anyway and the best thing to do was to see that they were looked after in institutions. Doctors who 'took up' psychiatry in the 1920s and 1930s were often discouraged by the hopelessness of the chronic schizophrenic and retreated from trying to treat psychotic patients into psychotherapy for neurotic patients which seemed more promising. Suddenly psychiatrists found that a drug, chlorpromazine, made it easier to relate with and rehabilitate schizophrenics.

Mental hospital psychiatrists at this stage were the poor relations of the medical profession—they had been left to look after the chronic psychotic patients for years and now found that they could improve their patients' mental states but at the same time they frequently had no facilities available even to follow up their patients. Psychiatry was given low priority in health care expenditure, as it still is, but despite this many hospitals began to develop follow up clinics and cooperation with doctors and social workers in local authority health services. And from this there arose the idea of planned community care where the hospital services, general practitioner and local authority services pooled their resources in terms of nursing and social work to look after psychotic patients, ensure that they took their medication, looked out for signs of relapse, helped them to find employment, in short by sensible collaboration tried to provide a rational programme of comprehensive psychiatric treatment and follow up. This is the *ideal* of community care; its realisation in practice is another matter and depends on available resources in terms of skills, money, manpower and goodwill. It is a fact that in terms of absolute priorities psychiatric community care still occupies a fairly low place in the wants of society and it is really no good pretending otherwise. This is regrettable since many areas have shown that effective community services can in fact be provided relatively easily and without the sort of expenditure that theory tends to discourage. At its best *community care* is the best way to plan psychiatric services; at its worst it becomes organised neglect.

I I

Normal and abnormal personalities, and psychopathy

PERSONALITY DEVELOPMENT

Most theories emphasise the importance of intrapsychic factors in the process of personality development and especially stress internal conflict set up by relationships with parents. This is reasonable, after all, the majority of people are first exposed to adults who are their parents and whether they imitate them or not they are imprinted with behaviour such that it would be surprising if they did not develop a mixture of feelings about them and end up with conflict about it all. So we are not surprised to believe that this key relationship influences the maturation and development of the personality. There is no clear understanding as yet as to whether genetic or family influences are dominant in moulding the personality. The consensus view favours an interaction of the two.

Defining the personality has never been easy. *Personality* is the sum of many different varying characteristics, intellectual, affective and physical, to name only a few, which gives to each person both an individuality and a resemblance to his fellows. These characteristics are present to some degree in everyone so that to speak of normal and abnormal personality is not to postulate end points separating the two categories, but rather to define an individual's personality as lying somewhere along a curve of normal distribution. In this way the abnormals are those who deviate markedly from the average and the normals are the bulk of the population. This method of considering personality has the great advantage of being experimentally valuable. Investigators can then go further and attempt to establish the psychological correlates of given personality characteristics. Much valuable work of this sort has already been carried out. The psychiatric approach to the study of abnormal personalities has in the main been a clinical one and has not been made easy to follow by the use of the term *psychopath*. In general, psychiatrists have tended to call psychopaths those patients with abnormal personalities but this is not universally so. The two concepts of psychopathy and personality disorder were most succinctly united by Schneider who defined psychopaths as *those abnormal personalities who suffer from their abnormality or cause society to suffer*. This definition is the one used in this book. It has one very important advantage, namely that it recognises that someone can have an abnormal personality without being regarded in some way as ill or antisocial, *i.e.* distinguishes between 'pathological' and 'non-pathological' abnormal personalities. This is important because the term psychopath has come to be regarded, in Anglo-American circles anyway, almost as a term of abuse.

There are a number of general environmental factors which influence personality development. Emotional security in childhood is founded first of all on the basic physiological needs of the infant and the ways in which they are met by the mother. This produces a straightforward dependence on the mother which is shown by distress when the infant is separated from mother for any prolonged period. We take for granted the helplessness of the infant, also its extreme vulnerability. It is thought that therefore the infant is at his most vulnerable at critical learning periods in early years, *e.g.* weaning and toilet training. These critical learning experiences can be made occasions of anxiety and insecurity for the infant if teaching is hard and rigid. So it is postulated that an infant can pick up rejection from cold and disciplinary parents who make the acquisition of dry pants a skill that rewards the successful baby with approval and the unsuccessful with outbursts of irrational impatience and anger.

Love is remarkably nourishing and a good fertiliser for emotional growth. Unmothered children, particularly those that are raised in the sort of orphanages and institutions that salved the consciences of the Victorian bourgeoisie, were exposed to discipline, homilies and exhortation, no fun and continual reminders of how fortunate they were to be where they were, admittedly materially better than starving in the gutters of London or Birmingham. Good descriptions of this type of early experience are found in the novels of Dickens, and in autobiographies such as those of Sir Charles Chaplin. But orphanages and children's homes are different now though contemporary accounts of institutional upbringing in England as recently as the 1930s plus the occasional scandals that have come from developed countries such as Italy, France and USA, still remind us of how people can persecute the defenceless.

Many studies have suggested that institutionally raised children may show emotional and other handicaps despite first class material care. A child's need for love is great, and the loss of love is a terrible blow to a child, perhaps the threat of the loss of love is as bad. So much for the credit balance of love—What about the debit? It is thought that parental love, if excessive and suffocating can be malign in its influence for example where the child is denied independence and kept in an infantile role. Staying a baby like this can persist to adult life, the adult whose selfishness, egocentricity and importunate irritability are a byword to his colleagues, may well have started out in life as an overprotected baby. Too much protection of a child is self-defeating. Growing up involves learning to find a separate existence, to take and accept risks and to make decisions for oneself. The parental emotional climate in childhood needs also to be consistent as well as loving. The child needs parents who communicate with him in a clear way and not in a series of contradictory flimsy signals. And the parents should be people worth identifying with.

It may be that cultural influences in personality development are overlooked. The needs and expectations of society find formal expression in laws, but the laws that influence human behaviour at a personal level are perhaps also more closely related to society and its needs and expectations than many would care to admit.

For a start people who develop in the same sociocultural setting are exposed to very similar social forces and very soon learn the varieties of behaviour expected and encouraged, those that win approval and those that don't. This process starts early—in primary school and throughout the educational process, whether the requirements are those of Eton or the local secondary modern school. Added to this, particularly in England a social class system still operates more forcefully than is realised; class oriented roles and prejudices are soon learned. So that in many ways when a normal personality is referred to it has to be acknowledged that 'normal' is time and culture bound. Normal behaviour of, say, the Barons in Feudal England would now be classed as deviant.

Recent history in Nazi Germany provides a clear example of how brutal sadism became normal. Normality is mainly defined by the culture in which a person is born and grows up. The requirements and attitudes, value systems and customs of a culture quite naturally influence a person's public behaviour, and to a measurable degree, his attitudes, feelings and view of the world. There are great differences between cultures and for that matter in the same culture at differing periods in time. To survive as an American Indian in the 19th Century normality meant being treacherous, a thief and murderer. A person who did not share this value system was not only regarded as a dangerous eccentric but his chances of physical survival were low. In fact each culture lays down fairly clear guide lines as to how people should behave, to control sexual and violent impulses and how to survive, in a highly specific way which starts at birth and follows each person to the end of his life.

For instance the basic crafts of child rearing are culture bound and expressed in highly specific forms. Parents learn how to relate to their young, how to feed them and all this comes from the culture nowadays in increasingly prolific ways, a flood of books, newspaper articles, television programmes and commercials etc., which tell the parent what to do. Often this advice changes quickly. The process of socialisation is lengthy and starts at around the age of six. From this age the child starts to move out of his immediate family and into the influences provided by older children, schoolteachers and so on. This means that he has new people to identify with and he is now beginning already to realise that his parents are not as omnipotent and omniscient as he had believed. This finds expression in adolescent rebellion and uncertainty.

AETIOLOGY OF DEVIANT SOCIAL BEHAVIOUR AND DELINQUENCY

The relationships of disturbed behaviour in childhood, juvenile delinquency and psychopathic disorder are important topics to clarify for a number of reasons. The first is that it might be possible to detect early disturbances that have a predictive value and the second is that finding characteristic early disturbances may illuminate the whole question of aetiology. No one would pretend that either of these questions have to date been answered but on the other hand there *are* long term prospective researches that help to clarify the picture as opposed to 'cross sectional' studies that are speculative in their interpretation.

Robins (1966) carried out a 30 year follow-up of 524 child guidance patients and 100 controls and was able to define the early clinical features and natural history of psychopathy based on the appearance of significant symptoms and behaviour in childhood. Psychopathy (sociopathic disorder) was diagnosed in adult life in 94 of the patients and was found to correlate highly with the onset of disturbed behaviour between ages 12 and 15. The predictive antisocial symptoms included truancy, lack of guilt, pathological lying, running away from home overnight, bad associates, impulsiveness, physical aggression and a poor work record and theft. Environmental factors were not clearly defined beyond being male and being exposed to inconsistent parental influence or having no parents at all.

This American study has been followed more recently by an English study (West & Farrington, 1973) of 400 London schoolboys from age 8 to 18. The following is a brief direct quote (Scott, 1974).

'Official convictions (based on police records and numbers of convictions) match well with self-reported delinquency and also with assessments made by teachers and by classmates; when a delinquency scale based solely on the boy's self-reports was substituted for the scale based on official records, the findings concerning the characteristics and backgrounds of delinquents remained substantially unchanged. A combined delinquency scale, based on both official reports and self-reports, demontrated two groups each including about a fifth of the sample the unusually good and the unusually bad boys, with the majority in the intermediate categories.'

'An unduly large proportion of the self-reported delinquent without juvenile convictions were subsequently convicted as adults. There is a tendency, among boys who indulge in similar delinquent behaviour, for those who have adverse background characteristics of a kind noticeable to authorities to acquire an official record, so that samples of official delinquents probably have an over-representation of unfavourable backgrounds.'

'Perhaps the most important result to emerge from this study was the undramatic and unfashionable conclusion that traditional criminological beliefs about the backgrounds and characteristics of delinquents are true.'

There were five background factors of particular significance: low family income, large family size, parental criminality, low intelligence, and poor parental behaviour. Each of these five factors, all of which were susceptible to reasonably clear definition and to careful measurement, remained significantly associated with delinquency after matching in turn for each of the others.

Background factors (even using any three of the five mentioned) are highly predictive of delinquency, yet the ratings of troublesome behaviour made by teachers and classsmates were in themselves as predictive of official delinquency as any combination of background assessments, and could be made at a very early age.

Sheldon's linking of mesomorphy with delinquency is not confirmed. Low performance on psychomotor tests of clumsiness (hitherto regarded as one of the most reliable correlates of delinquency) is linked with low intelligence rather than delinquency.

Eysenck's theory that neuroticism and extraversion correlate with delinquency is not confirmed, nor is minimal brain damage at birth an important factor.

Particular secondary schools do not foster delinquency (but perhaps the range of schools was not so wide as in the East of London where Powers reached a different conclusion). Shyness, timidity, and neurotic symptoms are possibly alternative forms of response to family stress.

'Altogether, the findings . . . strongly support the concept of a typical delinquent, in the sense that most delinquents display a behavioural syndrome which encompasses far more in the way of deviant conduct than the limited range of illegal acts for which they are apt to be convicted.'

PSYCHOPATHY AND ABNORMAL PERSONALITY

People who behave in an odd or eccentric way, or in a persistently anti-social way but who are neither psychotic nor mentally retarded tend to puzzle society, on the one hand they are not *ill* but on the other they are abnormal and this is something that may cause them distress, whilst if they are antisocial then society will suffer. Such people are usually des-cribed as having psychopathic personalities, a term which many find confusing, but which can perhaps be better understood with a clearer idea of the development of the concept of psychopathic personality. The first description of patients who behave in a persistently antisocial way, without regard for the consequences is usually ascribed to Prichard (1835) who coined the term 'moral insanity' which in fact covered mental illness though later he modified the term to denote people who 'display no lesion of understanding . . . and whose disease consists of a perverted state of the feelings, temper, inclinations and conduct'. Earlier Benjamin Rush (1812) had described 'persons of sound understanding and some of uncommon talents who are affected with this lying disease in the will', and stressed their innate lack of conscience and sense of responsibility.

The German descriptive psychiatrists of the 19th Century took up this problem with expected thoroughness and Koch (1889) suggested the term 'psychopathic inferiority' to denote a collection of constitutional disorders including the neuroses. Kraepelin (1909) listed seven types of psychopathic personalities, the unstable, the excitable, the swindler, the liar, the antisocial and the quarrelsome, and the eccentric, while Kahn (1931) listed 15 types. However Schneider (1934) restored order to the scene by suggesting that psychopathic personality should be defined as 'all those abnormal personalities who suffer from their abnormality or cause society to suffer'. In addition to this he proposed a theory of personality disorder based on deviation from the average, since many of our difficulties in the use of the word abnormal in psychiatry have arisen because normality is taken to mean an ideal of perfection rather than its more appropriate use in a statistical sense, *i.e.* the 'normal' personality approximates to *average* behaviour, and is to a large extent determined by the standards and expectations of the society concerned. Hence 'abnormal' in psychiatry should be used to designate deviations from accepted norms and not as a value judgement. Sometime in the 19th Century and early 20th Century confusion about the use of the term psychopathic personality seems to have begun, probably because the word was used in a different way in Europe to its use in the UK, and in the USA. Amongst English speaking psychiatrists it is quite definitely used to categorise abnormal personalities but particularly those who are repeatedly delinquent or less than competent socially.

Henderson (1939) suggested their classification into the *predominantly aggressive*, the *predominantly inadequate* and the *creative psychopath*. Curran and Mallinson (1944) suggested *vulnerable personalities*; *unusual* or *eccentric personalities*; and *sociopath* (*asocial or antisocial*) as three basic categories. These lists could be extended but the point will by now be taken, namely that it is one thing to define abnormal personality, it is another to provide a typology. In practice psychiatrists tend to use Schneider's definition and use the word psychopath to mean 'sociopath' and also refer to inadequate and explosive psychopaths and more or less leave it at that. It should be remembered too that it is possible to be excessively pedantic about the use of words. The meanings of words are, like it or not, influenced considerably by common usage.

The important clinical aspect of personality disorder is that it is not like psychiatric illness but rather a persistent, early onset handicap in the field of behaviour and life experience, something that always emerges in history taking where a seemingly acute problem turns out to be another landmark in a life of persistent problems since youth.

In England psychopathic disorders are defined in the Mental Health Act 1959 as 'a persistent disorder or disability of mind (whether or not including subnormality of intelligence) which results in abnormality or seriously irresponsible conduct on the part of the patient, and requires or is susceptible to medical treatment'. This is a definition which effectively restricts the use of compulsion in treatment of the antisocial psychopath. Scott (1962) has criticised the concept of psychopathy and points out that many of the seemingly definitive features (egocentricity, opportunism, affective coldness) do not differentiate from the normal and that in fact the term is most useful in describing recidivist criminals, repeatedly antisocial offenders, *i.e.* using it in a forensic rather than a purely psychiatric sense.

For the purposes of this work psychopathic personality is used to denote a special type of abnormal personality characterised by repeatedly antisocial behaviour.

Aetiology of psychopathic personality

The search for aetiology has covered genetics, brain damage, early childhood and family background, and theories of learning.

Genetic factors

Genetic factors are difficult to demonstrate as a significant influence in schizophrenia, less difficult in affective disorder, but in psychopathic personality the problems are immense since, as we have seen, the definition of psychopathy is very far from clear. For this reason genetic studies in psychopathy have concentrated on twins and the incidence of criminality in uniovular twins separated at birth and reared away from each other. However such studies are few. Lange (1931) examined 13 criminals with a living uniovular twin. Ten of the discovered twins turned out to be criminal but Lange was cautious in interpreting the findings.

Rosanoff (1934/1941) reported on 340 sets of twins but found equivocal incidence of criminality whether the twins were uni or biovular. Slater (1948) examined 300 sets of twins but concluded that although genetic influences were relevant in personality development nevertheless *symptoms* and maladaptation were more definitely related to environmental influences. Gibbens (1956) has commented on the high incidence of mesomorphism in Borstal lads suggesting a 'delinquency' factor. However Borstal lads show a social class skew so that it becomes very difficult even to assess the body build in Borstal lads beyond noting the incidence of a particular type; assigning to it a special significance is not easy.

Brain damage

A number of authors have noted neurological abnormalities, a history of meningitis or encephalitis and non-specific EEG abnormalities in adult criminal psychopaths and juvenile delinquents. Row (1931) found a 72% incidence of diffuse neurological defect, Thompson (1945) showed a 60% similar incidence in 500 juvenile delinquents. However, follow-up studies on postencephalitic children have been unrewarding in terms of later criminality (Puntigam, 1950; Essen-Moller, 1956) despite early confidence in epidemic encephalitis as a strong influence in producing adult criminality. Epilepsy has long been regarded as a factor in antisocial personality, yet the evidence remains conflicting (Ferguson, 1952; Brandon, 1960; MacFarlane *et al*, 1954; Harrington & Letemendia, 1958; Bridge, 1949; Grunberg & Pond, 1957). It appears that there is as much evidence linking the fact of being regarded as handicapped, *i.e.* abnormal with later criminality, as there is with epilepsy. The current tendency in assessing persistent criminality is to try and encompass the possible influences of fits, brain damage and early experience within a larger context, *i.e.* to imply a multidimensional aetiology.

Early childhood experience and family background

There have been a number of reports on the bad effects of separation from parents at an early age (Gesell, 1941; Davis, 1940; 1947, Willis, 1959; Lowry, 1940; Goldfarb, 1945) however all of these early reports were about 'wild' children reared in sheds, very deprived children. In short, they were generally extremely biased samples from which no really useful conclusion may be drawn beyond the somewhat naive one that if you treat a baby like a wild animal you must not be surprised if he fails to become a member of the stock exchange.

Separation from the mother was set on the map as a bad influence by

Bowlby (1951) who suspected that early separation from the mother would lead to the child becoming withdrawn and asocial, and that this would carry over in to adult life in an irreversible fashion. And he was quite uncompromising over this. However, other workers were not quite so confident of the special influence of the mother, and perhaps slightly more confident in the sustaining influence of a consistent parental type of influence in childhood where one or both parents were lost. Lewis (1954) found that separation from parents in 500 children was not significantly associated with delinquency or with the child's ability to be an affectionate person. Similar findings were reported by Rowntree (1960) and Pringle (1961). Bowlby's assertions remain unproven. Of course no one *wants* children to lose their parents but the end results are better than has been suggested. Family influences are hard to evaluate though many suspect that hostile rejecting and inconsistent parents provide a bad start (Goldfarb, 1945; Karpman, 1951). The usual comment has been that 'broken homes are relevant,' however the McCords (1959) point out that family discord may be more relevant than actual break between parents whilst Wooton (1959) has reiterated the real difficulties of *measuring* family influences. Lewis (1954) noted that children removed from bad family situations usually improved in all respects; a finding overlooked by those who strive to keep the parents of battered babies together.

Gibbens and Walker (1956) and Zuckermann *et al* (1960) also failed to relate intraparental problems to delinquency in the children. Perhaps the most relevant findings are those of the Gluecks (1956) who found that parental separation is less important in predicting later delinquency in children than is parental inconsistency in attitudes towards the children. Children it seems, can tolerate a good deal, mainly because they have time on their side but they cannot tolerate parents who blow hot and cold emotionally and who send out ambiguous signals.

Studies on the natural history of psychopathic disorders are thin on the ground though Robins (1966) has reported a 30 year follow-up of 524 child guidance patients and 100 controls, from which it was possible to delineate a fairly clear picture of psychopathic disorder and its antecedents. Robins' studies suggest onset before age 15 and in cases where a full history is available probable onset before age 12. Robins notes the diagnostic relevance of the beginning of serious antisocial behaviour relatively early in childhood. The symptoms in childhood that were found to be most significantly associated with adult diagnosis of antisocial personality included theft, persistent truancy, absconding from home, staying out late, having undesirable friends, aggressive behaviour and a bad job record etc. All these are in line with common clinical experience. An interesting finding was that antisocial symptoms in childhood were such a good predictor of adult antisocial behaviour that not one child in the follow-up developed an antisocial adult personality without having displayed antisocial symptoms in childhood. Also severely antisocial children seemed to have a bad prognosis regarding adult mental illness. Even allowing for transcultural differences. Robins' study confirms the general clinical impression that severely maladjusted truanting children who abscond from home are badly at risk in terms of later development of psychopathic personality.

Antisocial personalities

One of the difficult problems that confronts society is that of the repeatedly antisocial individual who seemingly learns nothing from either punishment or general life experience, who seems to be without conscience or any sense of social obligation, who lacks foresight, is egocentric and quite ruthless in pursuit of what he wants. This type of psychopathic personality, often referred to as sociopathic is one who is identified merely by his persistent delinquency since society passes the social judgement 'if he's as bad as that he must be ill'. And this is where we stand with the sociopath.

The key to understanding what the antisocial psychopath is really all about may be that he is basically immature in his whole emotional life and life style. His needs have to be gratified immediately or he explodes into rage or violence and he is as demanding as a child. He is always very demanding, in fact this is one of the most striking of his attributes. And he cannot see anything remotely unusual in the way he goes on. He has really no ethical or moral sense at all and the only guiding principle he has is to get whatever it is he wants. As a child he is usually unruly and rebellious and may show early signs of severe disturbance involving sadistic acts to animals and other children. Again early in childhood his emotional responses are sudden, impulsive and extreme. His schoolmates and friends soon learn to be wary of his outbursts.

Throughout childhood and adolescence he fails to adapt to the obligations and requirements of society in the normal way. He gets into trouble at school, truants and is often expelled. He gets into trouble with the law at an early age and repeats his offences unlike the 50% of juvenile offenders who never commit more than one offence. When he does come before the courts he is soon recognised by examining psychiatrists at remand homes as being curiously disturbed and maladjusted, though they would be understandably reluctant to label them as psychopaths at an early age. Early brushes with the law persist and such people began a dreary progress through the penal system; probation, detention centre, approved school, Borstal, young prisoner and adult prisoner status.

The range of antisocial activity displayed by the sociopath is wide and can encompass any type of criminality or social deviancy. At the emotional level he is cool, even callous. Feeling little or no affection, he can yield none, but whatever field he chooses he remains the classical recidivist offender. Drugs and alcohol are a danger to him for he will be unable to deal with them in a controlled sociable way. His interpersonal relations are unstable and short lived. He may have an easy superficial charm with often a brilliant and attractive quality to it that initially conceals the underlying vulnerability and emotional shallowness. His sexual life may be promiscuous or perverse or barren, depending on how his tastes lie. He cannot remain married or support a wife and children; he is too self-centred to be able to do this. Truth and honesty, loyalty and any sense of personal or moral obligations are alien to him and may seem to be attributes that he can recognise but in no way feel influenced by to any degree.

If he has a violent potential then he is a highly dangerous person who can kill without remorse, pity or any shred of feelings unless they are sadistic feelings. These are the sort of men who can become professional killers, mercenaries. Some of the most grisly examples of such people were found in the staffs of Nazi extermination camps in World War II murdering people by the thousand with callous brutal inhumane efficiency.

Other sociopaths may be thieves and swindlers and the classical confidence men. The latter are excellent examples of sociopathic disorder since their psychopathic brilliant charm and supreme self-confidence enables them to deceive even the most hard headed. Others may be pathological liars whose lying often has again a brilliant quality to it.

Certainly many of the most recidivist criminals, violent and nonviolent, are sociopaths and they are often in the headlines particularly when the crimes are sexual.

A good example of a pathological liar was provided by the following patient. A 40 year old man was referred for investigation of analgesic dependence. He was described as a doctor of science by his practitioner and when seen at the hospital spoke quite convincingly of his work in the higher echelons of pure scientific research. His drug dependence had started after an injury and on the face of it he was a good example of 'therapeutic dependence'. In fact his drug problem was a top dressing which overlaid a most picturesque and convincing collection of fantastic lies including a title forged on a marriage certificate, a non-existent inherited fortune in South America—in all a grandiose and inflated account of himself that was carried off with breeze and charm.

Schizoid personality

Many schizophrenics have been found to have displayed abnormal personality traits before the onset of their illness and this observation has prompted psychiatrists to speculate about the possibility of there being some variety of constitutional defect in the make up of people who later become schizophrenic. Particular personality traits have been noted and commented on and the whole picture fits into what has been labelled the schizoid personality. This is supposed to be a personality which it was thought by Kretschmer (1936) would be a precursor of schizophrenia. He described three types of schizoid individuals with clusters of personality traits

1   Asocial, quiet, reticent, serious, eccentric
2   Timid, shy, delicate, oversensitive, nervous, excitable, bookish
3   Well behaved, dull, consistent, good hearted

Actually these lists of adjectives are probably a good example of the serious limitations of the descriptive method of categorising personalities. Most of the terms are based on subjective judgement, and many have limitations that are influenced by the culture. For instance one may ask how keen a reader does someone have to be described as bookish etc. In this instance too it should be noted that a good 50% of people who develop schizophrenia have no signs of a previously schizoid personality. The general picture that emerges of the schizoid personality probably could be summarised in a list of the traits commonly noted in such people. In general behaviour the schizoid person is likely to be rather shy and unsociable, avoiding company because he prefers to be alone or because he feels uncomfortable or self-conscious with other people. This style of behaviour usually starts in early childhood where they are noticed to be less at ease with their playmates, less outgoing, less involved with the general run of activities than their peers. With hindsight no doubt parents etc. recall that in childhood the person was timid, unsociable, rather

K

dreamy and withdrawn. This is a state that is often regarded as being a sign of latent talent in childhood than of abnormality—'he's very imaginative'. In adolescence these traits become more marked, the quiet shy, even model child seems to be rather vague, the imaginative qualities now seem eccentric, withdrawal from others becomes very noticeable. The person is described as being rather aloof and cool; he lives absorbed more and more in his own thoughts and fantasies.

The emotional life of the schizoid is flat or at least flatter than that of his more responsive fellows. He is relatively unmoved by feeling, emotion and passion; detached from the general run of emotional life.

Often the schizoid person is hypersensitive, easily wounded and touchy to the point of being avoided by others. This is important since there is likely to be a vicious circle of withdrawal, avoidance by others, withdrawal etc. The schizoid person is not able either easily to reveal his feelings or talk about them.

Paranoid personalities

The basis of the paranoid personality is a tendency to be suspicious and oversensitive with an overriding predisposition to refer trivial events to the self and to rely on projection as a basic mechanism governing behaviour. Projection is an experience common to all—a simple example that is traditionally and correctly regarded as illustrative is the common experience, immediately distressing and usually later embarrassing, of going into a room full of people who become silent as one goes in and thinking that they have been talking about one (Mayer Gross *et al*). When this happens one has instant conviction that one is the subject of comment and discussion and unfavourable at that, but very quickly one realises that this is a false impression related to such simple things as being shy or having just bought a new tie or the uncomfortable suspicion that the trouser buttons are undone, or just plain lack of self-confidence.

Again in the case of someone who has paranoid delusions the situation is much clearer, for the deluded person has convictions of grandeur, of exaltation or of persecution. While one does not share his delusions they can be recognised by their extent and conviction for what they are as highly abnormal beliefs.

But the person with a paranoid personality disorder is in a different situation. He is not deluded but is highly oversensitive and above all oversensitive and egocentric in a way that has a certain deadly rationality about it.

The paranoid personality refers everything to himself and everything that happens to him convinces him that he is right. He is eternally defended against the world and against his own feelings and the feelings of others. Ever suspicious, always touchy and quick to take offence, he is at one and the same time convinced of his own importance as he is of being persecuted and put upon.

Paranoid personalities tend to be rigid, humourless, tense and insecure. They are always ready to interpret any comment as malignant and ill directed and a constant reminder to them that everyone is likely to reject them. Such people tend to be petty and quarrelsome and always affected by the feeling that no one likes or values them. There is some justification in dividing paranoid personalities into two sorts: the first being over-sensitive and excessively vulnerable to criticism who tend to blame others for their misfortunes and the second, a tougher breed whose vulnerability shows itself in an abrasive continued defence against fancied wrongs and slights, usually vociferous and always persistent.

The asthenic or inadequate personality

In every mental hospital and every prison there are found people who just cannot get on, they are ineffectual, disarmingly helpless in a way that would be hard to emulate. No doubt in a less urban society they are able to survive in village communities where they are accepted for what they are, namely people who find it very hard to cope with life, cannot hold on to a job, are easily influenced and are likely to drift into incompetent delinquency.

Such people are often recognised as having inadequate or asthenic personalities. Their main personality characteristic is that of inertia. Their energy interest, emotional response and general psychological set is less than adequate. They drift, are unstable, easily led and have no persistence. They are unable to plan for a future for which they have no concern anyway. They fill the ranks of the chronic unemployable as opposed to unemployed and many of them settle down as more or less institutionalised hospital or prison inmates or drift about as harmless vagrants. They are quite frequently rather likeable individuals.

12

Alcoholism and drug addiction

DRUG ADDICTION

Spread of drug abuse in the UK

In the early 1960s doctors, psychiatrists, officials of the Dangerous Drugs Department at the Home Office and others concerned with drug problems began to note a disturbing pattern in the increase of dependence on dangerous drugs such as heroin. The background to the growth of these problems has been reviewed by a number of authors (Bewley, 1966; James 1967; Willis, 1967; Spear, 1969; Glatt *et al*, 1967)

For years the UK had been regarded by countries such as the USA which had expanding problems of drug dependence as being particularly fortunate in that the drug problem was relatively small. Though morphinism had been prevalent in the latter part of the 19th Century, as also had the sporadic misuse of stimulant drugs such as cocaine, on the whole the casual use of narcotic drugs had been limited and there was little use by youth. Over the years the Home Office had kept careful watch over the number of people involved by the simple means of inspecting pharmacists' records of dangerous drugs prescribed for patients. When a name began to appear frequently in a particular pharmacist's list it was easy to check on what was happening and to identify the pattern of drug dependence.

Up to World War II the majority of dangerous drug addicts were people receiving prescriptions for morphine. There had been a rise in the use of morphine and cocaine after World War I, when cocaine was added to the regulations controlling dangerous drugs. This happened because soldiers on leave from the Western front had been obtaining cocaine in London and taking it as a stimulant. After World War I a number of notable examples of morphine and cocaine use appeared in the national press from time to time, but on the whole the problem was kept under control.

In 1926 the Rolleston Committee looked into the accepted medical practice of prescribing dependency producing drugs for known addicts. They reached the general conclusion that prescription was a humane medical practice that was suitable to those addicts who had a clear history of repeated treatment failures, and who could not be weaned from a particular drug but could be 'maintained' on it. It is probable that many of the drug users during the interwar period may have developed their habit in the late twenties, and were more likely than not to have been solitary neurotic drug takers. In addition there was a high percentage of people who had developed their dependence during the course of medical treatment that is to say 'therapeutic addicts'. Further, a small coterie were known to be involved with morphine and heroin in a non-therapeutic setting. The numbers were so small as hardly to present a social problem that was in any way serious. Cannabis usage was relatively infrequent and confined mainly to merchant seamen in seaports. During the war cannabis offences showed a rise but again these mainly involved merchant seamen.

With hindsight it can now be shown that the first sign of change in drug usage in the UK occurred shortly after the 1939–45 war when there was a rise in cannabis offences. These involved members of the West Indian immigrant population and various professional jazz musicians. But there was no immediate rise in the numbers of people taking morphine and there remained, as ever, a small quota of dangerous drug addicts who were physicians, nurses, and others with access to drugs.

By 1950 it was clear that cannabis usage was on the increase. An important case of drug trafficking occurred in 1951 (Spear, 1969) following a break-in at a hospital pharmacy. Large quantities of heroin, cocaine and morphine were stolen and subsequently it was discovered that these drugs were being sold illicitly in the West End of London. Some months later the man concerned was arrested and was found to have been formerly employed in the hospital concerned. His arrest and the identification of his customers revealed 14 heavy drug users previously unknown. His subsequent imprisonment led to the identification of 63 other drug users.

By 1960 the trend was alarming, for in this year the Home Office first got to know of someone under 20 who was addicted to heroin. During the years that followed although the numbers of morphine takers remained fairly steady the increase of young heroin addicts showed a steady growth rate.

There is little evidence to suggest that the average 'pre-war' drug user tended to congregate in subcultures, but by the 1960s this position was entirely reversed. Certainly there had been a small group of artists and intellectuals just before the war who were known to be heroin users, but there is little evidence to suggest that they spread the habit. By the 1960s London in particular, saw the beginnings of subcultures formed by young drug users. Many of these youngsters had drifted away from home and lived in parts of London where transient dwellers were commonplace.

Heroin could be obtained on a doctor's prescription comparatively easily. Doctors who took on such youngsters often found their surgeries swamped by large numbers claiming to be addicts. Hospital beds for the treatment of drug users were hard to come by and various predictions were made about the likely outcome of the general trend. The report of the Interdepartmental Committee then recommended the setting up of treatment centres in the hospital service where the heroin addict could have heroin prescribed for him on a 'maintenance' basis by licensed doctors. The object was to achieve rational control of the situation and to discourage the production of an illicit drug market.

While heroin was daily being proclaimed in the various media as the most difficult problem of all, there was an expansion in the taking of central stimulants orally and by injection. It soon became clear that inject-able methylamphetamine was a major source of psychosis and also because of the fact that people intoxicated with methylamphetamine went around in an excited, often irritable and aggressive manner, or became depressed when the drug was unobtainable. Since the amphetamines do not produce any physical dependency it hardly seemed justifiable to continue pres-cribing them, and it was agreed with the Ministry of Health that the prescription of methylamphetamine be discontinued. This proved to be a successful manoeuvre; although patients were very unhappy at the time the majority survived well enough. However, it is likely that some changed from methylamphetamine to either heroin or methadone.

The growth of the whole problem has, of course, to be viewed clearly in the context of expanding drug use involving drugs of all sorts. Since 1968, at least, self-injection with crushed sleeping tablets and the contents of sleeping capsules of the barbiturate and non-barbiturate type became another problem of drug dependence. In general the population involved today are predominantly young. It is also becoming apparent that in the UK, as in the USA, a younger generation is becoming more 'drug oriented'.

Since the increase in the problem subsequent to the late 1950s there have been many reports describing demographic details of drug users studied in hospital and in prison. These include those of Bewley (1966), Hewetson and Ollendorf (1964) and Gillespie *et al* (1967).

It is perhaps striking that a study carried out by Schur (1962) in England tended to confirm early speculations about the nature of the English drug using population. The author looked at occupation, social class, age, sex, marriage, sex-life, onset of drug habit, occupational adjustment, delinquency and so on, and commented on the high representation of people in the medical and allied professions. He also pointed out that a high proportion of the addicts studied came from social classes 1 and 2, and that addicts tended to be aged over 30. This is now no longer true.

Definitions

There is no general agreement about the meaning of the word 'addiction'. Medical men stress its physical aspects, sociologists its social aspects and lawyers its legal aspects. Nevertheless the term is so widely used that it is unlikely to be discarded. There is a tendency to use the word dependence which has been defined by the World Health Organisation in a way that qualifies each type of dependence by the generic name of the drug involved. However the majority of drug users take many drugs to satisfy their personal needs. Basic World Health Organisation definitions include:

Drug: any substance that when taken into the living organism may modify one or more of its functions.

Drug abuse: persistent or sporadic excessive drug use inconsistent with or unrelated to acceptable medical practice.

Drug dependence: a state, psychic and sometimes also physical, resulting from the interaction between a living organism and a drug, characterised by behavioural and other responses that always include a compulsion to take the drug on a continuous or periodic basis in order to experience its psychic effects and sometimes to avoid the discomfort of its absence. Tolerance may or may not be present. A person may be dependent on more than one drug.

Clearly the term 'drug' covers a wide range of substances, but in drug abuse and dependence the drugs involved are generally characterised by being 'mind altering'. Firstly, drugs which have a depressant effect on consciousness; these include narcotic analgesics *e.g.* opiates and opiate-like drugs and the hypnosedatives. Secondly, drugs whose action is primarily stimulant *e.g.* amphetamines, amphetamine-like drugs and cocaine. Thirdly, drugs whose effect is hallucinogenic *e.g.* LSD, psilocybin and mescaline. Cannabis is often included in this group, though strictly speaking cannabis produces its own pattern of dependence and abuse.

A distinction is made between *physical and psychological dependence*, and though the distinction may appear to be arbitrary, it has practical uses. Physical dependence is the end result of neurobiochemical change, no doubt transient, possibly prolonged, which creates in the taker a real physical need to continue taking the drug to avoid physically determined abstinence symptoms. Abstinence syndromes are often heavily overlaid with psychologically determined symptoms, but the consensus of opinion favours certain abstinence symptoms with a physical basis, *e.g.* many opiate withdrawal symptoms and barbiturate withdrawal confusion and convulsions. Psychological dependence covers not only subjective pleasure but also the emotional drives that lead the taker to persist. It includes relief of feelings of distress within the taker, *e.g.* anxiety, depression or general discontent. Psychological dependence extends into those extreme degrees of personal involvement in drug use that frequently occur. Such a state is found when a drug user radically alters his life style so that his life may come to revolve around drug taking. He spends all his time in the company of drug users who reinforce his dependence and bring about important social changes in him. He adopts a shared value system based on drug use and comes to regard himself as alienated from society not only because of society's apparent rejection of him, but because he comes to overvalue the state of being totally identified with drug use.

Thus drug use provides him with a life style and a career, albeit deviant, and a career that is hard to alter. The drug user may become a member of a subculture of drug users whose behaviour has important consequences for its members and society at large, particularly when they offend against the norms of society. A heightened sense of alienation from society tends to be self-perpetuating and to lead to the rejection of the customary goals, such as earning a living. Special modes of dress and speech may become badges of the subculture, far removed from the drug effects but important consequences. Though they are social consequences they are part of the overall picture of psychological dependence since membership of such a subculture may meet psychological needs related to drug use.

History

Descriptions of the actions of cannabis and opium go back as far as 2000 BC, but in the UK the history of drug misuse relates to the past two centuries. The abuse of alcohol in the 18th and 19th Centuries is well documented. It showed a decline from the mid 19th Century following the Temperance Campaign. These reforms were based on social necessity, since alcoholism had become grotesque in its extent, constituting a public and national disgrace.

Drug abuse, of opium and tincture of opium (laudanum), dates in England from 1700 when the virtues of opium were described by Dr. John Jones. After this, oral opiate preparations became so common that by the mid 19th Century there were very few people who had not taken them. This was particularly true for the poor, and thousands of deaths were caused by the use of opiates for ailing children. Many notable literary and public figures were opiate takers.

The invention of the hypodermic needle and syringe provided a more potent method of administration. Morphinism became a fashionable upper class disorder in the 19th Century. But control of opiate use was achieved by laws, so that by the beginning of the 20th Century—indeed until after World War II—the number of known opiate addicts in the UK was rarely more than 500. Of these 85% were therapeutic addicts using morphine, were middle aged and scattered all over the country, 10% were doctors and nurses and only 5% were non-therapeutic addicts—a special group of deviant people who kept their drugs use to themselves.

A dramatic change has occurred since the 1950s with the unexpected emergence of a youthful population of non-therapeutic heroin users. It is this change that caused public concern and re-examination of 'the British System'—the system by which any doctor could prescribe narcotics for an addict if he felt that cure of his addiction was impossible. The Brain Committee related the spread of heroin addiction to overprescribing and recommended, amongst other things, the limiting of the prescribing of heroin to specially licensed doctors. Spread of dependence, however, cannot entirely be explained in terms of 'epidemic spread'. Evidence to date suggests that drug users are likely to show psychiatric and social pathology before drug use.

A field study

The difficulties of accurately estimating the numbers of drug users in a population have already been touched upon. Its importance became crucial when the increase of drug use amongst young people began to attract public concern. The problem of numbers was frequently the subject of comment, much of it informed but some of it rather sensational. References in the daily Press were made to the possibility that figures produced by the Home Office Drugs Department might well represent 'the tip of the iceberg'. A number of rather bold assertions were made, often on the basis of interviews with a handful of young drug users. Many of these drug users may well have been exhibitionists, and only too ready to paint a highly coloured picture of the situation.

By 1969 there had been a number of reports published (Glatt, 1967; James, 1967; Bewley, 1966; Willis, 1969), all of which were based on drug users studied in hospital or in prison. A good example of an alternative method of study was provided by Kosviner *et al* (1968). The method used in this latter case involved a team of research workers investigating the extent of heroin use in a relatively compact area. The object was not so much to count heads but rather to try to draw a picture of the subculture of drug users and also tentatively to look into possible social influences contributing to their habit of drug use.

The town studied was small with a population of under 100 000. It had a university and, as the authors commented, 'an unusually high proportion of middle class people'. Members of the university were excluded from the study unless they happened to be local residents. The term 'heroin user' was employed to refer to people who had been taking heroin regularly during any of the preceding 3 months of the investigation's duration. At first contact was made with four users who attended a group directed by a local psychiatrist. Other drug users were then introduced through these initial four. At the same time the researchers rented an office and an apartment in the centre of the town and it became an informal meeting place for people with drug problems where they could feel free, in a non-institutional setting, to talk about anything whatsoever to a research team that was very much of their own age group. There was no occasion for fear or constraint.

The team collected the names of 47 people suspected to be heroin users. Thirty-one of them were found to be authentic users, 10 were not, and 6 had gone elsewhere. They also managed to find 6 heroin users who were not known to any official agency. The investigators made careful case histories of those involved with drugs and also collected information about the social and family backgrounds of the subjects, their education and occupational histories, their health records and delinquent behaviour. It was possible to verify the subjects' accounts from official records, hospitals, social workers and other sources.

One of the team's more striking findings was that they were unable to demonstrate a single common characteristic shared by all the users they interviewed. This tended to confirm their previous suspicion that the 'typical' addict does not exist. They commented that perhaps the most common characteristics of the group were that in general they came from backgrounds with a relatively high social status and also that they tended to show a pattern of academic failure despite having had good opportunities. It was suggested that middle class youngsters influenced by academic pressure and high family expectations might possibly turn to heroin as a means of escaping from stress. It was also suggested that, for some youngsters, taking heroin was something positive, an act of rebellious defiance. Further speculation was offered as to whether drug taking was a more attractive form of illicit gratification for some than for others. On the other hand there was no evidence that the group resembled in any way the aimless, purposeless drifting youngsters, basically delinquent, that had been described by Chein *et al* (1964) in a study in New York.

Perhaps one of the most valuable aspects of the study was that it was timely, thorough and essentially a prospective one in which the collection of data was, and is, an outgoing process; people initially contacted could be, and were, followed up. Reports were made one year later. A number of lessons were learned. A containment unit was set up in the town to control the quantities of heroin prescribed by licensed doctors. This unit became the only licit source of heroin supply. From early 1968 it was concerned primarily with heroin takers, so that although the total number of daily heroin takers did not rise in the year it proved impossible to make any accurate comment about changes in the misuse of other drugs in the area. No doubt many changes did occur, for patterns of change in drug use are normal in most areas. Overall, they reported on 14 newly discovered heroin users in the year, including not only chronic addicts but occasional heroin takers.

This type of investigation is of value because it contributes positively to the understanding of what we may call the 'natural history of drug dependence'. Hitherto there has perhaps been undue emphasis on taking cross-sections of drug users, describing the characteristics found, drawing conclusions and more or less leaving the matter at that.

Basic information of course is needed since it contributes to the central body of knowledge, but in the long term study of a chronic disorder it is time that counts. It is easy to speculate on data obtained by the cross-sectional method; this is rather like looking at a school photograph and predicting what is going to happen to the group. However, knowledge about a complex social problem is gleaned over a period of time, and it is a laborious process. Unfortunately because of the emotionally charged atmosphere that surrounds drugs there is a background clamour for as much instant information as possible, in the hope that this will illuminate a dark area and give the answer to the problem. Prospective research is time consuming, often wearisome and tends to lack the superficial attractiveness of hastily amassed data. Nevertheless in the long term it is more rewarding.

Drug dependence is a complex disorder related not only to the conditions of modern urban life, but to the further complexities of psychological disturbance. Supposed drug effects need to be regarded cautiously for they are related not only to known pharmacological action, but also to the mood of the taker and his expectations.

Patterns of drug dependence

Drugs with depressant action

1 *Narcotic analgesics: Morphine type* The type of dependence produced by these drugs is categorised by the World Health Organisation as *drug dependence, morphine type*. Some drugs included are morphine, diamorphine, methadone, pethidine and all analgesic drugs that are opiate derivatives and synthetic opiate-like drugs. This type of dependence is characterised by severe physical and psychological dependence and tolerance. This means the user may crave the drug, though this is not inevitable. Abstinence symptoms include restlessness, rubbing the face and body, irritability, apprehension, yawning, salivation, nausea, vomiting, abdominal cramps, joint pains, running eyes and nose, diarrhoea, and, in later stages, elevated blood pressure, raised blood sugar and spontaneous ejaculation or orgasm. The dependency producing potential of these drugs is high, probably the highest of all. The pleasure caused by opiates does not persist and as tolerance increases euphoria decreases. So that the ultimate

reason for continuing is the avoidance of withdrawal distress. Morphine-like drugs render people passive and inert with the social consequence of failure to function adequately as social beings. Though the hazards of these drugs per se are not spectacular (apart from death from overdose), there are real hazards from unsterile self-injection including abscesses, thrombophlebitis, septicaemia, jaundice, pneumonia, endocarditis and, rarely, tetanus and malaria. Also there are the major social hazards of drug use as a way of life, associated with the criminality and inertia—an impressive catalogue.

2 *Barbiturate type* Properly speaking alcohol is included here since dependence on alcohol and barbiturates are very similar.

Under barbiturate type dependence are included dependence on non-barbiturates, sedatives, hypnotics and tranquillisers. This type of dependence when mild is mainly psychological probably most commonly seen in the person who has been taking doses of say 300 mg of a barbiturate nightly for years and who cannot stop. If a dose of 700 mg of barbiturate per 24 hours is exceeded for a period of over 6 weeks, the taker is likely to become physically dependent. This leads to chronic intoxication (ataxia, dysarthria and nystagmus). Mild symptoms of physical dependence include nausea, dizziness, orthostatic hypotension and trembling. The major hazards of physical dependence are barbiturate withdrawal fits. These can be fatal if vomit is inhaled. States of confusion and delirium may also occur.

Stimulant drugs

1 *Cocaine type* Psychological dependence is often severe. There is no physical dependence and true tolerance does not occur. The subjective stimulant effect is often highly valued and large quantities may be taken. Psychotic excitement with hallucinosis and paranoid content can occur.

2 *Amphetamine type* This may be caused by all amphetamines and amphetamine-like drugs. It is characterised by severe psychological dependence and the slow development of tolerance. There is no physical dependence. Excitement, hilarity, restless irritability and repetitive over-activity are found, as are outbursts of aggression and depressed mood when the drug is stopped. A serious hazard is the amphetamine psychosis which is schizophrenic in form and characterised by paranoid content, loosely held fleeting delusions and hallucinations. The euphoria of amphetamine taking is short lived and self-criticism may be impaired by leading to antisocial acts.

Hallucinogenic drugs

The most commonly used hallucinogen is lysergic acid diethylamide (LSD). Other commonly used preparations include psilocybin, mescaline, dimethyl tryptamine (DMT) and Ditran.

Dependence is psychological, physical dependence does not occur. Psychological dependence often leads to radical alteration of life style. Tolerance to LSD and psilocybin occurs but develops only slowly with mescaline. Hallucinogenic activity is stressed but in fact is not the main action of this group. Emotional changes are more marked and include ecstasy, anxiety, terror, nameless dread, even depression. These are often followed by perceptual changes including not only hallucinations, but also distorted perceptions. A feeling of cosmic revelation is often described, of a sense of awareness of metaphysical union with the universe etc., these effects are often found and highly valued by the user. It is likely that a consequence of such experiences is that the user overvalues the effects, sometimes with disastrous social consequences to himself and family. Adverse reactions to hallucinogens are well documented, particularly following LSD. These include periods of intense psychotic excitement, often schizophrenic in form, also depressed mood, prolonged anxiety reactions and persistent feelings of unreality (depersonalisation).

Hallucinogenic drugs are substances which have as their most striking property that of producing severe perceptual disturbance including hallucinations. A number of names have been applied to this group including psychedelic, *i.e.* 'mind altering', and psychotomimetic, *i.e.* 'able to mimic the manifestations of psychosis'. Experimental studies, however, suggest that the term hallucinogenic by no means accounts for the bulk of the activity of these drugs, though hallucinogenic activity may be most striking. In fact the activity of such drugs is influenced not only by the user's personality structure but also by his mood and his expectations of the drug effect. This is true of all mind altering drugs, including alcohol, the opiates, barbiturates and the amphetamines. The use of naturally occurring substances with hallucinogenic properties is frequently recorded in history. The taking of hallucinatory mushrooms by tribes in northern

Siberia and the use of the sacred mushroom by Mexicans, the latter in the setting of religious observance, are well documented. Also the suggestion has been put forward that the state of 'berserk', described in Nordic myths, may well have been caused by intoxication with *Amanita muscaria* which contains the hallucinogen bufotenin.

The actions of hallucinogens are dramatic and remarkable. They include profound affective change, with feelings of fear, anxiety, dread and tremor, followed by disturbances in perception. These take the form not only of hallucinations but also quite bizarre changes in the quality of perception, intensification and distortion of images, and considerable preoccupation with the nature of the perceptual experience. In addition to this there are found feelings of altered reality of the self (depersonalisation) and of the enviroment (derealisation) and the subject's thinking is altered. Thought processes become more diffuse and show a dream-like quality.

A convenient classification of hallucinogenic drugs includes

1 *Tryptamine group* This group contains substances which are straightforward tryptamine derivatives and substances which contain the tryptamine nucleus in a complex ring structure. The simple tryptamine derivatives include dimethyl tryptamine, diethyl tryptamine, serotonin, bufotenin and psilocybin (the active principle of the sacred Mexican mushroom). Other hallucinogens with the basic tryptamine nucleus in a complex ring include LSD, harmine and ibogaine. Harmine is found in *Peganum harmala*, *Banisteria caapi* and *Haemadictyon amaconicum*, used by South American Indians. Ibogaine is the active principle of the plant *Tabernathe iboga*, used in West and Central Africa.

2 *Phenylethylamine group* These are all related to the sympatheticomimetic catechol amines, of which the best known is mescaline, the active principle of peyote derived from the leaves of the cactus *Lophophora williamsii*. It is used in tribal and religious ceremonies in America. Other substances in this group include TMA, trimethoxy amphetamine, and MDA, methylene dioxyamphetamine.

3 *Mixed group* The third group is mixed and includes ditran which causes total loss of contact with the environment and total amnesia; also tetrahydrocannabinol, the active principle of cannabis, and phenylcyclidine (sernyl), which may cause marked loss of skin sensation, body image disturbance and confusional states. Of all the hallucinogens, LSD 25 is the most widely known, and it has been used in psychiatric treatment and research, although there is little concensus of agreement about its place in therapy. Many claim it as a useful treatment for alcoholism, but its real place in treatment is not clearly defined. Research interest in the hallucino-genic induced states is based on their resemblance to psychoses, *i.e.* 'model psychoses'. Though it was thought that investigation of model psychoses might throw light on the aetiology of psychoses such as schizo-phrenia, it is a fact that as yet there is no clear evidence linking the action of hallucinogens to the causation of psychoses, though tantalising similarities between the syndromes exist. The casual self-administration of hallucinogenic drugs has found favour, but informed medical opinion rightly deplores such use as being yet another example of the use of drugs for hedonistic purposes in situations where the illusory gains of spurious insight are offset by the hazards of adverse reactions which are unpredict-able in onset and duration and sometimes tragic in outcome.

Cannabis dependence

There is no physical dependence or tolerance but severe psychological dependence may be found. In the latter there is a strong drive to continue taking the drug. There is no unequivocal evidence of permanent damage following long term cannabis usage, but states of chronic cannabis intoxi-cation are associated with deteriorated social behaviour, apathy, indolence and inertia. The heavy user becomes preoccupied with cannabis effects to the exclusion of all else. Short-lived psychotic states with paranoid content have been described though there is disagreement as to whether or not they are cannabis related or released by cannabis. The effects of cannabis in mild concentration are those of hilarity, jocularity, a carefree attitude and flippancy. On these grounds some regard it as a harmless intoxicant. But this ignores the real states of psychological dependence that can occur. There is no pharmacological reason linking cannabis to progression to other drugs, but social links may be present by association.

Cannabis is obtained from the flowering tips and leaves of *Cannabis sativa* plant. The resin extracted from the plant or dried leaves may be used as source material. The active principle of cannabis are chemically members of the tetrahydrocannabinol group of substances. Dependence of cannabis type is characterised by psychological dependence but no physical depen-dence. The effects of cannabis include tachycardia, raised blood pressure, conjunctival injection, pallor, faintness and later headache and nausea. Cannabis users look for effects such as insouciance, loquaciousness and mild hilarity, but in high concentrations excitement and hallucinosis can occur.

Acute reactions to cannabis have been described and these include unreality feelings, disorganised thinking and schizophreniform psychoses. Whether these are direct cannabis effects or whether they are reactions triggered off in unstable people is open to question but does not devalue their potential seriousness when diagnosed.

Permanent long term effects of cannabis have not clearly been demonstrated, but there is evidence to suggest that in the short term it can lead people into states of disorganised inertia. In the UK it is subject to the Misuse of Drugs Act and internationally is controlled by the Single Convention of which the UK is one of the signatories. The relationship of cannabis usage to crime is far from clear. Certainly its use is common amongst delinquent subcultures in the USA, but for that matter it appears to be widely used by 'normal' individuals there. There is no clear evidence to suggest that cannabis per se causes violent and antisocial behaviour in unstable individuals.

Again whilst there is no evidence that its use leads to progression to opiate use there is some evidence to associate its use with progression to the use of hallucinogenic drugs.

Aetiology

There is much evidence linking drug dependence with pre-existing severe personality disorders. Also many American studies link drug dependence with social pathology, social and material deprivation; blocked opportunity and membership of low status racial minority groups. This combination of social and personal pathology provides fertile soil for development of dependence. In the UK recent research shows a high incidence of personality disorders in opiate users but no clear pattern of social pathology is noted. It is found in all social classes and a wide range of family backgrounds, though the presence of parental alcoholism, psychiatric disorders, delinquency and separation is noted in a minority. A minority of drug users appear to develop their dependence against a background of pre-existing anxiety or depression relieved by the drug. Men outnumber women in the ratio 5:1. The links of drug dependence with criminality, though demonstrable, are not easily defined.

The diagnosis of drug dependence is based on history and examination. Supportive evidence of drug dependence includes the finding of injection marks, needle tracks, thrombophlebitis, abscesses, ulcers from self-injection and sometimes abstinence symptoms.

Final proof that the drug is being taken is achieved by thin layer or gas chromatographic examination of the urine. Urine should be collected whenever the patient is seen.

The ultimate goal of treatment is total abstention from drugs based on total social and psychological rehabilitation. This is so often a near impossibility to achieve that many regard total abstention as a primary treatment goal as unrealistic whilst acknowledging it as an ultimate goal. Relapse rates are very high in the first 6 months (90%), but follow-up studies in the USA suggest that heroin users may show a remission rate of up to 30% at 5 years.

With this in mind initial treatment is often directed at the medical and psychiatric complications of drug dependence. Long term support is then aimed at gradual re-education to more stable habits of living, and ultimately to total abstention. The most difficult task is to get the user to realise the real dangers of drug dependence and to accept a drug free life as worthwhile. Withdrawal from drugs and abstinence syndromes are easily treated in hospital. With opiate dependence, methadone is the most useful substitution drug because of its slow excretion and prolonged action. Withdrawal programmes vary according to preference of individual doctors, but most use methadone with or without tranquillisers. Some employ intramuscular heroin for a few days at the beginning of withdrawal. Phenothiazines are not without hazard as they may cause barbiturate withdrawal fits where barbiturate use is undetected. The opiate user who arrives in a surgery or casualty department with abstinence distress is best treated with oral or intramuscular methadone. Withdrawal from barbiturates carries the special hazard of withdrawal convulsions. In practice the simplest regime is to maintain the patient in a state of intoxication to a level characterised by slight dysarthria. Medication consists of pentobarbitone in divided doses every 4 hours and the dose is reduced by 100 mg every day. During any withdrawal the patient will need adequate feeding, rehydration and vitamin supplements.

Barbiturate induced delirium is usually treated by temporary re-intoxication though this is not necessarily successful. Withdrawal from amphetamines should be abrupt. This is usually followed by prolonged sleep, after which the patient is usually depressed and irritable. Weight gain is rapid with the return of appetite. Cocaine withdrawal is managed in the same way.

The main serious problems of withdrawal are found where there is physical dependence. This is not to minimise the pleadings, cravings and frank belligerance that often go with psychological dependence. The most difficult problems are encountered after withdrawal. These consist in the problem of maintaining abstention. Drugs provide for the user a ready escape from the problems of everyday life, an escape which is for the user too often far more effective and immediate than many treatment methods, however sophisticated they may be. Where dependence is a symptom of an underlying depression the outlook should be better for relief of depression should reduce drug-seeking drives, but such cases are not common. The bulk of patients are suffering from personality disorders, and will initially have used drugs for pleasure or as a barrier between themselves and the difficulties of existence, so that the problem becomes one of treating a personality disorder. This is not an area of resounding psychiatric success. Compulsory admission may be life saving, but its universal application though superficially attractive may be a euphemism for imprisonment.

At the present time there is considerable interest in the use of former drug users in the rehabilitation of the addict. There is increasing evidence that this may be a valuable manoeuvre. Patients put in a drug free environment and put under strong pressure to abstain, appear to respond more favourably if the pressure is exerted by former drug users. This form of rehabilitation based on self-help by reformed addicts has shown promising results in special communities in America. The former drug addict knows well the self-deceptions etc. that drug users employ and can confront the patient with these in dramatic fashion. In such communities the new entrant is given a low role and status, and is soon made aware that he has to contribute to the community and is responsible for his actions and feelings. Group encounter sessions are used and vigorous interaction is the rule. These approaches though lengthy and expensive, offer promising methods of total rehabilitation. Conventional psychiatric approaches, individual and group therapy have to date not been of any lasting value. The free use of tranquillisers and antidepressants for drug users carries the real hazard of further abuse.

A totally different approach to opiate addiction has been adopted in the USA by Dole and Nyswander. This discards a psychogenic view of drug dependence and emphasises the importance of long term physical dependence. Methadone is used as a pharmacological blocking agent, to reduce craving and to prevent euphoria should an opiate be taken. The method has had good results in America in centres where recidivist users maintained on methadone have been enabled to live productive and socially acceptable lives. Also the methadone programmes encourage group morale giving the user the sense of belonging to a successful venture, so that social forces play their part in the rehabilitation as well. It is likely that in the future, *pharmacological blocking agents will play an increasing part in the treatment of all varieties of drug dependence.* Until then, rehabilitation of drug users should profitably include a wide range of methods. There is little information about the rehabilitation of barbiturate and amphetamine users. Common experience suggests that severe barbiturate dependence is very difficult to treat. Amphetamine abuse also presents difficulties. The drug is attractive and relatively easily obtainable. Motivation to abstain tends to be low.

Heroin dependence may be self-limiting—the user no longer achieves euphoria with the passage of time and relies on it to avoid abstinence distress. Ageing brings psychological maturity and increasing awareness of the hazards of drug use. Therefore a patient with a relatively recent history may show less motivation to abstain than a patient with a much longer history. But this should not deter from vigorous attempts at treatment.

Drug dependence is a chronic and relapsing disorder, and the treatment of such disorders is commonplace in medicine and psychiatry. Thus, while the long term support and supervision may appear to be limited as goals they remain for the drug user the most practical way of helping him until he is capable of achieving more fundamental degrees of change.

In the UK the maintenance prescribing of heroin and cocaine is limited to licensed doctors. Prescribing heroin is fundamentally a social rather than a strictly medical measure, and this treatment approach is currently being evaluated. In general, however, it is unwise to prescribe dependence producing drugs for addicts—exceptions are the use of methadone to relieve opiate abstinence distress and the prescription of barbiturates in an emergency to the severely barbiturate intoxicated patient. This last measure will prevent withdrawal convulsions.

Legal aspects of drug dependence

The development of legislation surrounding the control of dangerous drugs goes back to 1868, since then a variety of Laws, Orders in Council,

Proclamations, Regulations and Acts—40 in all—have been passed. While it is not possible to review these in detail, a brief résumé of some of the more relevant aspects may be of interest.

1 1868 The Pharmacy Act was passed. This was a fairly straightforward legal attempt to impose some degree of control over opium and opium derivatives.

2 1912 The UK was one of the signatories of the International Opium Convention (Hague Convention). This was the first major concerted effort to establish a reasonable degree of control over the production, sale and distribution of opium. The object was to limit opium production for medical purposes only and to eradicate illicit channels of distribution. Britain, it will be recalled, had a somewhat murky reputation in this respect following the Opium Wars in the 19th Century when Britain had virtually reimposed the importation of opium into a reluctant China, since opium came into China from British-owned India and was a valuable source of income to the British Empire. Settlement of the Wars gave Britain Hong Kong as a bonus!

3 1916 There was concern about soldiers on leave in London who had obtained cocaine from prostitutes. As a result of cooperation between the police and military, cocaine and opium were controlled by Defence of the Realm Regulation 40 B. In fact the legal control of dangerous drugs remained in a rather confused state until 1920.

4 1920 In this year the Dangerous Drugs Act 1920 was passed. This was a fairly comprehensive law aimed at the control of dangerous drugs by regulating their manufacture, prescription, storage and dispensing. It was amended and modified over the years that followed. Originally it controlled opium and opioid drugs etc. However, with the passage of time new synthetic drugs came under its area of control. Also various further legislations were passed regulating prescriptions etc. In 1923 the penalties for infringement of the Act were increased.

5 1925 The UK was one of the signatories of the Geneva Convention. The Dangerous Drugs Act 1925 extended legal control to cocoa leaves and India hemp. The inclusion of Indian hemp as a 'dangerous drug' (UK) or 'narcotic' (US) is clearly very relevant to the current controversy over cannabis. It appears that the main pressure for its inclusion came from Egypt and South Africa, two nations where cannabis taking was widespread. The impression was created that cannabis was as dangerously dependency producing as the opiates and this impression was uncritically accepted. The consequence was that cannabis became subject to the same legal sanctions as opiates. Present thinking would suggest that cannabis is less dangerous and should therefore be subject to less punitive sanctions.

6 1926 Publication of the report of the Inter-Departmental Committee on Morphine and Heroin Addiction (Rolleston Committee). This report reviewed the practice of prescribing narcotic drugs for established addicts and recommended that though in general this could be regarded as a reasonable practice it should be restricted to addicts who had repeatedly failed in treatment.

7 1964 The Drugs (Prevention of Misuse) Act. This Act made it an offence to import or to possess without authority substances listed in the schedule to the Act including methaqualone. Infringement of the Act carried a penalty of unlimited fine or 2 years' imprisonment or both on indictment or, on summary conviction a fine not exceeding £200 or imprisonment for a maximum of 6 years, or both.

8 1965 Dangerous Drugs Act. This Act codified earlier legislation and extended control to all substances listed in the United Nations Single Convention of Narcotic Drugs, 1961. The Act was in four parts. Part I prohibited growth and import of all cannabis preparations and made it an offence to permit premises to be used for cannabis smoking. Part II dealt with opium in the same way Part III empowered the Home Secretary to extend or withhold control of drugs subject to decisions of the UN Commission on Narcotic Drugs. Part IV codified the offences and penalties involved, fixing maximum penalties as follows: On indictment, fine not exceeding £1000 or 10 years' imprisonment; on summary conviction, a fine not exceeding £250 or 12 months' imprisonment.

9 1967 The Dangerous Drugs Act, 1967, empowered the Home Secretary to regulate notification of addicts and regulate prescription of drugs to addicts. In effect this means that anyone suspected of being addicted to a drug covered by the Act must be notified to the Chief Medical Officer of the Drugs Branch of the Home Office and limits the prescription of heroin and/or cocaine to addicts to licensed doctors.

10 1968 The Medicines Act 1968. This Act provides for the control and clinical trial of therapeutic substances and for their development and manufacture under proper supervision.

11 1971 The Misuse of Drugs Act 1971. This Act, which came into action on 1 July 1973, supersedes the Dangerous Drugs Acts of 1965 and 1967 and the Drugs (Prevention of Misuse) Act 1964. It may be regarded as a response to the increased problems of drug usage in the UK and as such is intended as a comprehensive piece of legislation to replace previous separate legislative items in much the same way as the Mental Health Act 1959 replaced several rather cumbersome pieces of legislation dealing with the mentally ill.

The main provisions of the Act include first, the fact that the Home Secretary is given the power to introduce control of drugs without having to await recommendations from an international body. Thus, he may by Order in Council add new drugs to the schedules to those already controlled. Second it introduces legal procedures to investigate and control irresponsible prescribing.

Third it separates drugs of dependence and misuse into three groups relative to their harmfulness and creates new offences to check trafficking, increasing the penalites for trafficking and smuggling. Also it maintains the power of the police to stop and search those suspected of illegal possession.

One may say that it is easier to be a drug user in the UK than in the USA but whether this state of affairs would persist if the UK had a massive drug problem is entirely another matter. The history of the development of drug-problems in various countries such as Japan, Sweden, France and the UK since World War II is characterised by increased legal activity as the problem grows. It is difficult to see at what point large scale legal intervention has ever been really effective except in reducing the availability of certain drugs—a situation almost inevitably followed by the emergence of an alternative form of intoxication. This is not a criticism of those who formulate the laws, administer and enforce them. If it is a criticism of anyone it is rather of society in general which tends to over-react against whomsoever are designated as members of an out group—drug users, those who seek termination of pregnancy, homosexuals and latterly, it may be thought, the young often credited with free drug use, idleness etc.—for no very good reason save public anxiety based on incorrect stereotypes.

Since 1960 the UK has witnessed the emergence of an increase in drug use by young people. The more dramatic aspects of this change have involved the discovery of subcultural heroin use, usually by youngsters with a higher than average incidence of severe personality disturbance. Study of these young people produces the not surprising finding that casual experimentation with cannabis and LSD, was and is on the increase. But there is no evidence to date to suggest a massive drug problem and no evidence to suggest a growth rate which would bring the casualty list of drug use to the same proportions as death on the roads, alcoholism or suicide. In fact the 'typical' English drug user is not a self-injector with heroin, nor a pothead, but one of the 500 000 people in England who take hypnotics every night of whom at least 50 000 are physically dependent on barbiturates.

Another important observation has to do with the real changes in medical practice in the last 50 years. For hundreds of years doctors had no remedies for disease save opiates for pain, reassurance and comfort and the use of swift, skilful and crude surgery. Since the 1930s we have seen emergence of a large range of effective drugs to treat infections, alter metabolism and halt previously untreatable disease. Since the late 1950s doctors have had access to 'mind altering' drugs which alter disturbed mental states without altering consciousness—tranquillisers, antidepressants, etc. People have come to take these for granted, even ask for them. It is therefore perhaps not surprising that a new generation has a more casual attitude to mind altering drugs and seeks pleasure in them. Drug taking may already have been incorporated into 'normal' adolescent risk taking behaviour, much of which receives adult approval, *e.g.* motor cycling, skin diving, mountaineering etc. It is often hard to know who should arbitrate about risk taking.

We live in a pill oriented age and our concern for drug abuse is rooted in a mixture of reason and unreason. Unhappily people who use drugs habitually display a remarkable tendency to go on doing so and if we are to make any sense of all this it seems pointless to single out one particular group. It will be more profitable to look at these problems in a larger context.

ALCOHOLISM

The term alcoholism is regarded as synonymous with chronic alcoholism and described the overall picture of disability associated with prolonged excessive drinking. Acute alcoholism or simple drunkenness is a dose related state of acute alcoholic intoxication which is characterised by predictable changes in consciousness and behaviour. Initial disinhibited cheeriness is followed by increased impairment of consciousness, coordination and motor function, proceeding to drowsiness, coma and death if enough alcohol is taken. Alcoholism, *i.e.* chronic alcoholism, is a much more extensive disorder which imposes on the sufferer physical, social and psychological handicaps often of great severity.

The World Health Organisation defines as alcoholics 'those excessive drinkers whose dependence on alcohol has attained such a degree that it shows a notable mental disturbance or an interference with their bodily and mental health, their interpersonal relations and their smooth social and economic functioning: or who show the prodromal signs of such development'. By definition then, alcoholism occurs after excessive drinking, though it is realised that there is considerable individual variation. The important point is that when a person becomes alcoholic, the amount taken is excessive for him. An important part of the definition is 'dependence on alcohol'. It can be said that while psychological dependence on alcohol is common, to the extent that many regular social drinkers may show it, for the true alcoholic psychological dependence is so extensive as to cause symptoms and above all to cause a progressive loss of control over drinking. Physical dependence on alcohol appears relatively late in the natural history of the disorder, but when it occurs indicates severe dependence.

In diagnosing alcoholism, the finding of symptoms of loss of control of drinking should be regarded as paramount. These include lying to the self and others about the amount drunk, preoccupation with alcohol and with keeping up supplies, taking extra drinks before parties or ordeals, hangovers causing loss of work and drinking earlier in the day. Once drinking is out of control dependence worsens and further symptoms emerge: these include blackouts, memory gaps, early morning shakes relieved by alcohol, feelings of nausea and weakness on standing, tremulousness and further signs of physical dependence and physical complications. It is important to stress not so much individual signs, but the necessity of finding out from the patient how much of his life is absorbed by alcohol in time, money and interest.

Jellinek proposed a classification of alcoholism based on the notion of alcoholism as a disease process in which various systems are progressively involved He suggested, too, that the aetiology varied with the pattern of alcohol use displayed by the drinker. His classification includes alpha alcoholism, characterised by a 'purely psychological continued dependence . . . to relieve bodily or emotional pain'. Alpha alcoholism is said not to proceed to loss of control. Beta alcoholism is said to occur when organic complications, such as cirrhosis or polyneuritis, are present, but where the dependence is either physical or psychological. Gamma alcoholism is characterised by progressive development of tolerance to alcohol with cellular change, abstinence symptoms and craving with severe loss of control over the amount drunk—a truly progressive and the most damaging variety. This is the predominant type in Anglo-Saxon countries.

Delta alcoholism resembles gamma, but instead of a loss of control the person has total inability to abstain even for a day or so without the appearance of withdrawal symptoms. Epsilon alcoholism is episodic excessive drinking, *i.e.* dipsomania. Whether or not Jellinek's classification is employed, the basic problem to be clarified in anyone with a history of alcohol abuse is the presence of dependence, and, even more important, to find out if loss of control of drinking has occurred.

The importance of *making the diagnosis* of alcoholism cannot be over-emphasised: it is a disorder which may be missed by otherwise capable doctors This is not just because some ignore its existence as a disease, but because of the moral overtones and social stigma which may obscure the diagnosis.

The true extent of alcoholism is hard to estimate. Jellinek's formula based on deaths from alcoholic cirrhosis though often employed, is thought by many to provide an underestimate of the true prevalence. The World Health Organisation estimates between 400 000 and 500 000 alcoholics in England and Wales using Jellinek's formula. Whatever the true numbers may be, the problem is large and an important aspect of the public health.

The aetiology of alcoholism is best described in multifactorial terms. One-factor theories of alcoholism do not account for the facts. Heavy drinkers tend to come from heavy drinking families. The children of alcoholics have a higher expectation of alcoholism than do children of parents not alcoholics. Whilst no genetic inheritance has been demonstrated, it could operate; though to date family experience seems to be more important. Certain races show clear cultural and racial links with alcoholism. The Irish appear to be highly vulnerable, Jews and Moslems nearly invulnerable. There are wide differences between countries in alcoholism prevalence. The complications of alcoholism are extensive. The alcoholic is more likely to become diabetic, to suffer from pancreatitis and to be more prone to chronic bronchitis (because of heavier smoking) than the non-alcoholic.

Aetiology

Alcoholism is more common in men than women in the approximate ratio 4:1. The disorder is usually recognised in the middle years probably because prolonged heavy drinking leads to loss of control of drinking and consequent dependence. In order to discover the prevalence of alcoholism it is helpful to know something of drinking habits in the general population. A recent example was an American study in 1966 that suggested that 70% of US adults had had at least one alcoholic drink in the preceding year while 20% reported that they had never had a drink. But this is far from indicating the extent of alcoholism. Jellinek (1957) put forward a formula for estimating alcoholism prevalence based on the number of deaths per year from hepatic cirrhosis. Later he discounted the value of the formula as being likely to give a low figure; but even on Jellinek's formula it was calculated that there were 400 000 alcoholics in the UK.

National drinking habits change with time; the heavy spirit drinking in 18th and 19th Century England produced little moderate drinking; people either drank heavily or not at all. Nowadays drinking is more widespread and in general more moderate though there are no grounds for complacency.

Certain races are more at risk than others; in the UK the Irish and Scots lead the field. Mental hospital admission rates for alcoholism are four times higher in Scotland than in England. In the US the Irish and Northern Europeans are heavily represented in the alcoholic population but the Scots are mysteriously absent. Again in the US the black American is highly represented—but is this an ethnic or an economic association?

Epidemiology

The first difficulty in establishing prevalence rates is that alcoholism tends to be under diagnosed by doctors since medical teaching emphasises the late stages of the disorder with severe physical dependence and physical complications ignoring the importance of a history of *loss of control over drinking*. Also patients are reluctant to admit to themselves or others that their problems are alcohol related—thus doctor and patient collude in avoiding the recognition of the disorder.

Moss and Beresford Davies (1967) studied the prevalence in Cambridgeshire using hospital records, psychiatrists records, general practitioners, the police, the probation service, Salvation Army, children's departments, AA, the Samaritans etc. as information sources. They found an alcoholism rate of 62 per 10 000 (males) and 14 per 10 000 (females), differing from Keller and Egron (1955) who estimated 110 per 10 000 of the general population and Parr (1957) figure of 11 per 10 000.

General population studies are rare except for Scandinavia where there is a long tradition of population health records and a stable population in terms of emigration. Fremming (1951) for instance examined records on Bornholm Island covering 5500 people. He calculated an expectancy rate of alcoholism of 3·4% (male) and 0·2% (women).

Other have surveyed drinking patterns of population samples: Mulford and Miller (1960) found 9% of 1185 Iowans to be 'heavy drinkers', while Bailey *et al* (1965) surveyed 4000 families in Washington Heights and found an alcoholism rate of 19 per 1000. A repeat study identified a further 10% as alcoholic.

Transcultural studies reveal national differences in drinking—also different definitions. Beverage choice varies, in the US and UK people prefer beer and spirits whilst in Italy, Spain and France wine is the main drink. Jellinek (1962) commented on different alcoholism rates in France and Italy, both of which have similar sized alcohol industries. The differences in alcoholism are probably due to different drinking habits, *e.g.* in France drinking is spread throughout the day, in Italy it is more confined to meal times.

Sociological views on alcoholism such as those of Bales (1946) relate alcoholism to social attitudes, *e.g.* if alcohol is regarded as tension relieving then it is more subject to abuse. Horton (1943) related alcoholism to *subsistence anxiety*, *i.e.* to a culture's basic fears of being unable to survive crop failure, floods etc. Mowrer and Mowrer (1945) related alcoholism to levels of social change and disorganisation—rootless, drifting people with social problems are highly vulnerable to alcohol as an escape from their situation.

Snyder (1958, 1962) and Glatt (1970) have reviewed the relative freedom from alcoholism of orthodox Judaism where children learn early to respect, fear and control alcohol intake but at the same time learn its rational enjoyment in a ritual setting.

Occupation is important. People in the liquor industry are highly at risk as are people in jobs where alcohol is used as a 'business lubricant'.

The same is true for people where tension and competition are easily soothed by a quick drink.

In 19th Century England alcoholism was obviously linked to severe *poverty*. This is hardly true now, in fact there is a bias towards higher incidence of and deaths from alcoholism in Social Class 1.

Suicide Numerous reports reiterate the correlation between alcoholism and suicide, Kessel (1965) showed this quite clearly in the UK, Batchelor (1954) found 21% of 200 consecutive admissions for attempted suicide in Scotland to be alcoholics. Similar findings were reported by Ringel and Rotter (1957) in Vienna and Saarenheimo (1952) found 25% of autopsies on suicides to be alcoholics.

Criminality There are definite links between alcohol and crime. In the USA Wolfgang (1968) found that in 600 murders only 36% was there no evidence of alcoholism in victim or assailant. The general impression of a link between alcohol and violence is beyond question. As regards theft the main links are with petty theft, *e.g.* by a penniless skid row drinker and not with competent skilful criminality.

Road accidents Despite the claims of those who drive better when they've 'had a few' the plain facts are that alcohol decreases driving skills and leads to accidents and fatality. Plymar (1955) found a 20% incidence of alcohol abuse in fatal accidents in California in 1951. Other general findings indicate a 50% implication of alcohol in road accidents after 10 p.m.

Actually the links between suicide, violence and road fatality with alcohol are really beyond question except by those who are determinedly blind to the realities of the situation.

Psychiatric syndromes associated with alcoholism

There are a number of clearly defined psychiatric syndromes associated with alcoholism. Delirium tremens, a state of disorganised confused overactivity, usually follows a prolonged drinking bout and is, perhaps the most well known. Wernicke's encephalopathy and the Korsakov psychosis are both related to thiamine deficiency in alcoholism. In the former a confusional state is complicated by oculomotor paralyses and in the latter the main manifestations are severe disorientation for time and place, gross amnesia for recent events and a tendency to confabulate answers (it is also associated with an alcoholic peripheral neuropathy). Alcoholic hallucinosis is a rare psychosis which occurs in certain alcoholics and is characterised by the occurrence of auditory hallucinations and paranoid content, in a setting of clear consciousness. This psychosis is causally related to prolonged alcohol use: it clears with abstinence. Paranoid states occur in alcoholics, and when they occur it is common to find delusions involving sexual jealousy. These may be related to the loss of sexual potency in the alcoholic ('brewer's droop'). Marchiafava's disease is a rapidly fatal form of alcoholic intoxication with demyelination of the medial part of the corpus callosum. Alcoholic dementia is an alcoholic specific dementia and like all dementias is characterised by progressive irreversible intellectual impairment.

Treatment

The treatment of the alcoholic patient starts once the diagnosis is made. Alcoholism, when recognised, commits the physician to a treatment programme which has total abstention as the main goal. The first step is to investigate fully the physical and mental status of the patient so as to treat any existing physical or psychiatric complications. For this, admission to hospital may be necessary not only for 'drying out', but also for the evaluation and treatment of impaired liver function, vitamin deficiency, diabetes and chronic bronchitis, all treatable, not irreversible conditions. In addition the specific psychiatric syndromes mentioned above will need hospital treatment. These complications, physical and psychological, are rare and their absence should not prevent the making of the diagnosis, for they are, on the whole, late events in the natural history of alcoholism. After assessment and 'drying out', it is necessary to find methods of encouraging abstention. In the case of alcoholism which is secondary to some underlying psychiatric illness, *e.g.* depression, the expectation is that treatment of the underlying disorder will relieve the alcoholic dependence. Unhappily, this is not quite the case. Too often what appears to be 'symptomatic' alcoholism is not, or if it started out as such, the process has somehow become autonomous. Thus in practice, treatment of alcoholism means treatment of a chronic and relapsing disorder. In many cases alcoholism may be related to personality disorder but this does not account for all cases without stretching to absurdity the meaning of the term 'personality disorder'. Traditional individual and group psychotherapy are of little value in alcoholism. Sedatives are to be avoided and tranquillisers used only in withdrawal. Antidepressants should be used if depression is present. Suicidal risk should always be considered, suicide is more common in alcoholics than in non-alcoholics.

Admission to specialised hospital units is of value where the patient meets the selective admission criteria of the unit concerned. In many of these the better motivated patients respond to a vigorous group atmosphere which is positive and optimistic, no matter what idiosyncratic techniques may be applied. But many alcoholics may show poor or ill-sustained motivation. They show a high relapse rate. And for this reason pharmacological aids such as disulfuram are employed. These drugs cause distress, often severe, if the taker drinks alcohol and are often effective where all else has failed. They should be offered to all alcoholics.

All alcoholics should be offered membership of Alcoholics Anonymous (AA). This organisation, founded by two ex-alcoholics in America, has given help to a vast number of alcoholics: probably much more than that available from 'official' treatment sources. It is founded on self-help and acknowledgement of disability. The AA member can count on help at any time from other members and AA meetings combine *esprit de corps* with commitment in the face of a shared problem. Perhaps the basic statement about the treatment of the alcoholic patient is that each is likely to present a long term problem in which continued support may be the baseline though more esoteric approaches may be tried. For the severely recidivist alcoholic who faces repeated prison sentences and social dereliction, many feel that treatment is impossible, but current experience suggests that even the most grotesque derelict can improve in a well-run hostel.

13

Mental subnormality

People who are found to have 'arrested or incomplete' mental development from birth are usually described as being mentally subnormal. Their fundamental defect is one of intelligence. However, they usually have other degrees of psychological and social handicap which may be accompanied by physical disabilities, often severe. It is important to be aware of the many problems and difficulties that may upset the subnormal patient. Failure to recognise this from the start can result in the subnormal missing out on the detailed attention, advice and treatment which he and his relatives need. This awareness of the complexity of the problems of subnormality has led to a more hopeful attitude in management and treatment.

However, it should be realised that although intellectual deficit is the basic handicap of the mentally subnormal, this does not mean that the problems of the mentally subnormal are exclusively the concern of psychiatrists, psychologists or teachers. The basic problems of their care and education are social and almost entirely determined by the attitudes of society. If society regards them as hopeless individuals unable to compete in an assertive culture then they are likely to receive custodial care, something that has occurred since the 19th Century and which has become intensified in the 20th Century when the less bright are automatically disadvantaged alongside their more quick-witted and competent fellows. Oddly enough this is yet another historical accident which started in the mid 19th Century when important influences in Europe and America favoured education as a solution to diverse social problems. Before then

L

the mentally subnormal had been regarded as freakish victims of malign fate as jesters in the Middle Ages and later as objects of persecution. But the more liberal climate of the early 19th Century encouraged an optimistic educational attitude towards them. Unhappily the educational attempts failed and so the mentally subnormal were herded into institutions aimed at their education and ended up as people caught up in a system that provided custodial care, often of poor or bad quality. They were looked after by doctors who were assigned the role of specialists in mental subnormality as a result of a series of arbitrary administrative accidents. By the beginning of the 20th Century mental subnormality hospitals were warehouses and little else.

Intelligence

An acceptable working definition of intelligence is that it is a general ability which enables the individual to learn from experience, form judgements, handle concepts and modify behaviour. Intelligence is not regarded as a fixed unvarying entity but as something modifiable by environment, *i.e.* by education and favourable upbringing. Also it appears that the extent to which people utilise their intelligence is influenced by their level of motivation, emotional stability and maturity.

Experimental evidence suggests that intelligence is multifactorial, that is to say a general level of ability subsumes certain special abilities all of which correlate highly with each other.

Measurement of intelligence

Tests have been devised which are tests of ability. They are standardised for large populations and are reliable, *i.e.* when repeated on the same person give the same answer, and valid, *i.e.* measure what they are meant to measure.

Intelligence quotient (IQ)

This is a numerical way of expressing the level of intelligence. Originally the IQ was estimated by the calculation

$$\frac{\text{Mental age}}{\text{Chronological age}} \times 100$$

since the first attempts to measure intelligence (Binet) took as their unit of measurement the mental age, *i.e.* the average level of ability that could be predicted for given age groups. It will be realised therefore that to a large extent the IQ may be an unreliable figure.

At the present time the measurement of intelligence is based on estimations of the deviations from the mean scores obtained by individuals in the same age groups as the person being tested. Tests are standardised by being given to a representative sample of a population, stratified by age. For any given age group, the mean score obtained is given an arbitrary value of 100, *i.e.* the average IQ is assumed to be 100, and the standard deviation of IQ levels is set at 15 points.

In this way, when the distribution of IQs is plotted it is found that, like the distribution of stature, the curve approximates to the so called 'normal' distribution. That is to say the majority of cases cluster around the mean, and cases which differ markedly from the mean are comparatively rare.

Using a standardised intelligence test, approximately one-half of the population will score between 90 and 110 points and about two-thirds between 85 and 115 points. Of the population 95% will have IQs between 70 and 130, *i.e* two standard deviations either side of the mean.

On the whole lower intelligence is rather more common than high intelligence or put in statistical terms the curve is negatively skewed. This suggests that while the majority of individuals of low intelligence are normal variants, there are a certain proportion whose intellectual defect arises as a result of disease, injury or metabolic disturbance.

However, it has to be recognised that since the IQ is to a large extent an arbitrary score, it is difficult to be precise about the true distribution of intelligence. With this in mind it can be seen that the intelligence quotient, particularly when the figure is low can be very misleading without a total appreciation of the psychological and social characteristics of the person being examined. The estimation of subnormality of intelligence is therefore made by measuring the IQ. At present the cut off points are that subnormality of intelligence is said to exist if the IQ is below 70 points and severe subnormality if the IQ is below 50 points.

However, the position is made somewhat more difficult by the Mental Health Act which defines both subnormality and severe subnormality without reference to psychometry.

In the Mental Health Act the subnormal are defined as persons suffering from a 'state of arrested or incomplete development of mind (not amounting to severe subnormality) which includes subnormality of intelligence and is of a nature or degree which requires or is susceptible to medical treatment or other special care or training of the patient'. This attempt at categorisation would include those patients formerly described as 'feeble minded'.

The severely subnormal are defined as persons suffering from a 'state of arrested or incomplete development of mind which includes subnormality of intelligence and is of such a nature or degree that the patient is incapable of living an independent life or of guarding himself against serious exploitation, or will be so incapable when of an age to do so'. This description includes patients who would formerly have been described as 'idiots' or 'imbeciles', in addition to the lower grades of those patients formerly termed 'feeble minded'.

Having said all this we are left with the fact that official definitions such as the Mental Health Act are fairly unhelpful in any consideration of the problems of the mentally handicapped beyond purely administrative considerations.

Though severe subnormality is officially diagnosed if the IQ is below 50 this applies only to a small proportion of the population. Children who are handicapped to this extent are unlikely ever to be able to work except in a highly sheltered environment. Of the total population around 3% are found to have IQs below 70, and about 3 per 1000 to have an IQ below 50. This means that the numbers of the severely mentally handicapped are small, but the modestly handicapped, *i.e.* 70 to 90 IQ are considerably greater and represent an important group for whom a good deal more can be done in terms of education and training than is generally realised. In the case of these mildly handicapped patients social factors are often as important as genetic or organic factors in causation (Birch *et al*, 1970) as opposed to the severely subnormal, most of whom have organic brain damage. The severely subnormal are more prone to psychosis, fits and behaviour disturbance in general (Rutter *et al*, 1971). However, the mildly subnormal present an entirely different set of social, clinical and educational problems.

Many subnormal patients are otherwise 'normal' people whose intelligence is in the extreme low ranges of the frequency distribution curve. Others, however, are individuals of potentially higher intelligence who have experienced brain damage. The latter would include those affected by rubella in the first 3 months of fetal life or head injury or encephalitis in infancy. Others include individuals with genetically determined metabolic disorders which inhibit normal brain development and function.

On the other hand there are individuals who are subnormal by reason of intellectual, emotional or social deprivation in early life. A child reared in a brutalising atmosphere is likely to score many points lower on IQ tests than another child of equal ability coming from a more favourable home. It should be remembered too that limited intelligence does not mean that the patient lacks commonsense. Clinical experience of interviewing the subnormal patient constantly reaffirms this fact.

In addition to all this subnormal patients are commonly weighed down by other handicaps such as poor vision or deafness which prevent them from making the most effective use of their available intelligence. Disturbances such as epilepsy or birth induced cerebral palsy are common and provide further handicap. Subnormal patients are often, but not always, emotionally as well as intellectually immature. Also the severely subnormal often has a dysplastic physique with a small brain and head and may display hyperkinetic syndromes in childhood.

Aetiology of mental subnormality

Some idea of the growth of clearer understanding of the range of causes of mental subnormality may be gathered from the fact that while in 1954 a standard textbook of psychiatry listed 8 syndromes of known aetiology, by 1968 another standard text was able to list over 45. This is probably a reflection of the enormous impetus to research into mental subnormality that has followed the diffuse influence of the realisation that the mentally subnormal had been neglected and the specific influence of key discoveries such as that of Lejeune (1959) who showed that Down's syndrome (mongolism) was associated with 47 chromosomes, instead of the normal 46. This stimulated interest in cytogenetic research into subnormality. Interest in inborn metabolic errors was stimulated by the discovery of phenylketonuria (PKU). Mental subnormality caused by inherited metabolic disorders is said to comprise less than 4% of the total population of the mentally subnormal, but this is in the light of presently available information. Better understanding of cytogenetics and cerebral enzyme systems may reveal further inherited disorders as yet unsuspected. The first metabolic disorder to be discovered as a cause of subnormality was *phenylketonuria*.

Phenylketonuria (phenylpyruvic oligophrenia) (PKU) is a disorder transmitted by autosomal recessive inheritance and is caused by a deficiency of the enzyme phenylalanine hydroxylase which normally converts phenylalanine to tyrosine. This deficiency leads not only to a raised blood phenylalanine and a corresponding urinary excretion of phenylpyruvic acid but also defective cerebral biochemistry usually resulting in severe mental handicap. The majority of patients have EEG abnormalities and around 30% have fits. Motor and coordinative symptoms are common as are restricted growth and speech disorders. Treatment is based on screening using urinary testing to detect phenylpyruvic acid. And the treatment consists of a diet free of phenylalanine. The best results are achieved if the condition is detected within 6 months of birth. The basic importance of phenylketonuria from a brain biochemistry point of view is that it causes a deficiency of tryptophan which is a precursor of 5-HT (serotonin), a known central transmitting substance, possibly implicated in schizophrenia and certainly implicated in severe depression such as is caused by reserpine. This suggests, but does not exactly reveal the way in which brain function is impeded.

Disturbances of protein metabolism causing subnormality include phenylketonuria, as already described and other rare conditions *all characterised by aminoaciduria*. They include *Hartnup disease*, transmitted by autosomal recessive inheritance. Often symptoms vary and may present in adolescence with personality change since symptoms can be mild. The basic manifestations include a pellagrinous rash, cerebellar symptoms and subnormality. The metabolic deficit involves tryptophan metabolism. *Maple sugar disease* is caused by defective metabolism of leucine, isoleucine and valine, all of which are excreted in the urine, producing a characteristic odour. Autosomal recessive inheritance is the mode of transmission and symptoms come on early with fits and organic deterioration. Dietary treatment, *i.e.* restricting the amino acids involved, is used and the results are said to be promising.

Other much rarer inherited metabolic defects involving protein metabolism include histidinaemia, citrullinuria, argininosuccinic aciduria, hyperglycinaemia, homocystinuria and others. Their importance lies in their recognition by chromatographic screening of urine and blood and in the fact that recognition of one such rarity may lead to another and suggest further lines of research.

Carbohydrate disturbances include *galactosaemia,* transmitted by autosomal recessive inheritance. The basic deficiency is the absence of the enzyme galactose 1 phosphate uridyl-transferase. The onset comes on with milk feeding and may be rapidly fatal or lead to severe subnormality, hepatic failure and fits. Dietary treatment started early, prevents the disorder developing, hence the importance of early recognition. *Von Gierke's disease*, a glycogen storage disease, transmitted by autosomal recessive inheritance, is characterised by generalised glycogen deposits, hepato-megaly, fits and subnormality. Other inherited disorders of carbohydrate metabolism include *hypoglycaemia, fructose intolerance* and *sucrosuria*.

Disorders of lipoid metabolism include cerebromacular degenerations—Tay Sach's disease, this is transmitted by autosomal recessive inheritance. The onset is early with weakness, failure to thrive, spasticity and macular degeneration (cherry red spot). The basic defect consists in the accumula-tion of lipids (gangliosides) in neurones. There are a number of clinical types, the disorder is chiefly found in Eastern European Jews. *Niemann Pick's disease*, again autosomal recessive inheritance, is found mainly in Jews and consists in sphingomyelin storage caused by enzyme deficiency, *Gaucher's disease* is caused by failure of the enzyme that acts on glucocere-broside.

Progressive leucoencephalopathies include *Schilder's disease* and *Merzbacher Pelizaeus disease*. Other metabolic causes include *cretinism, hypoparathyroidism, idiopathic hypercalcaemia, Hurler's disease*, caused by accumulation of mucopolysaccharides, and *Wilson's disease*. But it should be emphasised that these are all *rare* and depend for recognition on *aware-ness of family history* and *proper screening*.

Chromosomal abnormalities leading to subnormality

Down's syndrome

In 1887 Langdon-Down described a syndrome of mental handicap associ-ated with various physical abnormalities and a supposed resemblance to members of the Mongol race. This was a mistake and gave rise to dis-content with the use of the term. The preferred name is now *Down's syndrome*. The incidence is approximately 1 in 600 births which makes it a relatively common type of mental handicap, the majority of those affected being severely subnormal. Patients tend to have a characteristic appearance with a 'typical' face—brachycephaly, short neck, epicanthic folds on the medial aspect of the eyes, short fingers, transverse tongue fissures, congenital heart lesions. In fact over 100 associated physical abnormalities have now been described.

In 1959 Lejeune, Gauthier and Turpin demonstrated the presence of an extra chromosome in Down's syndrome (47 instead of 46). The extra chromosome provided 3 at 21 instead of 2, hence the name *Trisomy 21*. This opened up a whole new field of research into cytogenetics and mental subnormality.

It is now generally agreed that there are at least three variants of Down's syndrome. The first is *Trisomy 21* as originally described by Lejeune *et al*.

This is the commonest variety of the syndrome and is accounted for by *non-disjunction* of unknown aetiology. The second variety is caused by *translocation*, with fusion of chromosomes 15 and 21. This is an inherited disorder, an important point when prognosis is under discussion. The third type 'partial Down's syndrome' is probably caused by chromosomal *mosaicism, i.e.* a mixture of trisomy and normal autosomes.

Other autosomal trisomic conditions and defects are also described these include:

Trisomy 13/15 (Patau's syndrome) There is severe subnormality, limited survival, scalp defects, polydactyly, narrow temples, septal defects, hypertelorism and epilepsy.

Trisomy 17/18 (Edward's syndrome) There is severe subnormality, micrognathia, hypertelorism, flexion of fingers, diaphragmatic hernia, kidney abnormalities.

Cri du chat This syndrome is caused by partial deletion of 5 chromosome. Severe subnormality is associated with many congenital defects and a characteristic cry likened to a kitten or a seagull.

Other cytogenetic abnormalities associated with mental handicap include sex linked disorders such as:

Klinefelter's syndrome The genetic constitution is XXY although XXXY, and mosaics of XX and XXY have been described.

The usual clinical picture is of testicular atrophy, girlish voice, tall angular build and gynaecomastia, usually recognised at adolescence. The syndrome is perfectly compatible with normal intelligence but *subnormality* can and does occur. Psychiatric problems are not surprisingly common in this syndrome.

Turner's syndrome Here the genetic sex constitution is XO and the syndrome includes dwarfism, webbing of the neck, ovarian agenesis and cubitus valgus. Mental subnormality is usually mild, normal intelligence is more common however.

The XYY syndrome This is associated with tall stature, mild subnormality and delinquent behaviour.

Other known types of mental subnormality associated with genetic inheritance include *microcephaly, tuberose sclerosis,* a triad of epilepsy, adenoma sebaceum and subnormality associated with renal and cardiac tumours. There are rarities also such as the *Sturge-Weber syndrome* with haemangiomata of face, retinal vascular abnormalities and cerebral calcification and the *Lawrence-Moon Biedl syndrome* where there is pituitary dysfunction, polydactyly, retinitis pigmentosa and subnormality.

But at the end of this list of known genetic causes *we are left with the fact* that once external causes such as maternal infection, especially *rubella, syphilis, anoxia, malnutrition* and *trauma,* have been excluded the *mass of the mentally retarded are normal variants* and that the recognition of handicap may occur at a wide range on the child's time scale.

For example the newborn may give rise to suspected subnormality because of small size, failure to thrive and fits. In practice, unless the baby has associated gross abnormalities, subnormality is unlikely to be detected in the first year of life. Poor progress in childhood is something that may raise suspicion, there again if the child has a biochemically identifiable lesion then the diagnosis is confirmed; otherwise it will depend on overall assessment of its abilities in *all* directions and will be largely determined as a case for investigation by the expectations of the family concerned. Failure of the development of speech is probably *one of the commonest presenting complaints.* Poor school progress comes later as a symptom to be evaluated. Kirman (1958) listed the times of appearance of the first symptom in 233 mentally handicapped children from birth to 48 months. They included physical features (61), eye defect (29), slow (43), not sitting (34), not walking (16) as opposed to much less common things, *e.g.* cerebral palsy (6), not crawling (2), destructive (1). In the first 5 years of life the child needs the fullest possible assessment by doctor, psychologist and social worker in order to establish the extent of the handicap.

The family of the subnormal patient

The handicaps of the mentally subnormal, as have been mentioned do not end with intellectual deficit. Many authors, especially Rutter (1972) and Rutter *et al* (1970) have pointed out that in the subnormal there is a higher incidence of neurosis, personality disorder, antisocial behaviour and developmental disorders. Also rare disorders such as hyperkinesis and infantile psychosis are more common in retarded children but they are not typical, *i.e.* peculiar to retarded children in whom there can occur a hetero-geneous distribution of psychiatric disturbance and behaviour problems. Rutter (1972) also emphasises that deviant behaviour is more common in children of average intelligence than in those of superior intelligence and more frequent in those of lower IQ than in those of average IQ.

Rutter relates the psychological disadvantages more to brain *mal-function* than to *lost* function and emphasises the importance of the adverse influences of social rejection, institutional treatment and adverse effects of medication. If we add to this the limited educational attainments and communication problems of the retarded child the spectrum of potential and real psychological disadvantage becomes complete. The management of the problems of subnormality is then a complex procedure which must always take into account not only the identification of special syndromes and the management of associated physical handicap but also the emotional, social and cultural disadvantages that may hinder his attaining the best possible level of achievement. And it is upon this sort of integrated approach to their problems that there rests the best prospects for at least adequate help for the problems of the subnormal and their families.

MANAGEMENT OF THE SUBNORMAL PATIENT

Children

Subnormal children develop better both from the point of view of intelligence and social ability if they spend their childhood with the family. Parents can accept the subnormal child as long as they are given sensible explanation and advice. It is vital to recognise that the parents may feel incompetent, helpless, resentful, frustrated, *i.e.* experience a wide variety of conflicting emotions when confronted with the realisation that the child is handicapped in this way. It is therefore particularly important that advice and support should be readily available when the abnormality is first recognised or when slow development is first suspected by either parent, doctor or health visitor. Full paediatric assessment is essential so that treatable metabolic disorders may be discovered. In addition sensory handicaps such as blindness or deafness should be recognised. And the problems of speech disorder, dyslexia and epilepsy may be recognised.

Educational requirements

The majority of children with IQs over 55 are 'educable' in that they will be able to learn the rudiments of reading and writing and attend schools run by their Education Authority. Those who are most backward in this group are classified as educationally subnormal and sent to special schools.

Children with IQs below 50 are excluded from school though the majority can benefit from education given in day training centres, run by the local authority. The majority of ESN school leavers manage to function as ordinary if somewhat limited people when they leave school and only a majority ever come to the notice of the local Mental Health Authority. Most of them settle down in time, find work, and present no great problem. A few may require institutional care which in every case should be on a voluntary basis to either residential home or hospital.

Severely subnormal children often make extremely good progress at day training centres and many achieve adult life able to work in sheltered surroundings. The most severely handicapped, and it must be emphasised that these are a minority, require to be fed and dressed and have long term care. After childhood, long stay hospital care will be necessary.

There are two definite indications for long term care of the subnormal or the severely subnormal individual away from home. They are:

1 Possibility of obtaining better education or treatment of a degree sufficient to outweigh the disadvantages of being away from home.
2 Where the patient's family is suffering from his presence in the home.

Thus it emerges that the criteria for admission to long stay hospitals for the mentally subnormal are largely social.

While it is true that a proportion of severely subnormal patients may require prolonged hospital care, it is increasingly realised that the basic needs of these patients are the same as those of their more generously endowed fellows, *i.e.* they need affection, warmth, social acceptance, education and employment. Given the right sort of environment any subnormal patient can find a more congenial and productive life in the community than he can in an institution. With this in mind day centres, occupational training centres and the like, are excellent examples of the sort of community orientated projects that foster enlightened care of such patients.

Subnormal patients can and do learn tasks that were previously supposed to be beyond their level of ability, providing that the teaching is carried out in a sensible patient way. Tasks may need to be broken down in various ways and the patient may need to learn via one sensory channel rather than by being given a variety of instructions all at the same time. Above all he needs a climate where failure is not penalised and where emotional outbursts are accepted with sympathy and understanding.

The family of the subnormal child need help if they are to keep him at home or if he has to go into hsopital. This help includes not only practical advice but also psychological support and understanding of the emotional problems posed by his very being. Guilt, resentment, anxiety, over-protection and denial are all common reactions and merit sensible accept-ance and free discussion between doctor and parents. This is one area where such communication can be of inestimable value.

In the past the mentally handicapped were described as 'idiots', 'imbeciles', and 'feeble minded', depending on their level of intellectual capacity as estimated by their degree of ability to look after themselves, attain any degree of independence etc. These terms are not and should not be used any longer since any meaning they may ever have had has been lost because of their continual use as pejorative terms. In the same way even the term 'mental subnormality', though given official recognition of its administrative usefulness in the Mental Health Act, is a term that carries an unnecessarily harsh tone, suggesting by implication something more than deficit based on psychometric assessment which is actually the only cut-off point that more or less arbitrarily separates the Nobel Prize winner from most of the population and from the 'mentally subnormal'.

Despite its great value, intelligence is not the only human attribute that gives colour to life and its lack does not disqualify someone from the right to a decent happy existence any more than having a high IQ would entitle someone to happiness, unlimited pleasure, a tax-free income and two or even three votes in the General Election. Intelligence is a human attribute to be used and valued but not to be worn as a badge of superiority as it too easily may be in a society that stresses achievement and material success as the ultimate in human experience. There are quite enough sources of human wretchedness and pain around without adding to them by classifying one group of people as inferior on the grounds of their place in a frequency distribution curve and herding them into situations of total or near total disadvantage.

In considering the various possible causes of subnormality it cannot be too strongly emphasised that the majority of cases are normal variants who form between 2·5 and 3% of all children and that the majority of such handicapped children have *mild defects* (Rutter, 1972) and that in their problems the aetiology is as *much social as biological* (Birch *et al*, 1970).

14

Disorders of childhood and adolescence

INTRODUCTION

It is not intended here to provide in any sense a comprehensive coverage of these topics since the psychiatry of childhood and adolescence is quite definitely a speciality of its own with an extensive literature. However, it is not possible to prepare any text on psychiatry without some reference to the general concepts of this branch of psychiatric practice. The difficulties of classification of disorders are here more perplexing. Obviously children whose handicap is one that is related basically to intellectual deficit occupy a special place of their own, as described in Chapter 13. However, it would be quite wrong to suppose that all children who appear to be intellectually dull necessarily are so. Such children's failure in performance may be attributable to emotional causes, to specific learning difficulties and also to disorders such as dyslexia.

The emotional difficulties of childhood, problems in relationships with parents and peers etc. have long been the subject of considerable interest in the field of child psychiatry and child guidance, and for many years it seemed as if children's psychiatric disorders were described in terms of emotional disturbances related to specific dynamic mechanisms. This rather simplistic view is no longer acceptable and its validity has been completely overshadowed by the finding of Rutter *et al* (1971) in their comprehensive survey of the physical and emotional development of children in the Isle of Wight. This work showed quite clearly that the 'disturbed child' in general has a high likelihood of associated parental

327

physical ill health, and in the case of the children it is poor physical health and disability often previously unrecognised including minor neurological defects and epilepsy.

Another important problem concerning classification is that children's symptoms do not occur in the same more easily recognisable clusters that are found in adult life, and in addition to this the various types of emotional problems and difficulties that they face vary fairly quickly with the passage of time, and also, their personalities are not established in any way since the child is maturing gradually towards an adult personality style. In addition to this there is disagreement about what constitutes the abnormal. Bedwetting, for instance, may be of little significance in a child of 3 or 4 but in an adolescent of 17 it is another matter altogether. In the past considerable attention was paid to behaviour such as thumb sucking or nail biting whilst it now appears from surveys in the child population these are hardly to be regarded as significant abnormalities at all.

However, some classification is needed: a relatively easy method is to list disorders *more or less related* to age whilst recognising that there may be considerable overlap.

CHILDHOOD

In childhood, *i.e.* up to 12, some of the most common disturbances apart from those related to epilepsy, specific learning defects and mental retardation, include disorders of *eating* and *excretion*.

Eating disorders

These include *refusal to eat* and *obesity*.

Refusal to eat

Children like food, whether from breast, bottle or plate. The baby is happy at the breast where he receives excellent nourishment, close bodily contact with mother and obvious stimuli associated with maternal care, in short a straightforward experience where feeding goes on in a positively reinforcing and enjoyable relationship. However, not all mothers *can* breast feed so bottle feeding is used. We need not make too much of this; anyone with any obstetric experience will have seen mothers made unhappy and exhausted by rigid overinsistence on breast feeding at all costs. Fortunately nowadays baby feeding has become a much more rational practice where the loving feeding of the baby is the object of the exercise. However, in the weaning period where the baby ceases to suck he then has to learn to feed in a way that is, emotionally speaking, more neutral. At this stage eating problems occur. Usually they are fairly straightforward and the baby learns to eat. In other cases, however, especially if the mother is herself a neurotic overdependent person, then the infant may refuse food, hold it in the mouth seemingly indefinitely or, worse still, vomit. This can then lead to a power struggle between mother and child that can be prolonged well into chilhood and may set the stage for later more severe syndromes such as anorexia nervosa.

Obesity

Obesity, which in adult life is associated with high degrees of morbidity and mortality, has now become a speciality in its own right. Contemporary evidence suggests that the obese child is one who has either been obliged to eat too much by over solicitous parents, the commonest type; or has come from a fat overeating family; or else has become podgy, the butt of his fellows and then overeaten to gain simple satisfaction in the face of his own depressed insecurity in the role of being a fatty in a society where slenderness is associated with energy, acquisitiveness and success and fatness equated with self-indulgence and sloth. And this is as true of the 10 year old fat boy as it is of the 30, 40 or 50 year old fat man.

Disorders of excretion/elimination

These tend to start at a later age where the reflex series of bowel/bladder evacuations are transferred from the casual demands of emptying into the napkin to fairly precisely defined and socially determined situations, first into the pot and then into the family bog. This fairly arbitrary change in behaviour however is not as precise as all that. Adults, even sober middle and upper class adults, sometimes urinate and defaecate in lay-bys, gardens or for that matter the street. The notion of regular unseen elimination has been reinforced by technology, building technology in particular. The Palace of Versailles after all was frequently befouled by the faeces of visitors, especially ladies who wore so much clothing that all they could do was evacuate bowel or bladder on the stairs. However, modern sanitation makes this unnecessary *and* undesirable; for humans that is. This is in sharp contrast to a society whose streets are fouled with animal excreta that contribute significantly to public health problems to an extent that has been only lately recognised.

In the child the two obvious elimination problems are *enuresis* (bed-wetting) and *encopresis* (faecal soiling).

Enuresis

Toilet training consists essentially of teaching the infant to learn to associate the stimulus sequence of pot/bottom with parental pleasure and a clean nappy. In learning bladder control the infant is faced with a harder task since bladder stimuli are often harder to perceive in sleep. One thing is certain and that is that fear and anxiety do cause unexpected bedwetting, *e.g.* a 10 year old boy, normally dry, was admitted to hospital after an accident. He wet the bed regularly in hospital and stopped as soon as he came home. This is a simple example as opposed to the cases where persistent bedwetting leads to all round family anxiety, concern and resentment. Simple causes such as infection (including worm infestation) and mental retardation need to be excluded and usually it emerges that the child is anxious and distressed, as are the parents. Reassurance all round is called for, the majority stop around puberty anyway and active treatment may include the use of antidepressants, such as amitriptyline, whose atropine-like side effects delay bladder emptying or else the use of conditioning methods, *i.e.* the pad and bell system where a bell is set off by wetting an electrical contact pad. The repetition of this experience causes the sufferer to awake if the bladder is sufficiently full. It should be remembered too that bedwetting can run in families, *e.g.* a 38 year old man became severely depressed and was treated with amitriptyline in the days when its side effects had not fully been appreciated. After 3 weeks he reported improvement but above all was delighted by the fact that he was now the only one of his adult 4 brothers who was dry at night. (A useful reminder too that nocturnal enuresis is more common in boys than in girls.)

Encopresis

This is defined as persistent faecal soiling beyond age 2. The investigation and treatment looks first of all towards simple causes such as cold, dank, dark and inaccessible lavatories as well as physiological rarities such as Hirschprung's disease.

Constipation may be caused by any of these, soiling occurs when the large bowel is overloaded and thus incontinent. Emotional factors *are* important. The child may have parents who are overfussy about regular bowel action as a sign of good health; or it may be found that their complaints of soiling are meaningless and based on their own overscrupulous obsessional concern with trivia.

However, *soiling does occur* and may be related not only to overrigid maternal insistence on child behaviour standards in all fields but also to the fact that the child may have learnt to use soiling as the only way in which he can show aggression. At all events the most useful treatment approach is to look carefully into the total picture and try to retrain the child's bowel habit in an atmosphere of calm good sense. The parents will need to understand how to learn to behave in a way that converts bowel evacuation into a normal and civilised activity like washing the face or brushing the teeth, and so will the child learn to empty the bowel without fear of punishment for mistiming nor eager anticipation of praise for a socially acceptable lump of faeces. Above all, everyone needs to learn that human survival does not depend on the daily passage of a 'well formed' stool and that there are considerable physiological variations in bowel habit. Some people defaecate once every 2 or 3 weeks and come to no harm at all. The medical profession has created bowel hypochondriasis and must not be surprised if its earliest manifestations occur in childhood.

ADOLESCENCE

Adolescent disturbances are more florid and more diverse. They come nearer to adult disorders, but being coloured by the intensity of adolescent experience and development they often present in a more dramatic and perplexing way.

Social withdrawal for instance is an important presenting symptom which may overlie disturbance ranging from fashionable adolescent discontent to a serious psychosis such as schizophrenia or the belated recognition of a syndrome such as *autism,* though the latter is usually recognised before the age of 12. Autism is the classical example of a *psychiatric syndrome* in that it is a term used to encompass defective social and interpersonal relationships from early childhood, speech disturbance and behaviour disturbance including impulsiveness, overactivity, repetitive behaviour and seeming unawareness or indifference to the environment—human or mechanical. It has long been a central issue in child psychiatry since the condition tended to be unrecognised, baffling and worst of all overlooked, since the autistic child tended to be included in the general categories of either psychosis or subnormality and end up as a long term inmate of an institution. Nowadays at least there is growing awareness of the special needs of the autistic youngster. The most important special needs are early recognition and adequate training and education towards comprehensible communication and easier relationships.

The aetiology is baffling though the rubric of autism may well cover a wide range of recognisable disorders varying from mental retardation to psychosis but always leaving a large group of children over whom rests the question mark ?psychotic ?cause. At least it can be said that child psychiatry has progressed far beyond the point when it was assumed that autistic children were always the offspring of neglectful, disdainful over-intellectualised 'refrigerator parents' who *made* their children autistic by lofty disregard and removing the inside door handles from their bedrooms. And yet we have to speculate about the effectiveness of parental hateful contempt of the infant in the aetiology of this very distressing condition. Present knowledge suggests a continuum of causes from brain damage and mental retardation to extreme parental rejection. Whatever may be the most important aetiological factor the barely concealed moralistic attitudes of psychiatrists and social workers about the rightness and wrongness of child rearing methods are never helpful.

The *withdrawn adolescent* always causes widespread concern, starting in the family and extending beyond it to school and/or job. This is possibly because in Western society people are expected to be outgoing, diverse in interest and activity and generally acceptable to the social group. Here we enter a delicate area since the varieties of acceptable social behaviour may easily be questioned. A surprising number of withdrawn adolescents turn out to have *depressive syndromes*. *Depression* is something that adolescents were supposed not to have, in fact they do. Often times it is related to real stress—fear of failure, fear of not being regarded as acceptable by peers of either real or fantasied sexual partners. Anxiety and neurotic disorders including hypochondriasis and obsessional problems can also cause the adolescent to seem either withdrawn or 'difficult'.

Adolescence can be and often is a time of stress and turmoil. Young people are subject to all sorts of pressure at this time of their lives. Normal adolescent development is a period during which strong emotions are easily aroused, emotions which the subject finds hard to channel. He is at an 'in between' stage of life where he is accorded neither adult nor childish status. He is often oversensitive and prickly, particularly about his appearance which is often gauche and pimply. It is hardly surprising then that emergent sexuality is tantalised by advertisements extolling the virtues of flawless skin or correct bust size.

The adolescent is full of doubts about himself—will he get the job?—the right sort of job?—will he get into a university?—is he going to be socially, sexually and in every other way competent when put to the test? All these sorts of questions are in his mind and it seems to him that everyone offers conflicting advice. In this setting he may develop anxiety symptoms. Often these symptoms lead to a near psychotic breakdown, sometimes mistakenly diagnosed as schizophrenia, which has been called the *adolescent crisis of identity*. This syndrome is really what the name suggests, a state in which the youngster becomes so uncertain of himself and his role that he breaks down into an overwhelming state of anxious uncertainty where contact with reality may apparently be lost. A good fictional description of this is to be found in the novel *Catcher in the Rye* by J. D. Salinger.

The adolescent crisis of indentity usually responds well to straightforward and sympathetic management. It is important that such patients are not mistakenly labelled as schizophrenic; on the other hand it has to be remembered that schizophrenia is a state which can and does begin in adolescence. But in schizophrenia the evidence for a more profound process should be sought for, personality change, thought disorder etc. (see schizophrenia).

Sources of anxiety in adolescence then are common; they may be social, personal or cultural. The symptom itself needs investigation and treatment since adolescence is a time of change and maturation. Sensible handling in adolescence may help the individual avoid chronicity of symptoms and the carry over of unresolved adolescent problems into adult life.

The *depressed adolescent* may present with mood disturbance, more commonly it appears he presents as a withdrawn apathetic youngster with suicidal feelings. Here it should be said, at the risk of seeming repetitious, that no suicidal remark, no matter how chance, lightly stated, nor seemingly trivial, should ever be ignored. The *schizophrenic* youngster, on the other hand, is often recognised rather late in the history of self-absorbed preoccupation with seemingly abstruse topics, day dreaming and odd eccentricity that are the common early symptoms of schizophrenia in adolescence—excluding, of course, fairly obvious *acute schizophrenic episodes.*

The diagnosis of schizophrenia is an important matter. On the one hand its early recognition and the start of vigorous treatment with pheno-thiazines should *it is hoped* prevent deterioration into chronicity. On the other hand, the too generous diagnosis of schizophrenia in young people may lead to disaster. Being labelled schizophrenic mistakenly can cause a youngster to lose the chance of employment, marriage and a whole series of life experiences that can only be summarised in the word misery. In fact for some it may be as effective as extermination by the administrative act of being apparently socially and ultimately excluded from the world of the acceptably sane.

School refusal is an important syndrome. It may arise in early childhood from a variety of causes. These may be obvious: an uncongenial scholastic ambience, playground bullies and the like, or it may develop because the child is neurotic and insecure or because the parent (commonly the mother) is herself a neurotic overdependent person who cannot bear to part with her equally overdependent child.

At its worst the syndrome becomes one of *school phobia* where the child is overwhelmed by anxiety at the threat of parting. *Truancy* is another matter consisting of a continuum of behaviour where truancy is normal, *i.e.* 'fine day' truancy to persistent truancy, one of the most important predictors of juvenile delinquency and later adult criminality. In *all cases* of school refusal an adequate assessment of the extent of the problem can only be made after the fullest examination of the school, the child and the parental and social background.

Aggressive behaviour in adolescents ranges from the truculent protest of near normal development to the impulsive aggression of the schizophrenic or the wilful destructiveness of the child who already has an impaired, ultimately badly damaged personality.

15

The psychiatrist in the general hospital

As psychiatry has moved further away from the mental hospital and more into the general hospital, so there are more requests for psychiatric opinion and advice. This has been noted by many (Crisp, 1968; Crown, 1973; Fleminger & Anstee, 1972) all of whom have commented on the fact that these referrals go beyond mere requests for clinical advice and that they are increasingly concerned with liaison between psychiatrist and colleagues, often involving group work (Crown, 1973).

The patients include not merely more obviously distressed patients, *e.g.* following suicidal attempts etc., but an increasing number of patients who have physical disorders with associated psychiatric symptoms and patients with illnesses that are badly understood. The latter group are mainly illnesses that respond capriciously to conventional medical treatment so that psychological aetiology is suspected—often called 'psychosomatic' though as Lader (1972) has noted, this term has many limitations. Finally there are those patients whose illnesses are intractable and are therefore supposed to have some unspecified psychiatric aetiology. It may be useful to list these groups with fairly typical examples.

1 Obviously distressed or disturbed: self-poisoning; states of excitement following surgery; myxoedema; myocardial infarct followed by depression
2 Physical disorders with associated psychiatric symptoms
3 Psychosomatic disorders: duodenal ulcer; asthma; ulcerative colitis
4 Disorders where psychiatric aetiology is suspected, rarely proved: atypical facial pain; migraine; cystitis

The first two groups are in a sense self-evident and can be properly evaluated and treated by sensible cooperation between the disciplines involved. The third group, psychosomatic disorders is more difficult and certain general aspects of psychosomatic disorders will be reviewed.

PSYCHOSOMATIC DISORDERS

Psychosomatic medicine is a term that should probably be dropped, since if it means anything at all it means the practice of medicine which acknowledges the interplay of many factors, physical and emotional, as causes and aggravators of disease which seems a long winded way of saying medicine. On the other hand the term psychosomatic *is* used to describe a diverse group of illnesses such as asthma, duodenal ulcer, and ulcerative colitis but has been extended to include coronary artery disease and rheumatoid arthritis. Much research has shown the importance of emotion in illnesses formerly thought to have an unknown physical cause but as Lader (1972) has pointed out, labelling an illness as 'psychosomatic' may be unhelpful since it implies that other illnesses are not so to be regarded, and this may divert proper attention from them. The other disadvantage of the term is that it suggests an unacceptable dichotomy between mind and body. There must be few illnesses where the emotions play no part.

The doubts about the usefulness of the term 'psychosomatic' are nowadays perhaps offset by the fact that in general doctors are more aware of emotional factors in disease. The awakening of interest in psychosomatic medicine in the 1950s was probably a reaction to the real neglect of the emotional influences in illness which had occurred with the real scientific revolution in medicine of the past 60 years. Nowadays scientific medicine and better understanding of metabolism is taken almost for granted. Medical and surgical technology have produced great improvements in the public health. It is hardly surprising that emotional factors were overlooked and large areas of illness are still badly understood.

History, as usual is helpful, the Ancient Greeks had a sensible regard for the interplay of causes epitomised in Socrates' comment 'As it is not proper to cure the eyes without the head, nor the head without the body, so neither is it proper to cure the body without the soul'. But as we have seen the good sense of this was lost in the Middle Ages, neglected by physicians in the Renaissance and in the 19th Century was obscured by the revelations of cellular pathology, *i.e.* if the disease is not in the cell there is no disease.

Interest in emotional aspects was awakened when neurologists such as Charcot began to study hysteria, reinforced by Freud's observations on the dynamics of hysteria, an illness where paralysis could be caused by emotional conflict. This was a novel idea at the time, greeted with derision, even vilification.

Much of the research on psychosomatic disorder has been influenced by Franz Alexander who introduced the idea that physiological changes accompanying emotional distress or conflict could be regarded as specific for some highly vulnerable people. He also observed that stressful experiences could evoke conflict which would evoke anxiety and a pathological physiological response. From Alexander's basic theory of psychosomatic illness other theories arose—many concerned with the organ or system involved, *e.g.* why does one person develop asthma and another duodenal ulcer? Other psychosomatic theories were influenced by pronouncements about symptoms and their meaning, thus vomiting in pregnancy signified rejection of the maternal role, diarrhoea could be caused either by letting out feeling or being unable to hold it back.

At the present time the basic model of psychophysiological disorder, *i.e.* a stimulus evoking stress, in turn leading to central nervous arousal with physiological accompaniments leading to symptoms, has been linked to three main hypotheses:

1 Alexander: stress produces unconscious conflict and regression to immature responses causing specific disorders
2 Mahl: the response is non-specific and is not linked to any specific stress and is the outcome of chronic anxiety, organ selection being determined by organ vulnerability
3 Lacey: the symptom response is specific but related to the internal arousal pattern rather than the stimulus.

The question remains unanswered as to whether psychophysiological symptoms are causally determined by specific emotional conflicts or whether certain people have a constitutional predisposition to react to stress by developing psychophysiological disturbances.

Cardiovascular disease

The effect of the emotions on the heart is so well known as to be almost axiomatic—quite apart from the ancient and still prevalent myths about the heart being the seat of the emotions. 'My heart stood still, my heart missed a beat, my heart nearly stopped when I heard the news, you're breaking my heart'—these are all well known phrases with the immediacy of colloquial language and are unlikely to be abandoned. Everyone knows what they mean, in fact they have a clarity which must seem enviable to many who have tried to elucidate the pathophysiology of the emotions.

In anxiety states tachycardia is a common symptom; similarly a person who gets paroxysms of tachycardia notices it and feels anxious and apprehensive.

A feeling of the force of the rapidly beating heart, palpitation is a common symptom of anxiety and one which causes a good deal of distress to patients. The same is true of extrasystoles which can occur in anxiety and also is a common symptom in heavy smokers and people who drink too much coffee or tea. Such symptoms are frightening and often interpreted by people as symptoms of organic heart disease and as such need to be the subject of very positive reassurance by the physician. In the case of extrasystoles caused by tobacco and caffeine, here again simple advice and reassurance should be given since 'give up smoking' is after all one of the most useful pieces of advice that any physician can give to any patient.

Uncomfortable sensations and pains in the chest may be both the cause of anxiety and apprehension in a patient as well as a symptom of anxiety and as such merits careful investigation and positive advice and reassurrance. Effort angina is a very frightening symptom and requires to be clarified.

The clinical features of effort angina have been clearly described in medical texts and authoritatively by Rose and Blackburn (1968). The wider aspects of angina have been reported by Tibblin *et al* (1972). They examined a random sample of men born in 1919 who were asked 30 questions about bodily and psychological symptoms. The men in question were part of a study aimed at screening for the development of myocardial infarction. Five hundred and seventeen subjects were divided into two groups (systolic blood pressure above and below 175) and they found a great difference between those who had angina and those who did not. In a word the angina group had twice as many *symptoms* as the other group. The symptoms were diverse and included joint pain, backache, visual disturbance, headache, indigestion, diarrhoea, dyspnoea, chest pain, poor concentration, depression, tearfulness and tiredness etc. On the other hand when hypertensive patients without angina were compared there was considerable difference in symptom reporting.

Anginal patients get more symptoms in general than straight forward hypertensives. The authors suggest that anginal patients may in fact be people with different perceptions of bodily discomfort than others. Whatever the real significance is it is clear that angina is more than an isolated symptom, is not easily understood but it is above all a symptom of immense psychophysiological significance.

Myocardial infarction

There is an enormous literature on the psychological aspects of myocardial infarction, the most recent review being that of Jenkins (1971) who summarised 160 papers. Much of the literature has dealt with premorbid personality and social aspects of the coronary patient. The general picture that emerges is of a man of young or middle age who is above all competitive, overcommitted to work, overpunctual, tense and overconscientious. General factors of neuroticism and anxiety are also common.

Others have commented that a coronary infarct often follows unexpected threatening changes in life style—rejection and loss of status being quoted as examples (Heijningen, 1966). Bereavement as a factor in coronary disease has been commented on by Parkes (1969) who found a 40% higher rate than expected of heart disease in widowers. No one can be certain as to *how* the emotions affect coronary disease but it is clear that they do. Finally the psychiatrist should always be aware of the real incidence of depression following coronary disease. Coronaries are frightening and the depression that may follow should not be as it were taken for granted but given adequate and sympathetic treatment.

Gastrointestinal disorders

Everyone knows that worry upsets the stomach and the gut. The experience of being sick with apprehension or having diarrhoea before an examination or an interview is familiar to the medical student and the doctor, but their certainty is not so easily shared by researchers into psychophysiology who have not been able to find absolute causal relationships between stress and disease even though ordinary emotional stimuli are reflected in the gastrointestinal tract.

Peptic ulcer

Though the aetiology of peptic ulcer is in general uncertain, one fact is certain, namely that its incidence in women is declining in Western society. In general duodenal ulcer is more common in men than in women in the ratio of 4:1. Duodenal ulcer tends to be associated with hyperacidity while gastric ulcer is associated with near normal gastric secretion. Psychic factors are said to be more important in duodenal ulcer than in gastric ulcer, but overall the incidence of both conditions is falling off, especially in women. The emotional aspects of peptic ulceration have been most intensively studied with regard to duodenal ulcer and these studies have produced little conclusive in terms of specific emotional states or personality types that could be regarded as firm evidence of causation. The most that can be said is that in states of 'stress', certain vulnerable people develop duodenal ulcer or if they have one it gets more troublesome.

These conditions of stress include general social and environmental pressure, the best known recent example being the high incidence of duodenal ulcer in bomber aircrew in World War II.

Psychodynamic formulations of the aetiology of duodenal ulcer have related it to conflict between dependency and independency needs, and its relationship to the frustration of oral gratification in early infancy. Other workers have related its fall in women to the changed status of women in a society which permits women easier modes of dealing with aggressive feelings. The summary of psychological findings in the aetiology of duodenal ulcer is that it may be associated with a dependent personality, poorly able to deal with his own internal aggression, resentment and frustration. However these findings can only be considered in the light of the poorly understood physiology of the stomach and duodenum.

In practice it is true that ulcer sufferers are often tense and anxious and that their ulcers fail to heal unless they are calmer. Often they are patients whose work makes their pain and tension worse, and unless they can come to terms with this, the healing of the ulcer is delayed. Another simple piece of advice is to encourage the duodenal ulcer patient to give up smoking.

Ulcerative colitis

Patients with ulcerative colitis have probably been victimised more by the quaint absurdities of the 'psychosomatic' approach than any other group of patients. We have been asked to believe that an obsessional personality, a strained mother ('unhappy, overactive, perfectionistic, martyred') and a life where special situations cause diarrhoea are entirely responsible for a condition that affects the entire colon, is associated with iritis and ankylosing spondylitis. This is in total defiance of the most important point about the uveitis–colitis–arthritis syndrome, namely its unquestionable genetic inheritance. Ulcerative colitis is an unhappy example of a disease that has sometimes led to nasty bullying of patients by doctors and nurses who take a dislike to a patient and justify their dislike on the basis of rather trivial research findings based on simplistic evaluation of equivocal data. A good example of the sad fact that patients who do not get better make doctors and nurses behave in an angry way and tell the patient that it is his fault that he is no better etc. These comments require elaboration. They relate to the author's clinical experience at a time when the stereotyped psychosomatic view of ulcerative colitis was that it was a disorder associated with a fussy, pedantic and rather unpleasant personality, and an equally unpleasant mother. This unjustified assumption was made the excuse for strikingly unkind treatment of patients.

Munchausen syndrome

This term was coined by Asher (1951) to describe patients with a history of repeated hospital admissions, often involving abdominal symptoms such as renal colic or '?pancreatitis' or obscure abdominal pain in whom the management of the disorder is made near impossible by the fact that the patient may simulate symptoms and more often than not become uncooperative and truculent when doubts are expressed about the 'genuineness' of their symptoms. The various cases that have been described contain a high proportion of patients who have undergone repeated laparotomy quite apart from extensive investigations and, as might be suspected, they are likely to be people with highly abnormal personalities. It seems that they become 'hospital dependent' in the sense that they are driven to obtain repeated admission to hospital in an unrelenting way. The syndrome is commoner than is thought and creates great problems in management. Blackwell (1965) in reviewing the syndrome in 10 patients seen in Guy's Hospital stressed its relatively frequent occurrence, its prevalence in men and the great determination to be admitted that such patients show. And related its pathogenesis to psychopathic personality, an abnormal desire to be ill and the importance of precipitating events—all comments with which few would disagree.

The importance of early recognition of such cases cannot be over-emphasised since once the pattern is started each new admission reinforces it and a prolonged sequence of investigation is established. The reaction caused by such patients calls for tolerance usually badly strained by the belligerence of the patient. For this reason it is wise to avoid public confrontations with the patient where he is unmasked and reviled, this only makes matters worse.

A typical example was a 50 year old man admitted following self-poisoning. He was found unconscious in an invalid motor tricycle. The ward sister was suspicious of his liking for pethidine and he was transferred to a psychiatric hospital where his history was pieced together. Twelve years before he developed severe headaches, thought to be sub-arachnoid haemorrhage. Thereafter he had over one hundred admissions to hospitals and neurosurgical units and developed a hysterical paralysis of the left leg with contractures ending up with amputation at the hip. He said quite definitely that over the years he had learnt to simulate headache in such a way as to lead to repeated AEGs, ventriculography etc. and of course once the chain of investigation was commenced it was inevitably repeated. He was a good example of Blackwell's observation that it is important always to try to discuss the patient's symptoms in a quiet interview and avoid 'scenes'. Where the patient is sufficiently disturbed it may be justifiable to detain him in hospital under S25 of the Mental Health Act in order to clarify the history. Asher's original description was colourful and to the point but the term 'Munchausen Syndrome' may ultimately be counter-productive by encouraging doctors always to regard such patients as tiresome psychopaths to be got out of the way as quickly as possible. It is better to try to contain such patients in the long term but it is conceded that to date no one seems to have been successful in so doing.

Anorexia nervosa

Anorexia nervosa is the term applied to a syndrome of eating disturbance, anorexia, weight loss and amenorrhoea. It was first described in 1868 by William Gull. Although it was formerly held to be peculiar to young women rare cases are found in young men.

It will be noticed that the definition above refers to 'eating disturbance and anorexia'—the reason for this is that many 'anorexic' patients have a normal, even an excessive appetite but the point about the patients is their refusal to eat even though they may be hungry. In fact episodic gorging and severe weight gain is a common antecedent in these patients whose central disturbance is a fear of being fat and gaining weight.

Amenorrhoea and lanugo hair, usually cited as diagnostic, are of course secondary to starvation. The amenorrhoea is caused by altered FSH secretion and oestrogen secretion, well known features of straight-forward starvation.

The syndrome is commonest in young girls though middle aged women may develop it, *e.g.* 42 year old woman was admitted for investigation of amenorrhoea, 56 lb weight loss and food refusal. She had a history of a similar episode at age 18, lasting for 2 years but had been in full remission until 2 years before admission since when she had consistently refused food, lost weight and developed depressed mood. In fact she turned out to have a depressive state which responded well to appropriate treatment, nevertheless her 2 year 'relapse' was remarkable in that whilst refusing food she had become obsessively concerned with the feeding of her family to the extent that her husband was 58 lb overweight and was refused life insurance and her children were overfed and overweight, as was the family dog which was so fat that it could barely walk; the family parakeet was similarly affected and sat fatly in its cage barely able to chirp.

This is an unusual example but a good example of the point that anorexia nervosa is probably *not* a unitary disorder. Some 'anorexics' turn out to be schizophrenics, others depressives, and others obsessionals, but the remainder are a group of patients of whom the most that can be said is that they are thin and refuse to eat. Speculation about psychodynamics has covered the relationship with either or both parents, rejection of the feminine role, problems in sexual identity etc. but in fact in many cases it is near impossible to say exactly why the condition has developed. Or this is how it seemed until it was pointed out that there is a significantly high incidence of body image disturbance in anorexic patients. The disturbance is one in which the patient sees herself as much bigger and fatter than she really is and this idea is held on to with conviction. To date this is the most impressive psychological finding, far out stripping earlier speculations about relations with parents, rejection of female sexuality etc., *e.g.* a 22 year old girl had been anorexic for 6 years. Psychotherapy and supervised feeding had failed to get her to a satisfactory weight. Her stated fear was 'I'll be like an elephant'. She was repeatedly tense and suicidal and underwent bimedial leucotomy. She gained weight but became obese and killed herself in a fit of angry self-disgust.

Treatment

The treatment is directed at restoring lost weight and to this end supervised feeding backed up by chlorpromazine and support remain the basis of treatment (Dally & Sargant, 1966). If depression or psychosis are relevant factors these are treated secundem artem but the majority of cases are non-specific except for the body image disturbance, no doubt reinforced by the peer group pressures of a society that equates beauty with slimness—a factor which is probably relevant in the apparent increased incidence of the condition. The mortality is high, up to 4%, so hospital admission is essential. Behaviour therapy has been tried with limited success. Recent work suggests operant conditioning as a good way of gaining weight quickly. Here the patient is asked to devise a list of desired goals after admission to a bare cheerless room. Achievement of the goals is contingent upon eating meals in a specified time (Bhanji & Thompson, 1974).

Whatever means are used to regain lost weight, all are agreed that relapses are common and follow-up difficult.

Puerperal psychosis and psychiatric disturbance

There is a large literature on puerperal psychosis but as Protheroe (1969) has commented 'most of it is incomplete in that rarely is any definition of the puerperal period made; frequently there is no attempt to differentiate between the various clinical syndromes seen when aetiology is considered, and little consideration is given to the extent of constitutional predisposition to psychiatric illness in the probands'. This is a very fair summing up of some of the difficulties that still surround the concept of 'puerperal psychosis'. For some time there has been disagreement as to whether the word puerperal should be used in an aetiological sense or whether it means 'occurring in the puerperium'. The present position in the UK at any rate is that in general, psychoses occurring in the puerperium are regarded as psychoses which should be capable of being classified either as affective, schizophrenic or organic. In other words occurrence in the puerperium is either coincidental or else has precipitated the psychoses in the same way that a major event such as a surgical operation might do.

The term therefore does not imply causality in the sense that childbirth is supposed to be specially provocative of psychiatric disorder either as a physiological and psychological event.

As has been pointed out by many authors (Mayer Gross *et al*, 1969; Engelhard, 1912) the puerperium is a time of psychological and physiological disturbance in which in fact the incidence of psychosis is lower than is predicted. This observation may be true for frank psychosis but the work of Pitt (1970) for instance has shown the prevalence of often unrecognised affective disorder passed off as normal 'blues'.

However psychoses do occur in the puerperium and their current status has been reviewed by Protheroe (1969) in a long term study covering the years 1927 to 1961. Case records of all patients who in that period had developed puerperal psychoses and had been admitted to St. Nicholas Hospital, Newcastle upon Tyne were investigated. Only those cases were included where the onset of the psychoses was within 6 weeks of labour.

The objects of the study were 4-fold—to look for possible changes in natural history of these disorders, to look for other psychiatric disturbances in the patients involved and in their first degree relatives, and to try and clarify the whole concept of puerperal psychosis and its general treatment.

A total of 134 cases were found to be acceptable for the study; three diagnoses were used, affective psychoses, schizophrenia or organic psychoses. The author found no evidence of change in the average age of onset (28·3 years). The study was divided into two periods: pre and post 1942. In the pre 1942 period 14% were unmarried as opposed to 2·25% after 1942. Of the whole group 66% developed a first puerperal psychosis after the first pregnancy. There was a preponderance of affective disorders (91) as opposed to schizophrenic (37) and organic (6). The author noted that this was in line with Hemphill (1952) who had also noted a preponderance of affective psychoses as opposed to others who claimed puerperal schizophrenics were becoming most common. He also noted the common finding of 'clouding of consciousness'.

Of the group 28% had had obstetric complications but these were on the whole not serious and throughout the series there was no evidence of any particular psychological trauma. This is actually quite an important observation since the psychoanalytic literature has laid great stress on the relevance of psychological trauma to puerperal disorders.

Only two of the pre 1942 patients (52) received any treatment and 25%

M

died in hospital from malnutrition and untreated infection. There had been only one death since 1942.

The most important treatment related finding was that physical methods of treatment had reduced the average period of admission from 8 months to 2·4 months for affective disorders and from 4 years to 3·8 months for schizophrenics.

The follow-up of the series traced 114 patients of whom one had been in hospital since 1941 and of the remaining 113, 104 were traced. The general finding was that the affective patients had on the whole made better progress than schizophrenic patients—two-thirds of whom had fared relatively badly, though 50% of the schizophrenic group who were discharged were in fact well as opposed to 86% of the affective group who were well.

Genetic studies were carried out on 98 of the patients and first degree relatives and these showed that the risk of psychosis amongst parents and sibs was no higher than for relatives of non-puerperal psychotics. The author drew the general conclusion from the study that there is no specific 'peurperal psychosis' on the basis of the clinical features of the illness, predisposition to non-puerperal illness and family history of mental illness.

Thus the term puerperal psychosis can probably be regarded as having the same significance as the term postoperative psychosis. Perhaps one of the most important features of the study is that physical treatment emerges as the most important factor which can be related to the much better outcome in the cases in the post 1942 era.

General clinical observations

From the above and other studies (Martin, 1958; Seager, 1960) the general clinical picture emerges of acute psychosis coming on within 6 weeks of labour. The psychosis may be affective, schizophrenic or organic and consciousness is often clouded.

The delusional content is related to the baby, *i.e.* someone has substituted another, or to the father. The diagnosis is unclear at first, no doubt because of the acute onset and seemingly mixed clinical picture. However in the affective and schizophrenic cases there is nearly always an excellent response to ECT and in the rare organic psychoses there should be a good response to proper treatment of the underlying infection plus the judicious use of psychotropic medication. Also it should be noted that puerperal psychosis is likely to occur in someone under stress, and the stress includes insomnia. Most mothers of new born babies do not get enough sleep. Other factors not helping the situation are blood loss, dehydration following excitement and food refusal plus a general feeling of anxiety and expectancy and instability of mood often found in mothers soon after childbirth.

In fact one is left with the general impression that psychoses in the puerperium are less common than one expected. Minor affective disorders in the puerperium are another matter altogether.

Suicide and attempted suicide

Suicide is a threatening and tragic event which distresses family and society alike. To quote Sainsbury (1972) '. . . it mystifies and disturbs us. Suicide also affronts society; opting out with such apparent scorn is seen as a vote of no confidence in the social order.' The personal causes of suicide though linked to physical and psychiatric illness are to some extent over-shadowed by growing emphasis on its relevance as an antisocial act. In this country attempted suicide was a criminal offence until 1961, it was an unforgiveable sin for the theologian and a seriously irresponsible breach of the mores of society.

The epidemiology of suicide and attempted suicide is important particularly as they involve different populations. Suicide is more common in older men whilst attempted suicide is more common in younger women. There is a growing store of information about both topics and it will be reviewed later. First a historical note, Judaism and Christianity were, and are, strongly against suicide as sinful and intolerable behaviour, on the other hand, Ancient Rome and Greece tolerated it. Nowadays though sanctions on suicide are more relaxed, popular opinion views it badly though contemporary philosophers, particularly the existentialists, regard it as a valid option for anyone to take up as a matter of responsible personal choice.

The sociologist Emile Durkheim (1900) was the first to look at suicide as a social phenomenon. He described three types of suicide: *egoistic, anomic* and *altruistic*.

Egoistic suicide is the suicide of a person who has never been a member of any cohesive social group. *Anomic suicide* is the act of someone who has become disaffected and alienated from his own culture, its needs, obligations and services. The term 'anomie' was coined by Durkheim to describe a state of rootless drifting taken up by someone who opts out, cuts himself off from customary activities or is forced into alienation by retirement etc. *Altruistic suicide* stems from the need to atone for the betrayal of the values of a social group—for example suicide by Old Style Prussian Army Officers rather than facing the consequences of cowardice or breach of a rigid code of behaviour.

Suicide

The suicide rate varies in different countries but tends to stay the same within individual countries, in England and Wales it is around 5000 per year and there are at least eight times as many attempts. There are a number of general observations about suicide, *e.g.* suicide rates vary inversely with homicide rates, and suicide is apparently less common in Roman Catholic countries.

Stengel pointed out that suicide correlates with

1 Male sex
2 Old age
3 Widowed, single and divorced state
4 Living alone in densely populated areas
5 Periods of personal or general economic hardship
6 Alcohol abuse
7 Psychiatric disorder
8 Membership of social classes I and II

as opposed to the general correlates of attempted suicide which include

1 Female sex
2 Relative youth (ages 15 to 35)
3 Living in overcrowded homes and bad social conditions (Kessel, 1961)
4 Poor work record
5 Drug abuse
6 Personality disorder and associated criminality
7 Poor health and neuroticism
8 Higher incidence in social classes IV and V

In the past 10 years the suicide rate has fallen. This has suggested to some that community services are more effective while others (Malleson, 1973) see the fall as related to the wider use of less toxic domestic gas. National suicide rates have been criticised by Douglas (1967) who regards official records as unrepresentative and misleading. This observation has been challenged by Sainsbury (1972) in a general review of suicide, dissenting from Douglas' view that official records are so inaccurate that they invalidate any research based on them since national definitions of suicide vary and coroner's records may be inaccurate.

Sainsbury and Barraclough (1968) examined Douglas' criticism and set up a simple experiment proposing that if the definition of and reporting of suicide were held constant and national suicide rates were found to be predictable then supposed deficiencies of definition and reporting could be irrelevant. They looked at the suicide rates of immigrants in America and compared them with the rates in their own countries of origin. They found the rank order of rates to be nearly identical, furthermore they found the same when they examined suicide rates in immigrants in Australia. They next looked at coroner's reports, reasoning that if coroner's reports were as unreliable as had been suggested by Douglas then suicide rates in certain areas should vary with a change in coroner. The suicides reported by coroners in 1950 and 1960 were recorded and repeated in a study of areas where the coroner had changed. Areas with high suicide rates remained so regardless of the coroner. Thus they concluded that neither national definitions nor coroner's practice affected regional suicide rates. Sainsbury (1973) has noted the changes in suicide rates in England and Wales since 1900, particularly the falls in both World Wars and the peak in the 1930 depression. Since 1900 there has been a general rise in suicide by men. Sainsbury stressed the importance of the following factors in the aetiology of suicide:

1 Psychiatric illness—identified in 93% of suicides studied by Sainsbury
2 Social precipitants—including moving house
3 Personal crises, particularly bereavement
4 Personality disorder particularly when associated with alcoholism, drug abuse and criminality

The clinical importance of this is that psychiatric disorders particularly depression should be recognised and treated and thus suicides might be prevented.

Suicidal feelings in the general population have been studied by Paykel *et al* (1974) who referred to previously frequently quoted studies such as those of Dublin (1963) on successful suicide and those on attempted suicide (Schneidman & Farberow, 1961; Mintz, 1964; Parkin & Stengel, 1965). He pointed out that there has been so far very little in the way of enquiries into the frequency of suicidal feelings in the general population. They interviewed 725 people in the general population and found that 8·9% reported 'suicidal feelings of some degree in the past year'. Such people tended to have minor psychiatric symptoms, *e.g. mild* depression, and were usually socially isolated with no cultural or religious ties and had to a lesser extent experienced recent life stresses and physical illness. This is a valuable study since it contributes facts to current speculation about the roots of suicide.

Psychiatric aspects of suicide and attempted suicide

There are a number of psychiatric symptoms and associated factors that are important warning signs of suicide, they can be listed quite simply as follows:

1 Depressive states, particularly where there is guilt and self-deprecatory feeling. Hypochondriasis and agitation are also bad signs.
2 Suicidal talk and thoughts. It is wrong to suppose that people who talk of suicide never kill themselves. Over 90% of successful suicides give clear indications of intent.
3 History of previous attempts and family history of suicide.
4 Persistent early waking and nightmares in depression.
5 Associated physical illness, alcohol and drug abuse.
6 Social factors such as unemployment and living with an unsympathetic family, in association with depression.
7 Suicide does occur in schizophrenia and personality disorder, in the former it tends to be impulsive—in the latter almost a chance occurrence in a sequence of personal disasters.
8 The suicide rate is higher in mental hospital patients than in the general population.

In England and Wales the suicide rates are higher in professional and managerial people (social classes I and II) also there has been a discrepant rise in suicide amongst university students.

Kessel (1965) has been among the first to review attempted suicide and has noted that the growth rate of 'attempted suicide' cases. Their apparent lack of suicidal intent entitles the behaviour to be re-named 'self-poisoning' particularly since overdosage is the preferred method. The Kessel 1965 study involved all cases admitted for self-poisoning to the Edinburgh Royal Infirmary. This covered 465 cases (151 men, 314 women) in 522 admissions. The general findings suggested a correlation with bad living conditions and overcrowding. Age specific rates differed between the sexes with high rates in teenage girls, though female and male rates were the same from age 50.

There was a high incidence of divorced men, and poor marital relationships covering infidelity, gambling, jealousy and debt. Major precipitating factors were tabulated (Table 15.1)

Table 15.1 Precipitating factors in suicide.

	Males (n = 165) %	Females (n = 350) %
Marital disharmony	68	60
Problem drinking	51	16
Money troubles	44	31
No job	34	18
Trouble with family	28	30
Housing problems	14	19

Diagnosis

Kessel found that conventional psychiatric diagnoses hardly applied to this mixed bag of unhappy people—depression tended to be mild and more common in women, as opposed to the men who had a significantly high incidence of personality disorders (see Table 15.2).

Table 15.2 Psychiatric diagnosis.

	Male (n = 165) %	Female (n = 350) %
Organic cerebral syndromes	5	4
Depression	26	43
Other psychoses	5	5
Other neuroses	5	12
Personality disorder	32	16
No psychiatric illness	26	20

The most important finding here was 'no psychiatric illness' in 26% (male) and 20% (female), this meant that psychiatrists were unable to detect *any* evidence of psychiatric disorder. Depression was more often than not linked to personality disorder overlapping with 'dysphoria' and 20% of the total series had seriously risked their lives.

Motivations for self-poisoning were diverse but Kessel pointed out one repeated finding, namely the insensitive husband who failed to notice his wife's need for support. In 23% of cases, no motive could be found, the act was impulsive. Kessel concluded that the term 'self-poisoning' is preferable to 'suicidal attempt' since the vast majority of these cases have no suicidal intent. He also noted that the risk of danger to life bears no relation to the need for psychiatric treatment. The study highlights the importance of assessing self-poisoning without prejudice and using a multidisciplinary approach in all cases.

Conclusion

Suicide and self-poisoning are important subjects where accurate data is now available. The collection of facts about these subjects may ultimately contribute to prevention. There *is* a difference between suicide and attempted suicide but this difference is not absolute—attempted suicide neither predicates nor prevents successful suicide. Doctors can contribute to prevention by simple means, first by learning to recognise depression and trying to treat it and secondly by being careful in prescribing sedatives and tranquillisers.

Aphasia

The psychiatric problems of aphasia have been reviewed by Benson (1973) who mentions that the simplest definition of aphasia is that it is 'loss or impairment of language caused by brain damage' and goes on to remind psychiatrists of their diffidence about its recognition and investigation. Benson's review of the psychiatric aspects of aphasia is timely and relevant. He notes that the main areas that concern the psychiatrist are diagnosis, specific psychiatric manifestations of aphasia and the psychiatric aspects of aphasia therapy.

Diagnosis

Benson (1973) points out that proper differentiation of aphasia from psychiatric syndromes is most usefully accomplished by the use of simple language tests which encompass the following.

1 Conversational speech
2 Ability to understand the spoken word
3 Ability to repeat
4 Naming objects
5 Ability to read and write

More formal testing is reviewed by Benson and Geschwind (1971) Goodglass and Kaplan (1972).

Specific psychiatric manifestations as noted by Benson range from under-standable anger and frustration at the inability to communicate to the real depressive states that often follow the prolonged obstructive despair that may overwhelm the aphasic patient.

The *catastrophic reaction* as discussed by Goldstein is an important complication, no doubt a global expression of frustrated futility and anxious anger at the limitations of the awful handicap of not being able to speak.

Normal people have no idea of how bad this must be, perhaps the nearest to it they ever get is in those nightmares where the dreamer knows what is going on, knows that something ghastly is imminent but cannot make anyone else understand it. Ordinary speech is greeted with blank incomprehension. Multiply this by 100 and we might appreciate the sub-jective distress of the aphasic patient.

Sometimes the aphasic patient appears much less aware of his disability, this is fair enough and no doubt related to more extensive parietal lobe damage. Practical aspects of aphasia can assume high degrees of import-ance, especially when the patient is involved in making a will, giving power of attorney to relatives, etc. There are no simple guidelines here. The most important thing is that each patient should be most carefully examined and evaluated as to his ability to comprehend and convey meaning.

Therapy

As in so many psychiatric conditions the most important tactic is the use of *active optimistic support* on a one to one basis. Depressive states may need antidepressant medication and paranoid reactions may need neuroleptic medication, but whatever may be the extent of psychiatric symptoms endured by the aphasic patient, his best chance of feeling better, improving his speech and generally gaining the suspicion that he has not been thrown on the rubbish heap will always follow concerned compassionate sensible support; and whether this comes from a first class speech therapist (best option) or from a speech therapist and psychiatrist is, in a sense, irrelevant. The main thing is that aphasic people need support and massive encouragement because mostly aphasia is their most important disability while their intellect remains unimpaired. Unhappily too many people equate aphasia with dementia—a cruel mistake.

16

Psychiatric disorders
in old age

INTRODUCTION

However the figures are examined there is no doubt that the medical and psychiatric illnesses of old age are a major sociomedical problem in this country and that they are dealt with inadequately. Not only that, if present population and survival trends continue, the forecast is that by the latter end of the century 73·5% of male hospital beds and 93·7% of female hospital beds will be occupied by people over 65 (Klein Ashley, 1972). This forecast is a simple extrapolation and may be incorrect but it predicts an obvious trend and a trend which excludes psychiatric illness. All are agreed on the inadequacy of services for the elderly.

Ageing and death are unacceptable realities in a society that is overwhelmed by the attractiveness of youth, bases its needs on material gratification and is overinvolved in the pursuit of leisure, pleasure and sexuality. At the same time it excludes the elderly from such treats on the rather parsimonious view that old people are 'past it' in the capacity to work, enjoy human relationships and be happy.

Elderly patients are unwelcome in hospital units geared to high powered technology, short stay admission and recovery. In such hospital conditions old people are an embarrassing reminder that medical advances have mainly benefitted young people and whilst prolonging life have not to date improved the quality of life of the elderly. Too often the hospital care of the elderly is aimed at 'disposal', one of the nastier contemporary euphemisms for getting rid of the unwanted. Death and the decline of function in old age are met with denial, total denial. A simple example is enough—when someone dies in a hospital ward an elaborate charade is played out. The ward is screened off and the body is wheeled away. When the curtains are drawn the patients see an empty freshly made bed and no one mentions the event except for oblique references directed as glossing over the fact of death. Junior hospital doctors hardly dare admit the elderly for fear of blocking a bed or of offending a consultant who might be put out by the spectacle of general deterioration and smelly incontinence. And all this goes on in the face of the increase in the elderly population and its growing unmet needs for treatment, support and rehabilitation.

THE AGEING PROCESS

In middle and old age people become more stable emotionally in the sense that they are less obviously influenced by their feelings; the turbulence of youth and adolescence have passed, ambitions are either fulfilled or not. The person is left with the realisation that radical changes in the life style are pretty unlikely and depending on their capacity for acceptance and resilience they make a good or bad adjustment. Sexual drives are less urgent and become the subject of compromise. Thus people often speak vaguely, even hopefully of the 'serene sixties' when life should seem less demanding and when anxiety and uncertainty should be replaced by a sort of confidence and wisdom based on experience, leaving behind the frustrations of middle age when unfulfilled ambition and desire may lead to irritable discontent. But, it is not as simple as that. The revered status of the elderly has declined in Western society and the ageing person runs into special physical, emotional and social problems directly related to the ageing process.

Physical changes are important. Joints and skin lose their elasticity, eyesight is troublesome, the cardiovascular system is more at risk for vascular and ischaemic disease. Bones become more brittle, the person becomes weaker and often shaky, everything seems to be slowing up. This is often associated with an increased concern over bodily health; a hypochondriacal attitude based on real physical decline.

The emotional changes of ageing are largely related to the person's general level of emotional stability. The person who has always been stable, independent and better able to get on with other people is better equipped to cope with ageing than is the person who is neurotic, egocentric or asocial.

It is usually said that an *increased emotional rigidity* is the hall mark of ageing but this seems to have been exaggerated—rigid people become more rigid but this does not include everyone. Certainly people tend to be less adaptable as they grow older and this is in contrast to youth which is very much a time for learning and exploration. Also as they grow older people become less interested in the outside world and more absorbed in themselves and their family circle. *Retirement* is often a critical event, since it means not merely loss of earnings but also a considerable change in social role so that the person feels useless and unwanted—'thrown on the scrapheap' is a common enough phrase.

Memory disturbance becomes a problem since short term memory for newly learnt material is not as good as it was though this *does not* imply that the person is dementing. There is slowness in coping and an undue reliance on experience which comes across as a rigidity of attitude. The fear of approaching death inevitably does cause problems but here again there is evidence that it is much more important in neurotic and depressed old people than in the stable who are better able to adjust to it.

It seems that retirement may be more of a bogy than we have been led to believe (Lorge & Tuckman, 1953) since people may dread it and then adjust to it. However, loss of a spouse is another matter (Cumming & Henry, 1961), in fact, it is suggested by Cumming and Henry that retirement and widowing are most damaging in the sense that they cut off the person from a wider range of social contacts.

In summary then we can say that poor health, poverty and social isolation, especially in a previously neurotic or ill adjusted personality, constitute the major stresses of ageing.

PSYCHIATRIC DISORDERS

The psychiatry of old age has only begun to be studied in any depth in the last 20 to 25 years. Roth (1955) reviewed the natural history of mental disorder in old age at a time when the problems of ageing people were belatedly starting to receive attention. He pointed out that the traditional classifications of psychiatric disorder were unsatisfactory for old people, since the natural history of illnesses changes and may be affected by physical treatments.

Roth's paper then reviewed diagnosis and prognosis of psychiatric disorders in old age which had hitherto been something of a ragbag with senile psychosis as an undifferentiated illness in some way associated with ageing. He had found a diagnostic/prognostic difference between elderly patients with affective psychoses (two-thirds still alive after 2 to 3 years). A further group of 464 patients were studied, and were assigned to six diagnostic categories:

1 Affective psychosis—a mental illness in which primary symptoms were those of mood disturbance
2 Senile psychoses—illnesses characterised by a typical picture of organic cerebral deterioration
3 Late paraphrenia—a well systematised set of paranoid delusions, with or without auditory hallucinations with a previously sound personality and emotional stability
4 Arteriosclerotic psychoses—patients with either dementia and focal signs or symptoms or a dementing process associated with any of the following: emotional incontinence, fits and the preservation of insight
5 Acute confusion—any state of rapidly developing clouding of consciousness from whatever cause and occurring in the absence of dementia
6 Other disorders—an important hypothesis was that psychiatric disorders in old age which started with mood disturbance were distinct from degenerative cerebral disorders, hitherto it had been said that affective disorders in the elderly were usually the prodromata of dementia. Roth ignored minor apparent organic changes, *e.g.* memory and slight clouding where symptoms were predominantly affective on the basis that such minor symptoms would be misleading and not indicative of serious organic pathology and that the outcome of affective psychosis would be real indicators of the disease process.

Late paraphrenia was regarded as a psychosis starting late in life and similar to paraphrenia as described by Kraepelin. All of the cases except 14 were placed in the five main categories, the remainder were a mixed bag including GPI, tumours etc. In fact *affective psychoses* accounted for over 50% of the cases. There was a significant difference in outcome between affective and senile psychosis. *Late paraphrenia* emerged as a distinct entity by diagnosis and outcome and there was a significant difference in outcome between *acute confusion* and *senile* and *arteriosclerotic psychoses* which emerged as different entities by diagnosis and by outcome at 6 months, though at 2 years the difference was less obvious.

The importance of this particular study was that it was the first clear demonstration that *affective psychosis*, *late paraphrenia* and *acute confusion* in elderly people are all separate entities entirely independent of the commonest causes of progressive dementia, *i.e.* senile and arteriosclerotic dementia.

The epidemiology of senile dementia

This is an important topic since an increasingly ageing population and a static birth rate has led to a situation where the needs of the elderly can only be met when the needs are properly appreciated. A hundred years ago the psychiatric illnesses of old age were comparatively rare since people lived shorter lives, thus questions about 'senile psychosis' were mainly academic. Actually nowadays in the UK one might be pardoned for thinking that the questions of psychiatry in old age are still academic if one used expenditure and interest as markers. The elderly and their social and health care have provided problems that provoke interest and well meaning lip service but little more in terms of planning and comprehensive service except for isolated examples that provoke admiration but little in the way of emulation.

The first factual landmarks on senile dementia are fairly recent. Roth (1952) differentiated between senile dementia, arteriosclerotic dementia and functional psychoses in the elderly in terms of diagnosis and prognosis. Kay (1962) reviewed elderly patients admitted in Stockholm in between 1931 and 1937 followed up to 1956 and found a significant reduction in survival time for senile dementia, while Corsellis (1962), using Roth's diagnostic criteria, examined the brains of 300 mental hospital patients and found that the diagnosis of senile dementia was clearly related to cerebral pathology. In the UK, Malzberg (1963) examined first admissions for senile dementia in New York State between 1919–20 and 1941–51 and found that the crude admission rate had risen from 6·4 to 16·2 per 100 000 population. There was a clear sex difference, male admissions went up by 75% and female admissions by 85%—the increase was entirely in the over 70 age group. These findings are in opposition to earlier findings such as Gellerstedt (1932) and Rothschild (1937) who said that senile pathological changes were common to the whole elderly population and that senile dementia was an idiosyncratic reaction developed by damaged people. A detailed prevalence study of psychiatric disorders in the elderly carried out by Kay *et al* (1964) on a census sample of patients in institutions and of a random sample of patients at home, showed a much higher number of patients at home with senile dementia than previously suspected (Table 16.1)

Table 16.1   Total prevalence rates for psychiatric disorders per 1000 population aged 65 and over.

Disorder	Institutions	At home	Total
Senile and arteriosclerotic dementia	6·8	38·8	45·6
Other severe brain disorders	0·8	9·7	10·5
Manic depressive	0·7	12·9	13·6
Schizophrenia—chronic	0·2	9·7 ⎱	10·8
Paraphrenia—late onset	0·9	0 ⎰	
Neuroses and allied disorders	1·9	87·4	89·3

The preponderance of senile demented patients living at home is striking, at the same time the high prevalence rate of neuroses and allied disorders is important, it is too easily assumed that elderly people are immune to neuroses and liable to only develop organic psychiatric syndromes.

In addition to their prevalence studies Kay *et al* (1966) found that a follow-up on their 1964 patients showed mild senile memory impairment was a highly sensitive index of later death from senile dementia, thus mild memory loss in the elderly person is never insignificant.

Bergmann (1969) commented on the possibilities of finding the cause of senile dementia by epidemiological means. Larsson (1963) for instance had noted that isolated, single and childless people were more at risk whilst Kay *et al* (1964) found that age was the discriminating aetiological factor in senile dementia and that apparent social factors were consequences rather than causes. Genetic studies in senile dementia are not especially helpful, in fact it is hard to see how they could be helpful or relevant. Kallmann (1956) was moderately sceptical about the usefulness of twin studies while Larsson *et al* (1963) examined the records of 378 patients and 2675 relatives. They found a higher risk for senile dementia in relatives of senile dements (4·3 times higher risk in sibs of dements than risk in general population).

We are left with the plain fact that the aetiology of senile dementia is unknown.

Classification of psychiatric disorders

The problems of psychiatric classification have already been stated. In the case of the elderly patient the problems are much the same except in that the elderly the commonest serious psychiatric disorders are either affective or organic. Minor psychiatric disturbance is often overlooked or put down to 'being old'; this may be more true of minor mood disturbance than anything else.

Post (1965) classifies psychiatric disorders in old age into four groups:

1 Organic syndromes
2 Affective disorder
3 Paranoid syndromes
4 Personality disorders

This classification is straightforward, based on traditional diagnosis and covers the range of psychiatric disorders in elderly people.

Diagnosis of psychiatric disorders

Though we rely on history taking and examination to arrive at a diagnosis in the elderly patient, just as we do for any patient, it will be realised that special factors will need to be taken into account. Psychiatric diagnosis is, as has already been stressed, entirely a matter of assessing probabilities, usually based on rather unreliable data in the ordinary adult patient but in the elderly the information is usually more difficult to obtain, also many elderly patients have some *associated physical illness* which may colour the abnormal mental state or underly it entirely. The patient's *social status* is important. He may be living on his own, eating a restricted diet, even near to starvation. He is likely to be living an uncomfortable life, short of minor luxuries or may be existing in total squalor. And whatever the social circumstances may be he is at a stage of life where he has little to look forward to in the sense of material things and usually few surviving friends. The point need not be overstressed. Old age is a time of decline and loss of the independence to cope on one's own for the vast majority of people.

The basic personality needs to be taken into account too—the more stable and well adjusted the person, the better able is he to cope with the problems of ageing be they emotional, physical or social or, as is usually the case, all three. With all this in mind it is hardly surprising that there is often a good deal of overlap in diagnosis, the syndromes are likely to be less *clear cut* than in ordinary adult psychiatry. This should not lead to a state of diagnostic hopelessness, it is important to arrive at as detailed a diagnostic formulation as possible taking into account all the considerations already mentioned. It is bad medicine and bad psychiatry to regard old age as a passport to wretchedness that is beyond alleviation and barely worth investigating. This is borne out by the experience of physicians and psychiatrists who specialise in disorders of the elderly who have repeatedly shown that careful all round assessment of the patient can lead to the use of a range of measures that can bring impressive degrees of improvement and well being to the patient and his family.

Proper assessment then includes:

1 History taking
2 Assessment of physical and mental states.

History taking needs patience and commonsense awareness of the fact that the patient is often unable to give a full account of the history either through the normal failure of memory of old age or through organic memory disturbance, so that the history must always be amplified by another informant, relative, friend or neighbour. In the examination of the mental state it is important to examine the patient's cognitive functions carefully, especially memory and orientation. Here there should not be a rush to judge, especially in the patient newly admitted to hospital. The old person needs time to settle down and become familiar with new surroundings. One cannot expect the patient to reel off a brisk stream of answers to questions about the date, or answer a set of memory tests.

Post (1965) recommends a series of simple questionnaires about general orientation, past and recent personal events, general events and orientation in the ward and recommends that they are given to the patient 3 to 4 days after admission. And the same is true of an interview at an out-patient clinic. The patient will need time to settle down in an unfamiliar, often frightening situation, especially if he is aware of his failing faculties, is anxious to 'do his best' and may be afraid that he may be bundled into hospital. This is where domiciliary consultation is of great value, since the patient is on familiar ground. Old people cling to the familiar and are easily bewildered by change and easily and understandably react badly to bossy people in an out-patient clinic. It is too often assumed that merely because the elderly may display little outward show of feeling that therefore they *have* no feeling. This is an assumption that is as incorrect as it is gratuitously unkind. It may seem unnecessary to mention these relatively simple points but clinical experience repeatedly show that they are overlooked at all sorts of levels in dealing with elderly patients. Overworked junior doctors afraid of 'blocking beds' may react with impatience, and this carries over to other staff members hard pressed to get on with the day's routine in a busy hospital ward, and a vicious circle of unstated but implied rejection set up leading to the patient becoming clinically worse in every sense of the word. Reasons for hospital admission may be obscured since admission may be requested in a state of crisis—agitated or confused behaviour often overlies a real situation where the patient's family are no longer able to cope with him at home, but are unable to say so explicitly.

The diagnostic classification already outlined (*organic disorders; affective disorders; paranoid syndromes; personality disorders*) provides a coherent basis for assessment. It is not proposed to describe the syndromes in detail since these syndromes have been already described in general, but rather for the purposes of diagnosis it is possible to offer a number of basic comments.

Organic syndromes

These include the syndromes already described, *e.g.* acute and subacute delirious states and dementia.

The acute and subacute delirious states are common in the elderly. They may be set off by obvious or less obvious physical causes such as bronchopneumonia, myocardial disease, uraemia, urinary infection, in fact any disorder that can cause cerebral hypoxia or metabolic disturbance (*e.g.* myxoedema; pernicious anaemia). These are causes that should always be excluded as are alcohol and sedative intoxication and vitamin deficiency, fluctuating subacute states altering with apparent lucidity are often associated with a subdural haematoma. Finally after all these possibilities have been excluded it may be that when the acute organic picture clears, the patient is found to have residual organic defect caused by a dementia.

Dementia in old age is usually either senile dementia or arteriosclerotic. The first type comes on more slowly with memory loss as the first sign. In the second type onset is earlier and there is usually a history of strokes, apparent recovery and fits. Dementia in the elderly is only rarely caused by tumour or general paresis.

Affective disorders

Here depression is the most common form and tends to be named according to dominant clinical features; *agitated depression* where there is weeping and restless semi-purposive movements, *senile melancholia* where there is profound sadness and despair often associated with delusional ideas. *Depressive reactions* are common in old age. Post (1962) found 67 of 100 consecutively admitted elderly depressives fell into this category since onset followed bereavement, physical illness, children moving away etc. *Mania and hypomania* are rare but can occur, the latter may be missed especially if symptoms are mild. Post (1965) comments on *organic depression* noting the usefulness of the term to denote the coincidence of depression and organic cerebral disease. *Unrecognised depression* in elderly people does occur especially where the patient complains persistently of vague physical symptoms.

Paranoid syndromes include late onset schizophrenia, paranoid reactions, following isolation or sensory-less organic mental states with paranoid colouring, and paranoid reactions in abnormal personalities.

Personality disorders lead to difficulties either in relationships with others, asocial withdrawal and irritability, or to neurotic symptoms, obsessional symptoms etc. that may be intensified by the special status of being elderly.

Management of psychiatric disorders

In theory it should be possible to avoid hospital admission for elderly patients by adopting a number of relatively simple measures. Macmillan (1960) for instance has noted that many of the clinical problems presented by senile dementia are aggravated by family and social factors and has suggested ways of dealing with them that minimise symptoms and delay, even avoid admission. The story is a familiar one—a person begins to dement and the relatives look after him, however gradually they find the task extremely irksome. The patient by this stage may have become the subject of family strife since one set of relatives resents the inactivity of another set. Then a crisis occurs, the patient becomes noisy or gets lost and becomes incontinent. From then onwards the patient is totally rejected. Once in hospital or institution he has little chance of returning to a family that cannot tolerate him any longer. Macmillan and others have suggested that if help is given *early*, *i.e.* before a crisis and total rejection, then the patient can be supported in the community for a much longer time. To this end day hospital attendance, brief periods of admission to give relief to the family are used. All this is excellent advice but depends on early recognition, good care of the patient's physical health etc. and such a service is not easily provided except where general practitioners, health visitors and community psychiatric nurses work as a team.

Admission

If admission is needed it is usually because there is associated physical illness, or the patient lives alone, is suicidal or his behaviour is unmanageable at home.

Admission to a mental hospital is undesirable for patients with senile dementia, on the other hand residential places for elderly confused patients are in very short supply. Like it or not, mental hospital admission still carries a stigma. Once admitted, the patient's chances of improvement or recovery are directly related to the competence of the nursing staff. This is something to which the psychiatrist can contribute much by explanation and support to the staff group meetings where problems and feelings may be freely aired. This is probably most needed in homes for the elderly where psychiatric knowledge is usually scanty and the standards of care good in a physical sense but rather dreary (Townsend, 1962).

Activity and supervision are important. Many writers have stressed the importance of activity as a simple way not only of slowing down deterioration but in many instances apparently reversing it, since much of the 'deterioration' of an elderly patient may be due to apathy and loss of hope. Nurses need support in this job. Looking after elderly patients is not cheerful and the work is hard and unrewarding. People react to old people either by writing them off as horrible, or by overidentifying with them in a sentimental way. Both of these extremes are absurd but represent ways in which people protect themselves from the unacceptable.

Psychotropic drugs are useful in calming agitation and paranoid tension, *antidepressants* are valuable in depression as is *ECT*, especially in the agitated patient with delusional ideas. *Psychotherapy,* mainly in the form of understanding and support, is valuable—too many old people feel overlooked and forgotten, and it is too easy for the doctor to walk past them. *Commonsense* is invaluable too. The confused patient needs to be spoken to quietly and needs to be told (a) where he is and (b) who is talking to him, two simple manoeuvres often overlooked, which help the frightened confused patient to find a reference point in an alien situation.

17

Psychosexual disorders

INTRODUCTION

Although psychiatry has been for some time associated with the identification of and treatment of sexual disorders it is now for question as to how useful and effective may be the role of the 'traditional' psychiatrist. To understand this it is necessary to re-examine the way in which psychiatry came to be involved in sexual problems. From a theoretical and practical point of view we can say that it all started with Freud's observations on the role of sexual drives in the development of the human personality. His observations, however modestly stated, led to a general assumption that not only were sexual drives prime movers in the determination of human behaviour but that because this was apparently the case then it must follow that psychiatrists not only knew, as it were, all about sex but were capable of identifying and *treating* all varieties of sexual disorder.

This was all very well until people started trying to define 'normal' and 'abnormal' in sexual behaviour and worse than that trying to find out the extent of 'normal' and 'abnormal' sexual behaviour in the population. Until then many psychiatrists, serenely confident of the rightness of Freudian theory not only tried to cure homosexuals but had caused a good deal of unhappiness to women who had failed to achieve the 100 megaton vaginal orgasm which Freudian theory postulated as not only necessary but also as rather a bad show if the lady did not experience it. However these confident psychiatric, not to say male chauvinistic, assumptions were shattered by experimental workers such as Kinsey *et al* (1948, 1953) and

Masters and Johnston (1966, 1970) who found that not only was the much prized vaginal orgasm a rarity but that varieties and modes of sexual gratification in the population showed a wide range of practice which far exceeded the traditionally approved twice weekly marital coitus in the 'missionary' position.

The world was ready for this scientific announcement, after all, to date, no one had become blind or mad through masturbation so presumably the commonsense of people in general had guided them through the maze of sexual behaviour that had been prescribed for them by psychiatrists and sociologists. On the other hand there is a good deal of unhappiness and misery related to sexual problems and sexual dysfunction whether the problems are related to failure to live up to prescribed expectations or related to 'abnormal' behaviour as defined by society.

At this stage then we badly need a definition of normal and abnormal sexual behaviour. Unhappily no one has provided an entirely satisfactory one though Storr (1964) has provided commonsense guidelines with which few would quarrel—'We should all, for instance, concur in regarding a man whose sexual desire is directed exclusively towards small children as abnormal (a view which would almost certainly be shared by the man himself); and we should probably all agree that the exhibitionistic exposure of the genitals is a deviant way of obtaining sexual gratification— but there would be disagreement upon homosexuality, since there are some who vehemently condemn homosexual behaviour, whilst others look upon it as perfectly normal.' This simple comment suggests that perhaps we should divide sexual behaviour into normal (*i.e.* expected) and abnormal (*i.e.* unexpected) on the basis of the prevalence of sexual behaviour in a given culture. Even this may be influenced by quite simple culture bound rules, *e.g.* in prison, on expeditions etc. homosexual behaviour may be determined by the absence of a heterosexual partner.

Even basic guides such as the Bible are unhelpful, *e.g.* 'Onanism' is thought to be the same as masturbation yet Genesis 38.8 clearly describes onanism as coitus interruptus—'And Judah said unto Onan, Go in unto thy brother's wife and marry her, and raise up seed to thy brother. And Onan knew that the seed should not be his, and it came to pass, when he went in unto his brother's wife, that he spilled it on the ground, lest that he should give seed to his brother. And the thing which he did displeased the Lord; wherefore he slew him also.' An extreme punishment for early attempts at family planning and one which led to much of the rubbish that has been talked about, written about and preached about concerning the supposed ill effects of masturbation which onanism clearly is not!

Unfortunately for mankind this sort of *ex cathedra* pronouncement about what constitutes normal and abnormal sexual behaviour has persisted and has led to endless unnecessary guilt, shame and even suicide relating to fancied sexual misdemeanours (Stekel, 1929; 1930).

However, though we acknowledge the difficulties that surround the definition of normal and abnormal sexual behaviour—it is in fact not quite as difficult as all that—some sexual behaviour is *very* abnormal (*e.g.* attaining orgasm *only* after murder) whilst most sexual behaviour is rightly judged to be normal. Perhaps the most difficult problems in sexuality arise when people feel that their sexual performance is (a) below normal or (b) are told that it is by their sexual partner. This leads to the consideration of the commonest sexual problems which are *impotence* and *frigidity*.

Impotence

Impotence means the failure of the erect penis to sustain intercourse before both partners achieve orgasm. At the most extreme it means total failure to achieve erection. Between these two end points there lies a wide range of relative failure. The commonest cause of impotence is straightforward anxiety since the anxious penis is obliged to droop. The causes of such anxiety are varied, ranging from the excited impetuosity of the novice to the exhausted and hidden fears of the self-styled virtuoso. Some fail to sustain erection because they fear that sexual performance will be judged in the same way that examination failure is judged, others fail out of sheer funk at attainment of the seemingly impossible. In either case the person is the victim of poor education. Sexual performance is enjoyable, or should be, and is not an athletic contest but unhappily many people approach intercourse with textbook standards in mind and no sense of fun or enjoyment. This has arisen because many books about standard intercourse have caused both partners to expect total ecstasy every time and anything less as at least partial failure.

The *impotent male* should always be examined carefully to exclude endocrine and neurological causes (*e.g.* diabetes mellitus), but the majority of cases turn out to suffer from psychogenic impotence. The causes here range from anxiety based on ignorance to deep rooted personality problems involving unconscious hostility to women and latent homosexuality. The *treatment of impotence* is not a matter for *any* psychiatrist—

rather is it a problem that should be dealt with by either a psychiatrist with special experience in sexual disorders, or probably better still *a psychologist* with such special experience. The common causes of psychogenic impotence may be listed as follows:

1 Anxiety:
   a based on ignorance
   b based on fear
   c related to personality problems and conflicts

2 Hostility related to:
   a aggressive feelings towards women
   b homosexual conflict

3 Psychiatric syndromes including:
   a depression
   b schizophrenia

However *anxiety* is the commonest causal factor and the treatment of this depends on:

1 Full appreciation of the extent of the disorder
2 Dealing with the anxiety and impotence by:
   a psychotherapy
   b behaviour therapy

Psychotherapy in impotence has traditionally been regarded as the basic approach. In this the object is to diminish anxiety by giving the person insight, awareness of the psychogenesis of his impotence—all in a climate of confident, reasoning psychotherapeutic support. In fact it seems that this approach is less successful than a *behavioural approach* in which the sequence anxiety—impotence is viewed as a learned disorder which is amenable to treatment by deconditioning, *i.e.* the person learns how *not* to be impotent and how to be potent.

The pioneer in this type of therapy was Wolpe (1958) who first employed the technique of reciprocal inhibition in the treatment of impotence. In this the object is to remove all fear and anxiety from the sex act. The girl is encouraged to handle and fondle the inert flaccid penis in an unchallenging fashion, *i.e.* not 'Why aren't you hard?' but 'I like you soft or hard.' This reduces tension and gradually encourages the timorous penis to stand on its own feet as one might say and hey presto— intercourse occurs, orgasms all round and everyone is pleased. The point is that this rather simple treatment not only works but has led to even simpler approaches to the treatment of impotence including not only penile splints to bolster confidence but also mechanical devices which promote clitoral orgasm and thus also encourage the fearful penis to become erect.

Frigidity

Frigidity is the term applied to encompass lack of sexual desire and failure to achieve orgasm in the female. Probably the latter is the most common. It has been unfortunately the case that psychiatry has been responsible for a good deal of misery by proposing that the vaginal orgasm is the summit of female sex life. This is not borne out by the findings of experimental workers such as Masters and Johnson who have shown that orgasm is related mainly to clitoral stimulation. In fact to the dismay of many men it has been found that women frequently obtain the best orgasms from mechanical stimulation.

In the treatment of frigidity much the same principles apply as have been described in impotence. Above all the situation has to be freed from the tension, bitterness and recrimination that have usually gone before. Understanding and support are paramount and this is true whether or not behavioural techniques are used. Perhaps the most controversial approach in recent times have included the use of surrogate sexual partners who encourage the impotent male or frigid female gradually towards adequate enjoyment and performance. Oral sexual gratification such as fellatio and cunnilingus are important aids to intercourse and for some are substitute.

Homosexuality

Homosexuality is usually regarded as deviant sexual behaviour though in many respects it is not so. In the author's opinion it has no place in a textbook of psychiatry except in so far as it may be pedophilia, *i.e.* where children are the preferred object. Many homosexuals, both male and female, suffer a good deal of misery, shame, guilt, and depression related directly to the negative attitudes of society and for this reason their problems call for compassionate understanding, counselling and help. Similarly the *homosexual* who *asks* for help to change to a heterosexual orientation is entitled to help whether by psychotherapy or by the use of behavioural techniques. Finally a distinction should always be made between homosexuality and homosexual behaviour. The latter is usually dictated by circumstance, *i.e.* school, prison etc. and transient. Again the immature adolescent may go through periods of intense personal crisis related to fears of homosexuality, uncertainty about sexual role and identity. A condition that merits sensible psychotherapy and guidance.

Deviant sexual behaviour

Deviant sexual behaviour is mainly identified by choice of sexual partner and includes:

1 Pedophilia, where sexuality is directed towards children
2 Bestiality, where sexuality is directed towards animals
3 Necrophilia, where sexuality is directed towards the dead

It also includes *fetishism* where sexual gratification depends on the use of garments etc., *e.g.* rubber raincoats.

Sado-masochism involves sexual gratification which can be achieved only through inflicting pain (sadism) or enjoying it (masochism). A few moments conversation with any London prostitute will provide a mine of information about the extent of this and fetishism.

These range from the bizarre, *e.g.* the eccentric gentleman who required a prostitute to run round the room naked with ostrich feathers in her buttocks while he masturbated to the frankly grisly ritual involving plastic sheets, whips and paper clips on the customer's nipples.

Sexual behaviour then is wide in extent and runs to extremes but for the majority it *should* be an enjoyable treat and the medical profession should learn to encourage this and help to remove Puritanism from a loving experience.

18

Management of psychiatric disorders

Here we consider the whole question of treatment in psychiatry. 'Management' of psychiatric disorders is a term that is unacceptable to many, but chosen here because the term 'treatment' implies uncritical acceptance of a medical model of psychiatry. Management seems to meet the needs of the psychiatrist better since so much of his work involves social manipulation, persuasion and psychotherapy—none of which quite meet the definitive needs of the term 'treatment' although in practice some of the most impressive results of psychiatric treatment/management involve the use of psychoactive drugs: hence the reason for starting with an admittedly cursory look at psychopharmacology.

PSYCHOPHARMACOLOGY

Though the *historical* aspects of psychopharmacology have been mentioned it should be realised that the word is used in a *relatively* restricted sense though Shepherd *et al* (1968) have defined it as 'the study of drug action in relation to the higher functions of the central nervous system both normal and abnormal'. By this definition psychopharmacology covers narcotic analgesics such as the opiates and hypnotics but modern psychopharmacology is concerned with drugs whose mind altering effects go beyond pain relief or altering consciousness and which are usually referred to as *psychotropic* or *psychoactive* drugs. They may be classified in a number of ways but most would agree with Rees (1972):

1 Neuroleptics
2 Tranquillosedatives
3 Antidepressants and central nervous stimulants
4 Hallucinogenics (considered under *Drug dependence*)
5 Miscellaneous

This classification is used here.

Clinical trials of psychotropic drugs are nowadays commonplace and it is in psychopharmacology that clinical trials have been most extensively used, and have effectively brought psychiatric treatment into a scientifically acceptable framework. Clinical trials are however not as new as many suppose. Hordern (1968) recounted their origins in 1747 when the Royal Naval Surgeon James Lind showed that citrus fruits were effective in treating scurvy which had killed a million sailors in 200 years. Lind took six groups of two patients who received randomly allocated treatments. The citrus treated patients recovered. Actually as Hordern (1968) noted James Lind's discovery was misused, an important lesson that is still relevant. After Lind's trial all went well until some sailors died on standard issue lime juice for the reason (later discovered) that economy minded bureaucrats decreed the issue of boiled (inactive) lime juice as opposed to the pure vitamin C in fresh lemon juice, (in those days the terms lemon and lime were interchangeable). The finer details of clinical trials will not be considered here. The literature is enormous. The main point is that trials depend for their usefulness on correct methodology above all, and by any criteria Lind's work was a good start.

Modern psychopharmacology has expanded enormously not only scientifically but also industrially and the end results have important sociological implications since such a large proportion of the population regularly take psychotropic drugs, often not realising what they are (Willis, 1973; Young, 1972) whilst often vociferously condemning those who use mind altering drugs casually.

The growth of psychopharmacology is related directly above all to the fact that psychotropic drugs have not only offered relief to patients but offered promise of better understanding of the biochemistry of mental illness. *Physical treatment* has gone beyond the shocks, whirls and showers of the 18th and 19th Century and became first established in 1917 when Werner Von Jaurreg used malarial therapy for GPI—at a stroke making 20% of the then mental hospital population treatable and impelling onwards the medical model of psychiatry. Later continuous sleep was used in psychoses, then in the 1930s Sakel introduced insulin induced hypo-glycaemia to treat schizophrenics. Though later this treatment was discredited it was an important start in that people began to see hope for patients previously supposed incurable.

This was reinforced by ECT introduced by Cerletti and Bini in 1937 as the first antidepressant treatment.

But the serious study of psychopharmacology remained fairly static until 1944 when Hoffman accidentally swallowed lysergic acid, experienced emotional changes and hallucinosis and started to investigate hallucino-genic drugs systematically. Further work on hallucinogens suggested that they had therapeutic possibilities, not only as abreactive agents but also as possible aids to deeper insights—'instant insight' etc. Lysergic acid (LSD) was the leading drug of this sort but its popularity waned since its therapeutic effectiveness was never properly demonstrated and also because of adverse reactions that followed its use. These adverse reactions, 'model psychoses', stimulated further interest in brain biochemistry and psychosis which, unhappily turned out to be a tantalising lead to nowhere. However a real milestone in psychopharmacology occurred in 1952 when Delay and Deniker used chlorpromazine to calm agitated psychotics after it had been discarded by anaesthetists looking for a 'lytic cocktail' to induce artificial hibernation and discarded because it had too wide a range of activity. Fortunately for psychiatry *chlorpromazine* turned out to be a drug that altered behaviour without diminishing consciousness—a real find at a time when mental hospitals were full of agitated and violent psychotics made stuporose by bromides and barbiturates that poisoned them.

Since 1952 over 50 million patients were treated in the 10 years after its introduction. Chlorpromazine and the phenothiazines are the largest group of *neuroleptic* drugs (major tranquillisers). Phenothiazines, chlorpromazine being the model phenothiazine, act on the mid brain activating system, and on the thalamocortical projections.

In experimental animals phenothiazines cause a general fall off in spontaneous activity, less aggression, loss of fear and diminished conditioned reflexes.

Neuroleptics (major tranquillisers)

The neuroleptics started with the demonstration by Delay and Deniker (1952) that an antihistamine, chlorpromazine, rejected by anaesthetists as having too wide a range of actions had a calming effect without impairing consciousness. Chlorpromazine, the first neuroleptic, transformed mental hospital life with its antihallucinatory and tranquillising effects. No one questions the value of neuroleptics in acute psychoses, the difficulties are in deciding whether the neuroleptics reverse a psychotic process or modify it by suppressing symptoms.

This is an important question since the proliferation of neuroleptic drugs which occurred from 1950 to the mid 1960s has now slowed and relatively few new advances have occurred except for the long acting neuroleptics. What has happened is that methods of study of drug action have improved and there is now a better understanding of the indications for the use of neuroleptics and more awareness of their side effects and limitations.

Phenothiazines

The biggest group of neuroleptics is the *phenothiazines* based on the phenothiazine nucleus: two benzene rings joined by a sulphur and a nitrogen atom.

Substitutions at the side chains R_1 and R_2 produce different types of phenothiazines as follows:

1 Side chains at R_1 produce three different series of phenothiazines: *aliphatic, piperidine* and *piperazine*.
2 Substitution at R_2 involves radicals which alter potency (Linford Rees, 1966; 1972).

The aliphatic and piperidine type are sedative, the piperazine type are stimulant but cause more extrapyramidal effects.

Phenothiazines in common use are given in Table 18.1.

Table 18.1 Phenothiazines in common use.

Type	Generic name	Trade name	Daily dose (mg)
Aliphatic	Chlorpromazine	Largactil (UK)	75–1000
		Thorazine (US)	75–1000
	Promazine	Sparine	75–1000
	Fluopromazine	Vespral	20–150
	Methotrimeprazine	Veractil	25–700
Piperidine	Thioridazine	Melleril	30–600
	Pericyazine	Neulactil	7·5–90
Piperazine	Trifluoperazine	Stelazine	3–50
	Prochlorperazine	Stemetil	15–100
	Perphenazine	Fentazin	6–64
	Thiopropazate	Dartalan	15–150
	Fluphenazine	Moditen	2·5–10
Long acting	Fluphenazine enanthate	Moditen enanthate	12·5–25 (monthly)
	Fluphenazine decanoate	Modecate	12·5–25 (monthly)

Though the phenothiazines are the biggest group of neuroleptics, they are not the only ones—there are now many others which include:

1 Butyrophenones
2 Thioxanthine derivatives
3 Rauwolfia and similar drugs
4 Diphenyl butyl piperidines

Butyrophenones

The tranquillising properties of the butyrophenones were discovered by accident when a potential analgesic was being investigated. The prototype butyrophenone is haloperidol which like all drugs of this group is excreted slowly and therefore accumulates; a bad effect which is offset by low doses given twice daily. Their main action is in slowing psychomotor activity, thus they are best used in mania and hypomania. However, their range of effects *is* similar to the phenothiazines.

The most commonly used butyrophenones are given in Table 18.2.

N

Table 81.2 Butyrophenones in common use.

Generic name	Trade name	Daily dose (mg)
Haloperidol	Serenace	2–20
Trifluoperidol	Triperidol	0·7–1·5

Thioxanthine derivatives

The thioxanthines are chemically similar to the phenothiazines but have as yet not been extensively used since they have not been shown to be superior to the phenothiazines. The best known are chlorprothixene (Taractan) and thiothixene (Navane). Taractan has been used in anxiety states because of its sedative action while Navane is said to have an alerting action on apathetic schizophrenics.

Table 18.3 Thioxanthines in common use.

Generic name	Trade name	Daily dose (mg)
Chlorprothixene	Taractan	30–90
Thiothixene	Navane	10–30

Rauwolfia and allied drugs

Reserpine (Serpasil) was one of the first antipsychotic drugs used. However the reserpine like drugs have fallen into disuse because of their high incidence of serious side effects.

Table 18.4 Rauwolfia and allied drugs in common use.

Generic name	Trade name	Daily dose (mg)
Reserpine	Serpasil	0·25–5
Tetrabenazine	Nitoman	30–150

Diphenyl butylpiperidenes

The diphenyl butylpiperidenes is a new group of neuroleptics of which pimozide (Orap) is the only one in general use. It has an alerting action on apathetic schizophrenics.

Table 18.5 Diphenyl butylpiperidenes in common use.

Generic name	Trade name	Daily dose (mg)
Pimozide	Orap	2–6

Use of neuroleptic drugs in treatment of psychoses

General comments

There are no clear findings to suggest a particular choice of drugs in treatment. The most that can be said is that the more disruptive and disorganised aspects of psychosis can be safely and sensibly controlled by using phenothiazines. Chlorpromazine was the first of the phenothiazines and really has stood the test of time in this respect, also more is known about its side effects and long term use than is known about any psychotropic drug. Neuroleptic drugs are used in an empirical way based on clinical experience and judgement and the safest rule is to use those which have the least likelihood of side effects. Extrapyramidal side effects can easily be controlled with drugs such as orphenadrine (Disipal) 100 mg tds. The acute extrapyramidal syndromes, *e.g.* dystonia and oculogyric crises can be abolished by giving antiparkinsonian drugs such as Kemadrin by injection.

While it is true that neuroleptics are relatively non-specific there is some evidence to suggest that phenothiazines with a piperazine nucleus have a more alerting effect than aliphatic phenothiazines. The butyrophenone group of neuroleptics are probably of most value in the treatment of mania and hypomania. Here again some have used butyrophenones in high dosage given intravenously in the treatment of manic excitement but again there is no firm evidence to suggest that this is a particularly valuable treatment method.

Side effects

Since the site of action of neuroleptics is on the mid brain it is hardly surprising that extrapyramidal side effects are very common with all of them, particularly the phenothiazines. Though the precise mode of action of the phenothiazines is not known, it has been shown that they act in two main ways, first by their anticholinergic action which blocks activity in the mesodiencephalic activating system, which is of course cholinergic, and secondly by action on the reticular activating system in a way that can be summed up as depression of hypothalamic activity.

Extrapyramidal side effects include parkinsonism, probably the most common of all, producing rigidity, facial masking and tremor. Less common but disturbing extrapyramidal side effects include dystonic reactions where there is repeated muscular spasm often involving face, head and neck which will often be associated with oculogyric crises. Involuntary movements of the mouth and tongue may occur and in some instances these occur in long term phenothiazine therapy where a patient develops involuntary chewing and tongue movements; these latter are usually irreversible.

In general, however, acute extrapyramidal syndromes associated with phenothiazines and neuroleptic drugs in general respond to antiparkinsonian medication. Another special extrapyramidal syndrome is akathisia in which there is restlessness and inability to keep the lower limbs still. This also reponds to antiparkinsonian medication.

Although the central nervous system side effects are the most common and may be the most disturbing to the patient, there are many other side effects caused by the phenothiazines in particular. They include postural hypotension, weight gain, atropine-like effects such as dryness of mouths and blurred vision and impotence. Agranulocytosis is fortunately rare. An obstructive jaundice, probably allergic, may occur in up to 4% of patients (highest record) or 0.1% (lowest recorded). There is great variation in the jaundice producing potential of phenothiazines. It was thought to be a possible coincidence of medication and hepatitis but has definitely been shown to be intrahepatic obstructive jaundice and its early onset (4 weeks) strongly suggests allergy as the cause.

Also it should be noted that phenothiazines are often epileptogenic. Psychotic and confusional states can be precipitated by phenothiazines, particularly in the elderly. Finally dermatitis and photosensitivity should be borne in mind as very common complications of phenothiazine therapy.

The neuroleptics may be described as drugs which in general have an antipsychotic effect in the sense that they either suppress or reverse psychotic symptoms such as delusions, thought disorder and hallucinosis quite apart from their overall activity of calming agitation and excitement without impairing consciousness. The proliferation of antipsychotic drugs in the 1950s and 1960s has settled leaving psychiatrists to try and define their indications and mode of action. Some have attempted to find drugs that are specific for patients and their particular disorder but large scale studies such as that of Hollister *et al* (1971) have suggested that apparent specificity of antipsychotic drug action is illusory and that their use is empirical, while Willis and Bannister (1965) found that psychiatrists' choices of antischizophrenic treatment was haphazard and influenced mainly by the presence of affective colouring, excitement or anergic symptoms.

The use of neuroleptics, however, is regarded as mandatory for acute schizophrenics whilst their value in chronic schizophrenics is disputable as they may control troublesome or unacceptable symptoms but hardly alter the natural history of the disorder. Or at least this is how it seemed until the arrival of long acting phenothiazines such as fluphenazine enanthate (Moditen) and fluphenazine decanoate (Modecate). Both these are injectable phenothiazines which act for 2 to 3 weeks and 4 weeks respectively. Fluphenazine decanoate has been known to be a highly effective antipsychotic drug which not only cuts down readmission rates but is significantly more effective than placebo (Hirsch *et al*, 1973) not only in symptom reduction but also in reducing social disability (Stevens, 1973). This is provided that the monthly injections are backed up by properly organised out-patient follow-ups and after care involving social workers and community nurses.

Other biochemical approaches to antipsychotic treatment have included the 'orthomolecular' therapy advocated by Linus Pauling (1967) which consists of high doses of niacin, ascorbic acid, B_6 and other vitamins. Despite the apparent impeccability of being supported by a Nobel prizewinner, the treatment has to date not been validated. The other vitamin therapy is the use of nicotinic acid and nicotinamide in high doses as adjuncts to neuroleptics in schizophrenia. However, well conducted studies (McGrath *et al*, 1972; Barr & Lehmann, 1970; Ramsay *et al*, 1970) have failed to show that adding these substances produces a better effect than neuroleptics alone in schizophrenia.

The phenothiazines are the most widely used neuroleptic drugs and though there are important structural differences between the three main types as already described, there is little to choose between them except that the aliphatic series are in general tranquillising and the piperazine series alerting. It is likely that the effects on thought disorder, hallucinosis and delusions are secondary to the tranquillising effect. Extrapyramidal side effects including rigidity, akathisia and dystonic reactions (oculogyric crises, neck retraction and tongue protrusion) are the most common, but other side effects include drowsiness and rarely intrahepatic obstructive jaundice. Sudden death due to cardiac arrest is rare and occurs mainly in chronic high dosage. Other effects include lactation, blurred vision, dry mouth, weight gain, impotence and skin rashes, these are usually dealt with by changing the drug or lowering the dose.

Lithium

Lithium was first recognised as a psychotropic drug in 1897 but its bad reputation for toxicity precluded further interest in it until 1949 when Cade noted its calming effect on guinea pigs and reasoned that it might be useful in mania. He found that it was, and this led to a gradual growth of interest in the drug reviewed by Schou (1959) who noted eighteen publications on lithium involving 370 patients and calculated that it produced a similar remission rate to ECT in mania, about 80%. Clinical trials of lithium in mania are of course extremely difficult because of the highly disturbed state of the patient although Maggs (1963) and Schou (1954) reported double blind studies in mania.

The present status of lithium has been reviewed particularly with regard to its prophylactic effect in manic depressive disorder. There has been disagreement about this in the past but it now seems established that it *does* prevent recurrences of manic depressive disorders. It is also used in chronic and recurrent depressive states as a prophylactic medication but its place here is much less certain.

Dosage and administration

The dosage depends on clinical response and the blood lithium levels. In practice this usually means giving 600 to 900 mg/day with the object of keeping the blood lithium level between 0·6 to 1·5 meq/l. The blood lithium should be estimated weekly at first, thereafter monthly estimations are sufficient in the patient on a maintenance dose. It is important to estimate the blood level at 12 hours after the last dose since top levels occur within 2 to 4 hours and may be misleading. It is also important to estimate the blood level if there are signs of toxicity, intercurrent illness or relapse.

Lithium should not be given to any patient with renal or cardiovascular disease, hypothyroidism or any state associated with sodium depletion. The importance of lithium toxicity is that it develops slowly, for this reason patients should be warned to report drowsiness, tremor, vomiting, diarrhoea or anorexia.

Side effects

These are *very* important as lithium is a highly toxic drug. Side effects are dose related. When the drug is started nausea, dizziness, fine tremor and thirst are common but usually settle down.

The serious side effects may be listed thus:

CNS
Dysarthria
Ataxia
Vertigo
Fits
Weakness
Muscle twitching
Choreoathetosis
Hyperreflexia

Endocrine
Non-toxic goitre

Gastrointestinal
Anorexia
Nausea
Vomiting
Diarrhoea
Weight loss

CVS
Arrhythmias
Hypotension
Peripheral circulatory failure

Renal
Polydipsia
Polyuria
Dehydration
Glycosuria

Congenital
Abnormal
  spermatogenesis

Changes in consciousness
From drowsiness to coma

The main point is that this highly toxic drug can be used safely as long as the patient has normal renal function and as long as the blood levels are monitored.

Tranquillosedatives (minor tranquillisers)

The benzodiazepines

These are the most commonly used psychotropic drugs, upwards of 16 000 000 prescriptions for them are written every year by practitioners in England and Wales.

They are effective in relieving the subjective distress of anxiety, also the associated muscle tension, and in hospital practice they are widely prescribed in departments of rheumatology. Their sedative action is relatively mild and their abuse potential correspondingly low, yet, nevertheless they *do* have an abuse potential and it should not be overlooked. Taken in sufficient doses they do produce drowsiness and stupor though cases of death from uncomplicated overdosage is extremely rare. They are anticonvulsants, hence the use of intravenous diazepam (Valium) in status epilepticus. They are mainly used in states of anxiety and tension, alcoholism and drug dependence, and they are widely prescribed in psychosomatic disorders and in combination with antidepressants in the treatment of affective disorders, though here their place is less certain. They act on the limbic system, inhibiting overactivity thus, it is thought, blocking the perpetuation of anxiety symptoms. They have no effect on midbrain or reticular areas. Common benzodiazepines are given in Table 18.6

Table 18.6   Benzodiazepines in common use.

Generic name	Trade name	Daily dose (mg)
Chlordiazepoxide	Librium	15–100
Diazepam	Valium	6–40
Oxazepam	Serenid	45–120
Medazepam	Nobrium	15–40
Nitrazepam	Mogadon	5–20 (nocte)

Side effects

In general they are well tolerated: nevertheless it should not be forgotten that they do cause drowsiness, especially in elderly patients and so the dosage will need to be varied. Similarly they do slow down reactivity and may thus impair driving and the operation of machinery.

Overdosage produces states of ataxia, dysarthria and impaired consciousness, and in cases of chronic intoxication with chlordiazepoxide and diazepam, withdrawal fits have been reported. An additive effect may occur with alcohol and patients should be warned about this just as caution should be used in prescribing benzodiazepines in combination with hypnotics, analgesics, antidepressants, antihistamines, central depressants of any sort, other tranquillisers and neuroleptics.

Severe overdose can lead to coma, respiratory depression though death from uncomplicated benzodiazepine overdose must be very rare.

Blood dycrasias and jaundice have been described while chlordiazepoxide was being given but the evidence linking it to these conditions is equivocal. In general the benzodiazepines are safe, well tolerated tranquillisers with a mild but definite abuse potential. They are very useful in suppressing anxiety and tension and diazepam is the drug of choice in status epilepticus. It is also given parenterally, to calm agitated psychotic patients and to violent aggressive psychopaths who are 'acting out'.

The tricyclic antidepressants

The tricyclic series of antidepressants are generally regarded as the safest and most effective antidepressant medications. Though their mode of

Table 18.7 Antidepressants in common use.

Generic name	Trade name	Daily dose (mg)	Comment
Imipramine	Tofranil	75–200	The first and, to date, the most effective
Nortriptyline	Aventyl	75–150	Mildly stimulant
Protriptyline	Concordin	15–45	Mildly stimulant. Higher risk of tachycardia and cardiac arrhythmias
Iprindole	Prondol	45–90	Mildly stimulant
Amitriptyline	Tryptizol	75–200	Sedative—hence often given in one dose at night
Trimipramine	Surmontil	75–150	Sedative—hence often given in one dose at night
Doxepin	Sinequan	75–150	Sedative, marked anxiolytic action
Dothiepin	Prothiaden	75–150	Sedative
Clompiamine	Anafranil	75-100	Sedative. Bad interaction with alcohol

action is not fully understood it seems likely that they act by increasing biogenic amine concentration through blockage of reabsorption of free amines. Carlsson *et al* (1969) have shown that tricyclic antidepressants act in specific ways: some inhibit the reabsorption of serotonin (5-HTT); amitriptyline (Tryptizol), imipramine (Tofranil) and clomipramine (Anafranil); while others inhibit the reabsorption of noradrenalin; desipramine (Pertofran), protriptyline (Concordin) and nortriptyline (Aventyl). Commonly used antidepressants are given in Table 18.7.

Though the side effects of tricyclic antidepressants will be listed in detail later, the main and most common effects are anticholinergic, *e.g.* dry mouth, constipation and drowsiness. Blurred vision and drowsiness are probably the most persistent and troublesome.

Uses of antidepressants

There is fairly general agreement that the tricyclic drugs *are* effective antidepressants, on the other hand the place of the MAOIs appears less certain. Davis and Janowsky (1974) reviewed antidepressant therapy covering the results of over 80 well conducted trials. Their results put imipramine and amitriptyline well in the lead though in studies where ECT is compared with imipramine it tends to come out as more effective, mainly in respect of speed of action, hence its continued use as the treatment of choice for suicidally depressed patients. Simple guidelines for antidepressant therapy are not hard to establish, providing they are based on commonsense and not on tenuous theory. The safest rule is to use one antidepressant at a time, also to avoid the simultaneous use of tranquillisers. Wheatley *et al* (1973) make these points very well in a review of psychotropic drugs in general practice where they note simple points about antidepressant therapy, for instance patients with dry mouths often stop taking tablets because they cannot get a glass of water at work.

Other authors have pointed out the high 'drop out' rate in psychotropic medication by out-patients (20%–30%) and day patients (10%–15%). This makes the once daily dose the easiest way to give medication. In the tricyclic antidepressants this is the method of choice, preferably at bedtime. There is no special merit in sustained release capsules, the ordinary oral preparations produce appropriate blood levels.

The duration of *antidepressant therapy* is still a matter for discussion; some authorities recommend that patients continue on medication for 12 to 18 months, others recommend withdrawal of medication as soon as possible. However there is already good evidence of the value of main-tenance therapy with antidepressants—the bulk of clinical experience backed up by trials suggest continuation for 6 months to 1 year (Kay *et al*, 1970; Mindham *et al*, 1972).

The monoamine oxidase inhibitors are generally regarded as being less effective and less safe than the tricyclic series though Davis and Janowsky (1974) concluded from their examination of the literature that the MAOIs were *nearly* as effective as the tricyclics. However the side effects of MAOIs preclude their widespread use in general practice and the plain truth is that the bulk of depressive states nowadays are treated by general practitioners (Wheatley *et al*, 1973)—a fact that cannot be overlooked. Its significance for the psychiatrist is that most depressives referred to hospital clinics nowadays are likely to be patients that have failed to respond to current treatment methods.

Another point about antidepressant treatment is that phenothiazines are useful drugs, often overlooked. Klein (1966) showed that chlorpro-mazine and imipramine are equally effective antidepressants; perhaps this is less surprising when it is appreciated that the chemical structure of the phenothiazines and the tricyclic antidepressants is remarkably similar. Raskin *et al* (1970) and Paykel *et al* (1968) also showed that the pheno-thiazines were similarly effective in the treatment of depression.

The general impression that is left after examination of well conducted trials of antidepressant therapy is as follows:

1   ECT is indicated in acute suicidal depression
2   The tricyclic series *is safer* than the MAOIs
3   Imipramine and amitriptyline are, to date, the best evaluated and safest tricyclic antidepressants
4   Phenelzine is the most effective and safest MAOI
5   Phobic states with or without depression respond equally well to phenelzine and clomipramine

Other interesting findings are that antidepressant drugs have no effect on 'normal' people but are only effective where there is primary mood disorder, *i.e.* they are *not* euphoriant.

Side effects

Since we live in an age in which up to 25% of medical admissions and up to 25% of new medical out-patients are suffering from manifestations of medication induced illness, hardly to be dismissed with euphemisms such as 'iatrogenic', it is necessary for the psychiatrist to know well the side effects of the drugs that he prescribes. Here it is possible to be definite, even dogmatic. We may be vague about definitions of psychiatric disorder but we can be very clear in our knowledge and understanding of the dangers of the treatment that we prescribe for ill defined illness.

Side effects should be listed comprehensively; there is no excuse for ignorance in this respect.

Side effects of tricyclic antidepressants

A wide range of side effects have been reported. Some of the tricyclic antidepressants tend to produce more side effects than others. The more common effects are in italics

1 **Cardiovascular:** hypertension, *orthostatic hypotension*, palpitations, *tachycardia*, arrhythmias
2 **Anticholinergic:** *dryness of the mouth*, nausea and vomiting, *constipation, urinary delay* and retention, *difficulty in accommodation*, mydriasis, *blurred vision*, sublingual adenitis, *sweating*
3 **CNS:** confusional states, states of excitement, agitation and restlessness, *insomnia*, paraesthesia and tingling, ataxia, tremor, fits
4 **Skin:** General and non-specific: rashes, photosensitivity, urticaria, oedema—especially of tongue and face unpleasant taste in the mouth, impotence, *drowsiness, feelings of weakness and fatigue*, weight gain, weight loss
5 Rarer adverse effects described include myocardial infarction, heart block, extrapyramidal side effects, paralytic ileus, depression of bone marrow activity, agranulocytosis, purpura, thrombocytopenia, black tongue, gynecomastia and testicular swelling, breast enlargement and galactorrhoea, alopecia

General precautions that should be observed when using tricyclic antidepressants

MAOIs There is fairly general agreement that they should not be administered in combination with MAOIs though some authoritative voices have claimed that the combination of MAOIs and tricyclics will succeed when one or other antidepressant has failed.

For the majority of psychiatrists however, combined antidepressant therapy is regarded as unhelpful and potentially dangerous. The dangers are recognised and emphasised by the manufacturers who in all cases caution strongly against combined antidepressant therapy.

Other psychotropic drugs There really is no justification either for using two tricyclic antidepressants together, a practice that has 'crept in' with no scientific justification. There should also be caution about using tranquillisers at the same time, something that is done quite commonly but with no good reason, there is not one trial that shows the superiority of a tranquilliser and antidepressant on its own.

Other drugs Central nervous depressants may produce an additive effect with antidepressants. Barbiturates may inactivate tricyclic antidepressants by their enzyme induction effect. Therefore it is sensible to discontinue barbiturates during antidepressant therapy.

Cardiovascular effects Tachycardia and postural hypotension may be dangerous especially in patients with a previous history of cardiovascular disease particularly hypertension and myocardial disease. The same general caution applies to their use in elderly people.

Pregnancy Tricyclic antidepressants should not be used in pregnancy or for mothers who are breast feeding.

Dosage and modes of administration

The dosage rates vary from one tricyclic to another. In recent years there has been a tendency to give a once daily dose, preferably at bedtime if the tricyclic concerned has a sedative effect. In the case of the tricyclics with an alerting effect it may be wise to give the last daily dose at midday.

Where a patient has been receiving a MAOI it is essential to allow a 14 day drug free period before starting a tricyclic and vice versa. The dosage of tricyclic antidepressants is probably more important than has been realised. In the case of imipramine and amitriptyline many recommend a top dosage level of 200 mg daily while others recommend a top daily dose of 300 mg on very little scientific evidence. There have been a number of claims that certain tricyclics act more quickly than others but to date there has been really little convincing evidence of this.

The blood levels of tricyclic drugs are important too since blood levels reach a steady state fairly quickly. There are however differential responses to similar doses and at the same time there are surprising differences in response seemingly unrelated to the drug blood level. This and other evidence suggests there are genetically determined individual metabolic differences (Burrow & Davies, 1971; Perel & Glassman, 1973). Certainly clinical experience suggests a wide range of response to tricyclic antidepressants and for this reason current research looks for ways of finding the particular drug to suit the particular patient.

The first choice of tricyclic antidepressants then lies between imipramine and amitriptyline. Clinical experience suggests that imipramine is slightly more effective in anergic depressives and amitriptyline is slightly more effective in anxious, agitated depressives. An important point to be remembered however is that there is no point in continuing an antidepressant indefinitely if there is no response. A good rule is to change to another if there is no significant improvement in three weeks.

The monoamine oxidase inhibitors should be reserved for patients who fail to respond to a fair trial of tricyclics.

Using other psychotropic drugs

Although it is not generally advisable to use combinations of psychotropic drugs, there are occasions when it is necessary. This is true for patients with associated severe anxiety symptoms or who have become more agitated after starting on antidepressants. Again this is true for depressed schizophrenic patients who may develop worsening of psychotic symptoms on tricyclic antidepressants.

Monoamine oxidase inhibitors

In a recent review of the use of monoamine oxidase inhibitors in pyschiatry Tyrer (1973) commented on the wide differences of opinion that surround the use of this interesting group of drugs. The difference of opinion go beyond the choice of patient most likely to benefit from them but extend into divisive opinions as to whether they should be used at all. On the one hand Sargant (1966) has shown that they are effective in the treatment of phobic anxiety and Slater and Roth (1969) recommended them as the drugs of choice in treating neurotic depression, whilst Hollister (1969) has prescribed them as last ditch antidepressants when all else has failed. This is backed up by Jarvik (1970) who comments on their relatively low efficacy and high toxicity as factors leading to a general decline in their use. The monoamine oxidase inhibitors (MAOIs) were used extensively before their dangerous effects were recognised.

The first indication of their possible antidepressant action was discovered in the 1950s when isoniazid, the antituberculosis drug, was found to cause euphoria. Iproniazid, another antituberculosis drug turned out to be even more euphoriant and also was found to act by inhibiting monoamine oxidase. This finding led to great interest in MAOIs as mood elevating drugs, unfortunately at a time when trials of psychoactive drugs were badly designed and led to inconsistent results.

The Medical Research Council trial (1965) showed that the MAOI phenelzine was no more effective than placebo in antidepressant therapy.

At the same time others have commented that MAOIs are useful in treating 'atypical depression' and 'depressive equivalents'. These are two badly defined terms: the former designates a mixed bag of phobic, unhappy and hypochondriacal patients who appear to be depressed whilst the latter describes patients who are *not* depressed but have inexplicable symptoms.

Recent investigations suggest that there is not one enzyme, monoamine oxidase, but several (Youdrin & Sandler, 1967; Collins *et al*, 1970) which might account for their varying and unpredictable clinical uses, while Pare (1962) suggested that differences in responses to MAOIs might be explained in terms of genetic differences as yet hardly demonstrated. Monoamine oxidase inhibitors in common use are given in Table 18.8.

Table 18.8   Monoamine oxidase inhibitors in common use.

Generic name	Trade name	Daily dose (mg)	Comment
Tranylcypromine	Parnate	30	Food reactions most common
Phenelzine	Nardil	45	Probably the safest
Isocarboxazid	Marplan	30	Probably the safest

Side effects

These include hypotension, states of excitement and elation, hepatoxicity, oedema, sexual impotence and failure of orgasm, dry mouth, blurred vision and constipation.

1   The most serious side effects are hepatotoxicity and interactions with food and drugs. MAOIs interact with most psychoactive drugs, particularly narcotics, including pethidine, barbiturates and barbiturate-like sedatives, tricyclic antidepressants, tranquillisers and alcohol. The drug interactions are usually described as synergistic but may be additive.

2   Food interactions. In the early days of MAOI use many clinicians were impressed by the frequency of severe, sudden and intense headache reported by patients taking tranyclypromine (Parnate). This phenomenon was shown by Blackwell (1963) to be caused by a sharp rise in noradrenaline which occurred whenever MAOIs were ingested in combination with foods that contained tyramine. The reaction was shown to be a hypertensive crisis caused by the release of pressor amines thus foods that contain tyramine, *e.g.* certain cheeses, broad beans, beef extracts and certain red wines are implicated as well as sympathomimetic amines, *e.g.* amphetamines and ephedrine which interact with MAOIs and cause hypertensive crises.

Therapeutic uses   The use of MAOIs is not clearly established and their toxicity is high. In carefully selected phobic patients and in certain neurotic depressives they are useful providing their use is carefully supervised.

PSYCHOTHERAPY

All psychotherapy is based on the communication that can go on between therapist and patient and the relationship that exists between them. The various types of psychotherapy are classified according to their underlying theoretical and philosophical framework. The general aims of psychotherapy are to alter personality as well as to relieve symptoms. To what extent the personality may be altered by therapy of any sort is open to question and in recent years the whole standing of psychotherapy has come in for considerable criticism and review.

Psychotherapy is influenced considerably by the prevailing culture, by social class and by economic forces. Also and perhaps more important is the question of who *receives* psychotherapy. The most likely people to get psychotherapy are young, intelligent and articulate, and as some have unkindly added 'attractive'. Many doctors have a rather vague idea of what exactly *is* meant by psychotherapy supposing it to be a highly esoteric form of treatment; vaguely linked with jokes about doctors with beards, foreign accents and a tendency to state the obvious in a series of solemn platitudes.

But psychotherapy is of course a serious matter and in covert or overt form very widely used in psychiatry although the *classical* forms of psychotherapy have been less *popular* in recent years.

It received its biggest impetus with the work of Freud and the psychoanalytic school who noted first of all the subjective relief experienced by the person who was enabled to talk about painful, shameful and guilt ridden topics without prejudice.

But it was soon realised that psychotherapy went beyond the familiar experience of 'confession being good for the soul' and that the relationship between therapist and patient was highly important, particularly in psychoanalysis where the patient was encouraged to bring out every idea, no matter how seemingly irrelevant or trifling in an attempt to reach material repressed below consciousness. This meant that the patient would not only go through a wider range of turbulent experience as he became gradually more aware of the real significance of his fantasy life but that he would invest the therapist with a good deal of feeling; frequently feeling that he had directed towards a parent—thus arose the concept of *transference*, central in psychoanalytic theory.

Whatever may have been the ramifications and developments of analytic psychotherapy the theoretical basis is founded on the importance of unconscious drive in shaping and colouring mental life and on a hierarchical theory of personality in which the presentation of the visible self is determined by the interplay of ego, superego and id and above all in the morbid influences of conflict in early childhood in laying down the basis of neurosis and personality disorders, all coloured by the ineffable forces of sexual conflict. Analytic psychotherapy stands or falls on the acceptability or otherwise of this deterministic philosophy. To some it is totally or near totally acceptable, to others it lacks the absolute conviction provided by testable hypotheses.

But whether proven or not the psychoanalytic frame of reference remains very potent in psychotherapy since it suggests at least a fairly commonsense notion namely that early experience and conflict shape the later development of the personality and emphasises the therapeutic potential of a one to one relationship that may become durable enough to withstand the raw emotions generated by the revelation of the meaning of symptoms in symbolic terms and the release of the anxiety concealed by symptoms.

It also has been effective in directing the therapist's attention to the individual rather than to the disorder per se. Unhappily however many feel that analytic psychotherapy has become less effective by being impractical and uneconomic in terms of time and effort.

An attempt to alter this came from group psychotherapy which originally started with tuberculosis patients where group discussions were found to improve morale in a positive supportive way. Group psychotherapy is most effective with groups of 8 to 12 patients who may find in the group a place where they can learn about the experiences and motivations of others and apply them to themselves.

This type of experience led to the concept of the therapeutic community (Maxwell Jones, 1968) in which the whole hospital community is regarded as a source of therapeutic or non-therapeutic influence and where every member of the community is expected to bear responsibility for his actions and the way in which they may impinge on others. The therapeutic community philosophy has benefitted psychiatric hospitals considerably by making patients and professionals more aware of the value of free communication at all levels and of a therapeutic climate in which *all* members of the community can share by being concerned and involved in what goes on in the community. No one would suggest that all psychiatric hospitals are run in this way; far from it, but in the English speaking world at least by now there must be few psychiatric hospitals that are untouched by a philosophy that rejects a totally authoritarian style headed by a benign dictator (physician superintendent) who delegates authority downwards in a community where patients are regarded as incapable of behaving like responsible beings and in need of care by being placed in a totally dependent role.

The therapeutic community principle suggests active roles for patients and staff in a climate of mutual trust and free communication. This is no doubt an ideal that has not been attained but it is a move in the right direction especially in that it helps to preserve the integrity and self-reliance of the patient.

It may be asked what exactly are the indications for analysis since the criticisms of analytic theory and practice have become more forceful. This is hard to answer. Most would suggest that a candidate for analysis needs to be intelligent and articulate and have enough personal commitment to embark on a lengthy process that may lead nowhere. This excludes all psychotic patients and most depressives since both these groups can derive more benefit from a combination of medication and time. But it leaves a small group of people with anxiety symptoms and with problems in their personality development *who feel the need* for such a lengthy process.

Shorter analytic type therapies are more commonly used and may be somewhat arbitrarily classified as *insight therapy* and *relationship therapy*. In each case the process is measured in months rather than years. In *insight therapy* the object is to help the patient to get better understanding of the meaning of his symptoms and encourage him to adopt effective alternatives in his life style, *e.g.* to live rather than be ill. In *relationship therapy* the object is to enable the patient to realise that his difficulties may be reflections of his inability to relate with his peers in a mature and stable way, since he may have carried into adult life an infantile way of relating with other people whom he sees as threatening parent figures etc.

In recent years there has been a general move away from *classical psychoanalytic* therapies towards briefer psychotherapies, many of which focus on specific areas in preference to attempting the global task of trying to change the personality.

Actually this change started quite early in what may be termed the immediate post-Freudian era in the 1920s and 1930s when many psychiatrists though impressed by Freud's theoretical position, soon found that analysis did not live up to its apparent promise, something that Freud himself was never slow to recognise. This was particularly true in America where Adolf Meyer's concept of psychobiological theory saw psychological development in terms of a life process where the individual and his interaction with the environment were examined in minute detail. Unfortunately this was in such fine detail that the practicalities of psychiatric syndromes somehow became obscured rather than clarified. Other Americans such as Harry Stack Sullivan and Karen Horney took Freudian concepts and seemed to make them more pragmatic in terms of explaining the influence of interpersonal relationships in shaping the personality whilst looking for ways of utilising this in therapy. In more recent times psychotherapy has moved more in the direction of counselling. A good example of this is the client centred therapy of Carl Rogers in which the person is regarded not so much as a sick patient but rather as someone capable of being responsible and self-reliant.

Thus therapy is directed at finding out what the patient may need in terms of how he sees his problem and of his view of the world in general and also of helping him via the therapist's recognition of the importance of his own attitudes as influences for good or bad—always relying on the client's (patient's) own phenomenology as the clues to fuller understanding of the meaning of his problem(s). The therapist needs to be honest and aware of himself and not afraid of his own feelings about the patient and his state and prepared to relate honestly with the client (patient) *i.e.* to be himself. This type of therapy, it will be realised removes the therapist from the often faintly ridiculous role of the omniscient physician-healer interpreting the sayings of the patient without fear of contradiction and backed up by a catch all theoretical system.

In Europe and in England this type of approach has been influenced by *existential psychotherapy* in which there is absolute recognition of the total integrity of the person as a real and valid being with a total right to his own thoughts and feelings. Thus in therapy he is encouraged to be his real self and to lose the constraints imposed by the special needs of family and society so that his personality may be liberated into a state of valid free existence and not continue as a series of acts designed to please or placate others or to assuage the individual's neurotic fears of not being himself.

All heady stuff and in general fairly far removed from the bread and butter of psychiatry which is *support*, *i.e.* the process of encouragement and assured reassurance in a non-judgemental setting which enables large numbers of people to be helped through crises, pain and suffering in an unpretentious way providing always the patient realises that he is not to be encouraged to be sick in a self-indulgent way but that he can count on finding someone who can help him to stand up to his problems and try and solve them. This is the *essence of supportive therapy*, that is to provide the potential for calm acceptance and help. And it is surprising in practice that people can manage very well with very little as long as they know it is available. It is also perhaps not so surprising how little support is often available to people and also it is very impressive to discover just exactly what are the burdens and stresses that people tolerate in an uncomplaining way despite the fashionable tendency to suggest that the human race is becoming overdependent and neurotic.

Psychotherapy then, is in a state of change and under considerable critical attention. It is, in general, not as effective as it has been claimed to be, neither however is it as ineffective as all that. It remains as a humane expression of a sympathetic individual to understand the psychological distress of another and by whatever method to try and improve it or eradicate it which is, after all, not bad.

BEHAVIOUR THERAPY

When anxiety is linked to specific stresses, (*e.g.* cats, heights, open spaces) and only triggered off by these, it is called phobic anxiety. These phobias may be single or multiple.

In recent years, psychologists studying theories of learning have pointed out that phobias are probably the result of maladaptive learning, *i.e.* the patient has become conditioned to experience anxiety at the sight or sound of a given object. They have reasoned from this that the phobias could be cured by a deconditioning process which desensitises the patient from the cause of the attacks. This has the advantage of being based on a rational theoretical basis. The most obvious drawback appears to be that its usefulness is limited by the fact that it may only be applicable to patients with isolated phobias.

Behaviour therapy has been criticised for the failure to take into account the existence of a therapeutic relationship between doctor and patient and its consequent effects in altering the course of the patient's illness. However, careful evaluation of behaviour therapeutic methods has shown that this need not necessarily be the case.

In general it may be said that the term behaviour therapy is applied to a variety of psychiatric treatment in which use is made of the principles of behavioural sciences in re-educating a patient away from abnormal behaviour.

The theoretical basis runs counter to a dynamic basis in that it rejects the supposed importance of unconscious processes and conflict, stressing rather the importance of symptoms as learnt manifestations of a neurotic disorder.

The beginning of behaviour therapy occurred in the early 1950s when Professor H. J. Eysenck and colleagues in the Institute of Psychiatry in London made serious criticisms of the value of conventional psychotherapy and suggested in its stead the use of behaviour therapy a treatment in which learnt neurotic responses would be replaced using learning and deconditioning techniques.

Typical methods of behaviour therapy include:

1 Conditioned avoidance
2 Reciprocal inhibition
3 Desensitisation
4 Flooding

Conditioned avoidance

In these techniques the behaviour to be extinguished, *e.g.* alcoholism, sexual deviation, is linked to a repeated aversive stimulus such as apomorphine causing nausea thus producing in the subject a state of conditioned aversion.

Reciprocal inhibition

This technique is based on the finding that some human behaviours are mutually exclusive, *e.g.* relaxation and tension. In practice use is made of this finding by endeavouring to replace an unwanted response by one which is incompatible with it. In time the subject responds with relaxation to situations which have previously caused fear.

Desensitisation

Here the subject learns to avoid responding to noxious stimuli by being exposed to the stimuli at such minimal levels that little or no unpleasant response occurs. In this way his tolerance to the stimuli improves and the response is lost.

Flooding

A newer technique in behaviour therapy is 'Flooding' or 'Implosion' in which the patient is not desensitised from the dreaded stimulus but brought face to face with it until the anxiety fades. It sounds terrible but it works!

Behaviour therapy has now been so extensively used that it is possible to review its place in psychiatric treatment. Early critics feared that it would be a dehumanised procedure or that isolated phobias if removed would be replaced by others, in practice neither of these criticisms is valid.

In general it seems to be most useful in phobic states. Gelder and Marks (1966) found that desensitisation was the treatment of choice for simple phobic disorders but that it was less effective in agoraphobia especially when accompanied by generalised anxiety. For this reason flooding has been suggested as a better alternative though the results to date have been conflicting (Barrett, 1969; De Moor, 1970). However Marks *et al* (1971) using a cross-over trial of flooding and desensitisation in agoraphobia found flooding to be superior to desensitisation. Gelder *et al* (1973) treated thirty-six phobic patients randomly assigned to flooding, desensitisation or control treatment, and carefully assessed and followed up for 6 months. They failed to show any difference in outcome between the flooding and desensitisation groups both of whom did better than the control group.

The theoretical basis of behaviour therapy is not as satisfactory as its more ardent supporters would wish. Nevertheless it is an important type of treatment which has the merit of simplicity and also does not commit the patient or therapist to the uncertain duration and dogmatic position of formal psychotherapy.

ELECTROCONVULSIVE THERAPY (ECT)

ECT has been used in psychiatry since 1938 when Cerletti and Bini showed that electrically induced fits were safer than chemically induced fits—it is as simple and as daunting as that. The idea of using fits as treatment started with the incorrect hypothesis that there was a negative correlation between schizophrenia and epilepsy and that the induction of fits might alter the course of schizophrenic psychoses. When it was found that this was not exactly the case, fits were tried as a treatment for affective disorder and to everyone's surprise depressives started recovering more quickly than could be explained purely on the basis of spontaneous remission. This is an important point—before ECT depressives died of starvation and neglect—nowadays this is extremely rare. Another interesting finding is the decline in the mortality associated with puerperal psychosis following the introduction of ECT.

As it happened ECT was the first seemingly really effective physical treatment in psychiatry, and therefore at first it was given to every sort of patient—this may seem absurd but has to be understood in the context of the time. Until ECT there was no way of altering the course of psychosis and then quite suddenly there was a relatively simple effective treatment which could, for days at least, restore a schizophrenic to normal contact with reality and in the case of severe depression bring about a remission after a few treatments.

Methods of giving ECT have remained fairly uniform despite early and irrelevant controversy over the question of DC versus AC. The standard method employs a simple machine that gives a 100v AC current across the head via two electrodes. The convulsion is *modified* by using muscle relaxants and the procedure made less frightening by giving the patient intravenous thiopentone/muscle relaxant and is something that is part of the training of a competent psychiatrist but on no account should a psychiatrist, however competent he may be, attempt to give ECT unless there is another doctor present. It is unwise to give ECT more than twice in a week though exceptional circumstances may require three ECTs in a week for instance in severely suicidal patients.

The use of *regressive* ECT is described. This consists of daily ECT given to schizophrenics. It produces an organic mental state (subacute delirium) and has never been shown to be of any use. It is beyond belief that it could be called treatment. In fact it is a deplorable 'treatment' which is barely above rendering a patient confused by repeated blows to the head.

The number of ECTs should be guided by the patient's response—there is no such thing as a 'course' of ECT. The patient should be assessed between treatments and the treatment stopped when the patient has improved. In practice depressed patients rarely need more than 10 treatments and any 'course' should never exceed 20.

Contraindications and complications

Absolute contraindications include pulmonary tuberculosis, thyroid disease, any space occupying lesion or organic cerebral disease, skull bone disease such as Paget's disease and recent myocardial infarction. *Complications* of ECT include:

> normal anaesthetic hazards
> cardiovascular hazards, *e.g.* arrhythmia
> injury to mouth, tongue, jaw and bones
> amenorrhoea
> burns
> memory disturbance and confusional states
> headache

Indications

Despite the apparent hazards of ECT it remains a safe and useful treatment for depression. Nowadays the tricyclic antidepressant drugs have become the first choice in depression but it should be realised that in fact the effectiveness of ECT as measured in comparative trials is still slightly ahead of drug therapy. About 70% of depressives treated with drugs respond but of the remaining 30% approximately half will respond to ECT.

ECT is also used in manic states mainly as a way of controlling excitement—nowadays this is usually more easily achieved by use of drugs such as haloperidol and lithium. The place of ECT in schizophrenia is debatable though most psychiatrists use it in combination with phenothiazines in the acutely disturbed schizophrenic patients and in schizophrenics whose illness has a marked affective colouring.

Mode of action

This is quite unknown though there has been considerable speculation about the neurophysiology and biochemistry of ECT. Some regard it with suspicion and consequently undervalue it, others are convinced of its neurophysiological action and probably overvalue it. There has never been a controlled trial of ECT, *i.e.* shock + anaesthesia *versus* no shock + anaesthesia, and attempts to set up such trials have been dismissed as inhumane. All that can be said is that it really seems to work in depression. Those who favour ECT as a treatment tend to subscribe to a neurophysiological/hypothalamus/biochemistry model of its activity and those who are against it tend to regard it as a crude blockbuster which appears to act by knocking the patient out and causing amnesia.

In recent years it has been suggested that unilateral ECT given to the non-dominant hemisphere may be more effective and cause less memory loss (Fleminger *et al,* 1969). This has been disputed but has been investigated but the results to date seem equivocal (Abrams *et al,* 1972; Volavka *et al,* 1972). Nevertheless, despite the doubts and misgivings, ECT is a very useful way of aborting depression.

PSYCHOSURGERY

Psychosurgery used to be called leucotomy since the first brain operations aimed at altering tension and agitated behaviour consisted of dividing fibres, this has now progressed to surgical procedures aimed at nuclei (Schurr, 1973; Falconer & Schurr, 1958). The whole topic of the use of brain surgery to relieve distress or alter behaviour is one that evokes strong feeling, first since there is a natural reluctance to destroy healthy tissue and secondly because many feel that it is an unwarrantable intrusion on the freedom of choice and freedom of experience of the individual. This moral dilemma remains unresolved and still provokes hot debate. Nevertheless psychosurgery is used and psychiatrists should be familiar with the facts such as they are.

The first leucotomy operations (Moniz, 1936; Freeman & Watts, 1942) consisted of blind surgery aimed at dividing fronto-temporal connections since it was reasoned that the frontal lobes probably caused exaggeratedly abnormal behaviour (agitation) or experience (tension) through some unspecified overactivity. However, these early attempts at altering behaviour through surgery were clumsy, the cases badly chosen and the effects overshadowed by bad side effects ranging from antisocial behaviour to incontinence. The anatomical possibilities of brain surgery had however been suggested by Papez (1933) and later by MacLean (1958) who thought that the limbic system was a modulator of the emotions and it is on these observations that present day psychosurgery is based. These have developed from the modified leucotomies (Scoville, 1949; Knight, 1964) to the more refined stereotactic surgical techniques aimed at removing defined areas of brain tissue. Thus Lewin (1961) described surgery on the anterior cingulate gyrus while others have pointed out the good behavioural consequences of accurate surgery in temporal lobe epilepsy.

Psychosurgery has passed well beyond early ill directed enthusiasm, and later uncritical total rejection to the status of a treatment procedure to be used in selected cases where conservative methods have failed but above all it is a treatment directed at symptoms rather than illnesses. The particular symptoms are tension and anguish whether they are affective, schizophrenic or obsessional in origin. Duration of symptoms is important as is the presence of a relatively stable premorbid personality.

The assessment of the results of psychosurgery is ever beset by the lack of controlled studies though Schurr (1973) argues the case of surgery based on sensible clinical judgement in a way that is unfashionable yet not to be dismissed.

SOCIAL PSYCHIATRY—THE INTERFACE BETWEEN SOCIOLOGY AND PSYCHIATRY

Some psychiatrists are unnecessarily perturbed by the fact that psychiatry seems to be moving away from a special concern with the individual and his symptoms, but patients can neither be studied nor treated in a social vacuum. There are very few people who are so isolated that their behaviour touches no one. A person's interaction with his environment is complex, admittedly, but there are many environmental causes which may be ignored by psychiatrists, possibly because of their universality. For a large segment of the population the physical environment and especially their social class determines childhood health, educational opportunity, job expectation, age at marriage, life style and health in later life and mortality. An obvious example of the latter being the higher smoking habits and consequent respiratory diseases in social classes IV and V.

In psychoses there are again simple examples of cultural influences, *e.g.* in influencing the content of psychoses. In England 100 years ago regular church-going and religious belief were established features of life and so it is not surprising that religious delusions were more common then than they are now when the deluded patient is more likely to believe he is influenced by radar, television, communists etc. (Hare, 1955). Tantalising examples of how culture colours mental illness are found in supposedly abnormal mental states in immigrants. The majority view rejects spells and witch doctors, yet psychiatrists are from time to time perplexed by an immigrant brought to hospital in a state of terror and apparent catatonic stupor only to find that the patient has consulted a witch doctor but has become convinced that the witch doctor has put a spell on him and the wrong spell at that! Storey (1967) summarised this well by saying that an Englishman who says that witches are persecuting him is likely to be psychotic but that in Southern Italy where witchcraft is believed in, the patient would need a more sophisticated evaluation.

These simple examples are mentioned to remind us of the necessity of being aware of the interface between sociology and psychiatry so that we can learn more about social influences in the aetiology of psychiatric illness. Social markers such as group membership, race, sex, occupation, and social class can influence diagnosis and treatment (Hollingshead & Redlich, 1958). These are sophisticated topics no doubt but sociology also deals with the straightforward practical realities of the life of group rather than individuals, for instance the effects of institutions on individuals (Goffman, 1968). The list of involvement of sociology with psychiatry is formidable, in fact psychiatric epidemiology and social psychiatry are direct outgrowths of sociology. With the passage of time people have realised that a purely one to one relationship with a patient in a consulting room state is a limited way of learning anything about psychiatric morbidity, and may well be a method of creating 'illness' that hardly exists at all.

The history of sociology is well beyond the scope of this book but psychiatrists should be aware of some of its early writers. One of the most intriguing early attempts at sociology, anecdotal no doubt, but vividly interesting, came from Mayhew in his work on London Labour and the London Poor, an example of indefatigable interviewing of hundreds of poor people in Victorian London. He produced a series of brilliant portraits of the underprivileged, submerged in a metropolis that combined ferocious capitalism with pinch penny charity. Apart from this Mayhew did something else, usually overlooked, he made a good attempt at a census of the underprivileged be they watercress sellers, street entertainers, whores, beggars, navvies or pick pockets.

Since then, sociology has become a science that increasingly uses surveys, screening techniques etc. plus refined statistical methods, in the examination of every conceivable aspect of population behaviour, social problems and pathology of all sorts—racism, voting habits, eating and drinking, purchasing, media influences, health, employment, educational opportunity, new towns, delinquency etc.,

Where does psychiatry come into all this? We may start with *suicide* as studied by Emil Durkheim in the 19th Century (1951). Suicide is very much the concern of the psychiatrist yet it took the 'father of sociology' Durkheim to produce the first large scale study on epidemiology and sociology of suicide in his analysis of 26 000 cases in France. He drew attention not only to differing national and religion bound rates but also to a sociological model of suicide in which the act was defined in terms of the individuals varying responses to the needs, ties and obligations of his culture.

Statistics of insanity studied in the 19th Century were mainly based on hospital cases and were related to occupation and social class etc. However their limitations were recognised and it has been mainly in more recent times that we have had data from community surveys—although in 1855 the state of Massachusetts mounted a community survey that showed that the number of 'idiots and lunatics' in the State was over 100% higher than predicted by hospital figures.

Surveys of prevalence, surveys of attitudes to mental illness, sociological studies of hospitals as mini-societies, studies on rehabilitation of long term psychotic patients are now all taken for granted as highly relevant topics to be clarified by sociological research. In practice the psychiatrist's involvement with sociological principles starts at the straight-forward clinical level.

Making a psychiatric diagnosis frequently involves making a judgement of behaviour and this is true whether the basic pathology is organic or dynamic, since it is the altered 'behaviour' that brings the patient to the psychiatrist. When we categorise behaviour as abnormal or sick, no matter how we dress it up we are making a judgement and not only that, our 'treatment' and advice/counselling/psychotherapy may have immense and disastrous social consequences.

It is said that 'mental illness' has lost its stigma, this is not as true as we are led to believe. The diagnosis of 'mental illness' can cause a person to lose his job, be dismissed from university or lead to divorce. Also the patient is someone who has little or no chance of ever again being regarded as normal. The process of social damage may be worsened by well intentioned treatments, *e.g.* drugs that slow thinking, ECT that causes memory loss or therapy that turns 'illness' into self-indulgent histrionics. In short the psychiatrist has a heavy responsibility to society and should always ask himself whether he may be doing the patient harm by casting him in the role of patient. Just because a person enters a psychiatrist's office this does not automatically confer on him the status of being ill.

In the early 19th Century days of descriptive psychiatry as we have seen the main social factors in question were occupation, education and social status. In individual cases factors such as overwork and strain, sexual excess, diet and masturbation were widely invoked as causes of mental illness. Masturbation in particular has been brilliantly reviewed by Hare (1954) as a topic that psychiatrists extolled as pathological to such a degree that even in 1938 in England a leading surgical instrument manufac-turer still advertised antimasturbatory garments for male and female patients.

The relevance of sociology to psychiatry was neglected when psycho analysis seemed to offer treatment and explanation of psychiatric illness in highly personal terms. Modest forays into social aetiology faltered when psychoanalytic theory emphasised unconscious motivation plus conflict in a way that contrasted dramatically with the hopelessness of 19th Century descriptive psychiatry. Unhappily these advances in the understanding of personal dynamics held back the development of social psychiatry by encouraging an excessive preoccupation with the individual. Psycho-analytic theory 'caught on' in a remarkable way, particularly since the whole theory was based on untested hypotheses derived from the uncontrolled study of a handful of patients. Freud was aware of these limitations but his followers were not.

Only one aspect of this untested set of beliefs needs be mentioned. Freudian theory emphasised the idea of 'penis envy' thus unwittingly discriminating against women who were supposedly traumatised by having no penis, and as if that were not enough a whole farrago of theory about the best type of female orgasm was set out by a man, leaving thousands of women thereafter not only feeling cheated but also regarded as ill if they did not achieve orgasm as defined by the psychoanalytic school. The myth was perpetuated until Masters and Johnson studied orgasms and found that the much prized vaginal orgasm hardly existed and the clitoral orgasm was the most enjoyable and not only that, some women found that their most enjoyable orgasms were set off by battery operated vibrators!

However this purely personal theory of mental life was not universally accepted, even in 1921 Adolf Meyer said:

'Much is gained by the frank recognition that man is fundamentally a social being. There are reactions in us which only contacts and relations with other human beings can bring out. We must study man as mutual reagents in personal affections and aversions and their conflicts: in the desires and satisfactions of the simpler appetites for food and personal necessities: in the natural interplay of anticipation and fulfilment of their desires, and their occasional frustration; in the selection of companionship which works helpfully or otherwise—for the moment or more lastingly throughout the many vicissitudes of life.'

Again in America, the move away from a purely personal view was influenced by Harry Stack Sullivan who emphasised interpersonal relationships but viewed them in a social context. But this process was gradual and in fact the most important advances have occurred where the techniques of sociological research have been used to study the prevalence, aetiology and treatment of psychiatric disorders. Case finding and prevalence rates are the bread and butter of contemporary psychiatric research.

INSTITUTIONS AND THEIR EFFECTS

Many studies of hospitalised chronic schizophrenics have suggested that the structure of a closed institution can affect a patient badly by denying him individuality and responsibility for himself. Russell Barton (1959) described this state very aptly as 'Institutional Neurosis'—a state of apathetic inertia in long term mental hospital inmates where the patient becomes a dull colourless person, unable to make choices, cowed by absurd rules and regulations, badly fed, shabbily clothed and with no individual badges of his own identity. This was taken further by the studies of (Wing & Brown, 1970) who showed how varying degrees of institutionalism existed in hospitals and how they could be measured by the fact that such patients had firstly lost contact with the outside world and secondly, had been processed by their environment into becoming acquiescent automata. The area that causes controversy here is to what extent this is due to a process such as schizophrenia, and to what extent it is caused by the institution. Wing *et al* (1970) have noted that 'institutionalisation' is also found in chronic schizophrenics in the community.

Erving Goffman, the sociologist, examined the 'inmate society' of large institutions such as mental hospitals and concluded that the bureaucratic stucture of these institutions is bad for patients as it exposed them to a muddled system of custodialism, neglect, and denial of responsibility for himself which effectively prevented rehabilitation. Goffman's observations have mainly referred to large state mental hospitals in America and also to the inmate culture in prisons. Their relevance in England is repudiated by some, mainly on the grounds that institutions here are smaller and less rigid in structure. This is fair comment but it is still a fact that patients *are* submerged and dehumanised in mental hospitals firstly because their illness makes their hold on reality precarious and secondly because the patient's role of subservient compliance and acceptance of a negative self-image and lack of responsibility very soon becomes a self-perpetuating system.

The process of humanising mental hospitals *has* flourished in Britain however, after a 100 year lapse things began to look up in the 1930s when hospitals such as Warlingham Park and Dingleton unlocked their wards and encouraged active occupation and social activities for patients and also started the beginning of community mental health services. All this was accelerated after World War II when psychiatrists found that they had been well able to treat patients in the services with relatively little of the traditional 'bin' atmosphere and questioned the rigid hierarchy of the hospitals they returned to. The Mental Health Act, 1959, was a great influence in changing the custodial role of mental hospitals by encouraging informal admission and cutting through the unwieldy net of legal procedures governing admission.

The patient role

Many sociologists have examined the patient role in mental hospital society (Goffman, 1968; Stanton & Schwarz, 1954) pointing out that a person's role changes substantially when he becomes an in-patient. This is also true even for admission to a general hospital ward where a person's awareness of his own identity is rarely affected, but nevertheless he may easily become quite institutionalised, though only for a short time. The day-to-day life of the ward often absorbs him to an extent that his visitors find amusing and when he returns home he is often vaguely tetchy and ill at ease after the ordered life of the ward. But for the psychiatric patient this is a more intensive process since by his acceptance of the patient role he is regarded as less than responsible for himself or at worst, totally incapable of taking any responsibility. This means that he is not encouraged to make decisions, loses personal privacy and loses social obligations and basic rights. He has to ask permission to move around the hospital, and here is an interesting point, the mental hospital patient may be restricted in this way for no good reason at all—the general hospital patient is not so restricted when in fact his heart may be more at risk!

In short, the mental hospital patient is no longer a free agent and soon becomes dependent on the authority and word of others to guide his actions. This is backed up by a life style that encourages identity loss, usually psychiatric wards have a clinical atmosphere despite the lip service paid to privacy by hideous furniture and multicoloured curtains. In long stay wards despite improvements there is little domesticity, no privacy, much dinginess and a good deal of well meant herding. This type of environment is justified in a number of ways, *e.g.* on the grounds of security ('he might kill himself or harm someone') or clinical efficiency ('this is the best way to treat patients'). So the patient's liberty and personal identity are gradually eroded in the name of clinical necessity dictated by bureaucratic need. For the long stay patient a bleak lack of common humanity gilded by eager attempts at rehabilitation can nevertheless be disastrous, since he is up against a system that he can never overcome. If he defies the system this may be interpreted as a further sign of psychosis or serious personality disorder, while if he complies with the system he may become dependent on a mini society that rewards boring trifling work with trivial luxuries and punishes 'uncooperative' behaviour with physical assaults such as ECT, excessive use of tranquillisers and loss of privileges.

Thus the long stay patient can melt into a corporate state of anonymous helplessness.

Sammer and Osmond (1967) commented on the mental hospital as a 'no society' where patients live in a society that has no recognisable cultural elements, *i.e.* sparse language and a climate where all needs are met by a system. Art and occupation are mainly superficial; even hospital newspapers are weak and ineffectual, religious observance is often a way of passing the time and the patient society does not even bury its own dead.

These observations on the sociology of patient life are provocative and convince by their repetition in too many mental hospitals that cope as best they can with the care of the socially disadvantaged with poor resources, low public esteem, short staff and all in the absence of brutality. In short, the medical model of psychiatric disorder is least convincing when applied to the care of chronic patients beyond availability and expediency.

The past was not all bad—the 'moral treatment of the insane' in the 19th Century went beyond mere removal of restraint, encouraged occupation and self-reliance. But the scientific rationalism of the late 19th Century overstated mental illness as 'illness' and led to neglect based on the hope that problems in human behaviour would be solved in the postmortem room. If we add to this a laissez faire attitude, socioeconomic disasters such as World War I, we find Western society ideally equipped to overlook people who could not earn enough to survive nor seem successful in a materialistic society.

But it is no longer justifiable to assume that mental patients are less than responsible, there is a need for hospital communities where an attempt is made to encourage responsibility. 'We know what is good for the patient' is not good enough and from the reaction against this philosophy we find the development of the concept of the *therapeutic community*.

Therapeutic community

The basic idea of the therapeutic community is simple—it is that everyone in a hospital is potentially therapeutic in the sense that their actions and attitudes may influence the patient for good or ill in ways that are not obvious but which are none the less effective. The concept of the therapeutic community seemed revolutionary when originally stated by Maxwell Jones, but with time his ideas have come to be accepted as part of the sociology of mental illness, even by those who profess not to

o

follow them (Jones, 1960; Clark, 1900). In psychiatric hospitals a thera-peutic community is one where hierarchical control of patient behaviour ideally is replaced by a general commitment to democratic participation in the running of the hospital. This means general acceptance of an ideology of the 'treatment process' based on interchange of ideas, acceptance of responsibility for one's actions and total ventilation of feeling in an attempt to discover the underlying significance of 'abnormal behaviour'. For example aggressive and self-destructive behaviour is usually 'treated' by medication or by controlling the patient as being irresponsible. In a therapeutic community the patient is required to be accountable thus his behaviour is examined in group discussion. He is confronted with his lack of responsibility and called on to account for it.

The community operates through group meetings traditionally the community day starts with a general meeting where administrative matters are raised and where day-to-day problems come up. Thereafter the com-munity operates on the basis of informed self-help, backed up by staff groups where staff reactions and attitudes are examined and modified. The most notable uses of the Therapeutic Community Scheme have to date been in special units aimed at treating people with antisocial person-ality disorders but in fact most progressive psychiatric hospitals employ therapeutic community methods.

The best lesson to be learnt from the therapeutic community philosophy is that patients are to be treated as equals and not to be cast in the role of being 'one down' as against their omniscient healers. This assumption is technically valid in much of general medicine and surgery but only in a *technical* sense and never in a personal sense. In psychiatry the assumption of superiority is misleading and immoral. Any patient should be able to enter any hospital without fear of the staff and a hospital which provides such a climate creates goodwill and patient cooperation that can barely be estimated and renders unnecessary and irrelevant questions such as 'Why is this patient so difficult?'

PSYCHIATRY AND SOCIAL WORK

This is no place to write about such a vast topic as social work. There used to be a special type of social worker, the *psychiatric social worker* who was a specialist in psychiatry, but this idea is now superseded by the *generic social worker,* a professional who brings to whatever task the special skills of basic social work. The question is what *are* the special skills of social work? No one quite seems to know though all agree that they exist. In psychiatry in fact the social worker probably has more to offer than in any other discipline since psychiatry and the social sciences are so closely linked.

It is easy enough to list at random the range of activities of the social worker in the psychiatric team, *e.g.* counselling, casework, follow-up, crisis intervention, rehabilitation, psychotherapy, support, advice, encouragement, etc., but hard to define exactly what they all have in common except in one sense; namely that the social worker is usually someone with a sense of professional committment to a personal involvement with the idea of helping the client, the patient to live more effectively and positively in the world. Many social workers feel their efforts frustrated by the ill-defined nature of their work and the lack of professional autonomy, although the latter has happily altered. Others have felt frustrated by social work which seems to consist of self-defeating efforts to patch up people beaten by a political and social system that seems to contribute largely to their ills. All these discontents are however not peculiar to social work—they exist to much the same extent in medicine and psychiatry—it is just that social workers are usually more aware and concerned about them.

REHABILITATION

Rehabilitation and treatment are inseparable concepts in the management of all psychiatric disorders. Admittedly it must seem to many that a good deal of psychiatric treatment consists in relieving or suppressing troublesome symptoms. On the other hand the majority of psychiatric patients are handicapped beyond mere symptoms by changes in their life experience and life style which extensively influence their ability to enjoy life, have relationships with others, earn a living—in fact to do all sorts of things that normally are taken for granted. For the depressed patient, for the anxious patient, rehabilitation usually consists in a process where he is enabled to return to familiar day-to-day existence untroubled by depressive self-doubt or worried indecision—in these cases the rehabilitation consists mainly of time and sensible positive support and encouragement.

For the *brain damaged* patient, rehabilitation means learning to make the best of available brain function, to tolerate a more limited range of abilities etc., and for the *schizophrenic patient* rehabilitation means the avoidance of institutionalism and apathetic deterioration so that he can live and work in the community.

There is no simple recipe for any or all of these objectives but there are a number of tactics and techniques that are available, and nowadays all are based on the use of *teams* of professionals involved aimed at producing the best possible comprehensive care for the patient. This is the theory and an excellent ideal; rarely attained in practice. In hospital, for instance, the patient may join in *occupational and industrial therapy*.

Occupational therapy

For many years it has been realised that work can be diverting and interesting to the disturbed patient. Nowadays the occupational therapist has a wide range of activities to offer the psychiatric patient. These include art and craft work which can calm the anxious patient or revive the interest of the retarded depressive. Tasks can be provided for the brain damaged patient which may afford him some degree of satisfaction.

Also the occupational therapist can assess the limits of such a patient's ability and help to provide him with a suitable environment. In rehabilitation the OT Department can help to plan a patient's daily round of activity and to prepare for the return home by helping him to acquire new skills or refurbish old ones. The housewife can be particularly helped in this direction by the provision of a kitchen in the OT Department. Ideally occupational therapy should be realistic and diverse and as far removed as possible from the traditional picture of basket making or the manufacture of useless ornaments.

Industrial therapy

This is an attempt to provide the patient with a working day, a regular wage and the prospects of working outside hospital. It provides a sheltered working environment for the chronic patient where he can learn, practise and gain confidence in new skills. In many hospitals light assembly work etc. is done on a contract basis with local firms and after a patient has 'proved himself', he can then go out to work.

Rehabilitation of chronic patients, particularly chronic schizophrenics, is a difficult task. Patients need graded tasks, encouragement and supervision. Many chronic schizophrenics are much more employable than formerly was realised *provided* they can work in a sheltered setting. Special techniques of rehabilitation developed in recent years involve the use of the Token Economy. This is a technique based on Skinnerian Learning Theory, in which a patient is rewarded for acceptable behaviour while unacceptable behaviour is ignored. In a token economy unit the chronic schizophrenic patient is rewarded for basic acts such as shaving, dressing, bedmaking etc., by a system of tokens used to buy rewards, *e.g.* cigarettes, etc. (though the use of a public health menace such as cigarettes as a reward seems pretty dubious!).

19

Rare syndromes—classifiable
and unclassifiable

MORBID JEALOUSY

Jealousy is an interesting and disturbing state which should be interesting to any thoughtful psychiatrist because jealousy encompasses not merely the delusions of the psychotic but is an emotion which can seep inexorably and understandably into the half verbalised fears of a normal person who suspects infidelity or betrayal and may alter his mental life and judgement to the extent of committing murder.

Morbid Jealousy as a psychiatric syndrome has been definitively reviewed by Shepherd (1961) whose overview remains the most comprehensive. Jealousy has been perfectly described by poets, novelists and philosophers but remains ill defined for the behavioural scientists. The origins of the word itself are clouded—the Latin adjective *zelosus* was transmuted from meaning zealous or keen into something less noble, more mean, and less acceptable or even tolerable since now the word means envious hate in a setting of amorous loss. Psychiatrists began to be interested in jealousy in the 19th Century; as did psychologists such as Ribot who found the passions complex and ineluctable, for Ribot jealousy was a 'complex state' compounded of 'pleasure, anger and chagrin'.

In more recent times attempts to understand jealousy in psychological terms have been hardly more successful. The problem is to distinguish between normal and morbid jealousy. Morbid jealousy is more extensive; it involves the person totally and ultimately is incomprehensible even though its beginnings may be understandable.

As a symptom morbid jealousy is important because it is found in a wide range of disorders—schizophrenia, organic syndromes, the neuroses, personality disorders and senile disorders. In every case of morbid jealousy there is a repetition of familiar themes that are not merely clinically interesting but are also warnings of personal disaster—in this lies the dramatic relevance of morbid jealousy.

Though jealousy is universal, this should not divert the clinician's attention from its general symptomatology. Delusional jealousy for instance is more complex than straightforward paranoid delusions since it is eternally intermingled with the search for proof.

The deluded schizophrenic who believes he is Christ, knows he is and needs no proof from everyday trivia but the morbidly jealous person, deluded or not, looks for proof in an accumulation of daily happenings that assume prime importance and a growing burden of certainty. A look in the eye, a fancied blush or catch in the breath, a certain smile, an uncertainty in talk, all become part of a catalogue of proven sin and betrayal. From this the jealous person finds cool embraces and discovers unexplained sexual excitement, *e.g.* vaginal moistness—an obvious sign of increased desire or recent intercourse. Consider the following case.

A 48 year old man was found to be morbidly jealous of his wife who had been referred for treatment of 'depression'. At interview after a guarded start he spoke at great length about his suspicions about his wife. He said 'Well I suppose many people would say I was suspicious but if they knew the whole story they'd agree with me and understand. My wife, well she's an attractive woman, too attractive in a way as I know too well. She's always liked men's company but now it's beyond that. Not just a flirt you understand. I first realised something was up when she came home late. Said she'd been out with a girl friend from work but it became obvious to me later thinking about it that she was obviously meeting someone. Who? God knows, I don't, but I know she is . . . well over the next few months it all began to add up . . . little things that all point to one thing . . . one night she came in all smiles and kind of flushed and I remember when we got to bed I touched her private parts and they were all moist and hot. So you see I knew. Well after that it was just a succession of things that proved it—stains on her clothes, a funny smile—you know. . . .'

It emerged that he had been questioning his wife nightly, sometimes all night, with threats, promises, blows, anything that would give him proof. This is important—the morbidly jealous patient seeks proof relentlessly and in a way that is absurd to anyone else.

Morbid jealousy *does not have to be delusional* to be morbid, often it is excessive suspicion founded on nothing and thriving on everything. Shepherd (1961) commented that the full evaluation of morbid jealousy should include taking into account:

1 Associated syndromes
2 Personality age and sex
3 Speed of onset and any tendency for jealousy to be phasic.

The diagnostic possibilities as listed by Shepherd include the whole spectrum of psychiatric nosology: organic psychoses, schizophrenia, affective psychoses, personality disorders and neuroses.

Organic psychoses

Here it is important to note the importance of intoxication with alcohol, the amphetamines, hallucinogenic drugs and cocaine as opposed to senile dementia and rarities such as Huntington's chorea and presenile dementia.

Schizophrenia

True delusions are nearly essential features in schizophrenia. It is always important to distinguish between delusions and delusional ideas or overvalued ideas which might be understandably developed by a suspicious oversensitive person.

Affective psychoses

Manic and depressed patients can develop delusional ideas and these may be jealous in type.

Personality disorders and the neuroses

The paranoid oversensitive personality is likely to become jealous, this is a recognised feature of personality disorders. In the neuroses jealousy is likely to be part of a diffuse view of the world where the neurotic finds compensation for his own deficiencies in envious hatred and mistrust.

Management of morbid jealousy syndromes

Clearly where a schizophrenic process underlies a morbid jealousy syndrome one can expect some improvement either through phenothiazines or natural remission, in the case of affective disorder causing morbid jealousy the outlook through antidepressant treatment is no doubt better. But above all the psychiatrist should always be aware of the real dangers of violence and murder in the morbidly jealous, numerous studies reiterate this (East, 1936; Brierley, 1932; Hopwood & Milner, 1940; Ey, 1950).

FOLIE À DEUX

Folie à deux is a disorder in which two or more people become psychotic and share delusional beliefs. It was originally described in France and is a rare condition more common in women than in men. Essentially the disorder consists of one paranoid schizophrenic dominating a close relative and imposing a delusional system which comes to be shared by the more passive partner. The syndrome develops slowly and insidiously. Separation of the two individuals usually causes improvement in the passive partner, this is based on the close emotional ties between a psychotic and a non-psychotic person the latter having become overidentified with the former. Despite the assertions of those who have commented on this in speculative terms the process seems little more than a highly specialised form of collusion. More extensive varieties have been described in primitive and unsophisticated communities.

GANSER SYNDROME

Ganser (1898) described a psychiatric syndrome characterised by altered consciousness—a 'twilight' state of apparent hysterical dissociation in which the main abnormality was a tendency to answer questions in a way that was 'past the point'. He called it the 'syndrome of approximate answers' as exemplified by the answer 'five' to the question 'How many legs has a cow?'—a question which many would suppose might well invite such an answer!

However Ganser's observations are not to be dismissed so lightly. Like most 19th Century German psychiatrists Ganser set out exactly what he had observed and kept speculation about aetiology to a minimum. Later authors have argued about whether the Ganser syndrome is or is not a hysterical disorder—an argument made at least partially sterile by the finding that a significant percentage of patients diagnosed as '?Ganser syndrome' turn out to be psychotic. The majority of Ganser syndromes *are* found in prisoners and may be regarded as atypical psychoses which cover a continuum that extends from malingering through hysteria to frank psychosis, occurring usually in patients of low intelligence in highly specific stressed situations such as imprisonment. The term 'Ganser syndrome' is therefore not a diagnosis but merely the first stage in a differential diagnosis and as such merits appropriate recognition and treatment.

KORO

This is another culture bound syndrome peculiar to the Malay Archipelago and Southern China. It consists of acute anxiety symptoms associated with feelings of unreality but the whole picture is dominated by the fear that the penis is shrinking and that if it goes the sufferer will die. This bad news causes intense family disturbance, panic, strings round the penis and general alarm. It is no doubt related to culture bound fears about the possible harmful effects of supposed sexual excess—something about which Western man need not feel unduly superior if the myths about masturbation, the large penis of the negro etc. are anything to go by.

The Koro patients described are inevitably heavily influenced by their culture and a general atmosphere of sexual hypochondriasis which finds expression in this rather dramatic syndrome. The Malay Archipelago is clearly an area where special cultural influences colour psychiatric syndromes in a dramatic way since this part of the world has provided the phenomena of *Latah* and *Amok*. In *Latah* a patient may develop echo reactions, echolalia, and automatic obedience or may develop severely inappropriate behaviour in response to trifling stimuli. In either case the syndrome appears to be a neurotic disorder triggered off by fright and heavily coloured by cultural beliefs in demonic possession, and the influence of malign spirits. *Amok* is an interesting culture bound phenomenon in which a person suddenly becomes homicidally violent following a spell of sullen gloom. It has only been described in Malays and its incidence fell sharply when it was designated as a criminal offence. It is best regarded as a culture bound and culturally permitted behaviour disorder of no real significance beyond its violent content. Perhaps its most interesting aspect is that it was controlled by the law!

COTARD'S SYNDROME

This is a good example of an eponymous syndrome which no longer has any meaning since the syndrome is now recognised for what it is, namely severe psychotic *depression*. In the 19th Century the French physician Cotard described 'delire de negation', *i.e.* a mental state in which the patient describes severe material poverty ('all my riches have gone') and loss of vital organs ('my heart and liver are gone. I have none'). Cotard was describing depressive delusional beliefs, usually found in elderly, often seclusive patients. The term was rediscovered a few years ago and made a brief appearance in the correspondence columns where it seemed to be hailed. It is mentioned only in the hope of protecting examination candidates from examiners who are bent on interrogating people about irrelevancies. The same comments apply to *Capgras' syndrome*, an eponym for paranoid schizoprenia, in which the central delusion is that a member of the family is an impostor either very like the original, or to be detected by close questioning etc. This schizophrenic content has usually been described in relatively unsophisticated communities influenced by superstition, belief in changelings, witchcraft etc. A grisly example occurred in 19th Century rural Ireland where a farmer caused a child to be murdered by the family persuaded by him that the child was a changeling. A good example of the force of paranoid schizophrenic's delusions in a closely knit circle just like folie à deux.

20

Psychiatry and the law

INTRODUCTION

Psychiatry and the Law interweave in many ways. In the first place psychiatry can deprive a man of his liberty on the grounds of mental illness, subnormality or psychopathic disorder and if this is backed up by a court order, in certain cases a person can be deprived of liberty indefinitely. This is probably the most concrete example of the interrelationship between psychiatry and the Law, others are less clearly defined, for example the psychiatric aspects of adult crime and juvenile delinquency. These latter are important topics because of their social and clinical importance, the psychiatric evaluation of an offender may largely influence a court's decision in applying the law. This is important since it means that the concept of illness is being used to modify the decisions of society's appointed representatives. And this is not a simple matter since it means not merely deciding whether or not someone is responsible for his actions but going beyond this and suggesting that *he needs or is amenable to treatment*. This provides at least legal recognition of a medical model of psychiatric disorder, but one which does not really measure up to society's expectations since the 'treatment' of socially deviant behaviour judged to be a manifestation of 'illness' is less successful than is hoped. On the other hand penal methods are in general no more successful. Part of the problem lies in the fact that a moral model of deviant antisocial behaviour has been abandoned in favour of a sickness model. But antisocial behaviour is more complex than psychiatric disorder, for a start criminality shows a wider range of definition than does psychiatric illness. These and other aspects of criminality will be examined.

Criminal responsibility

In ordinary life a person's responsibility for his actions is hardly ever called into question. It is generally assumed that adults control their behaviour and feelings, indeed, learning to do this is a basic part of personal and social development and maturation. In civilised societies the assumption of a man's responsibility for himself and his actions and for his obligations to his fellows is to some extent recognised in laws which codify society's limits of tolerable behaviour. In this country the law assumes that a man is responsible for his actions in that he intends and expects their result. In fact from the legal point of view the whole question of responsibility is tied in with intent and the ability to form intent. For legal purposes, therefore, concepts of guilt, responsibility and punishment are fairly clear. Criminality is based on criminal intent, *i.e.* the person is a completely free agent who has chosen to behave badly. He is responsible for what he has done and must take the consequences.

This may seem an oversimple way of looking at human behaviour and it is certainly one that has been questioned by legal scholars as well as psychiatrists and psychologists. The concept of free will and free choice is basic to the legal system but at some stage it has to be clarified as to what is meant exactly by free will, quite apart from any philosophical or theological considerations that arise. Very often when jurists and psychiatrists disagree over responsibility they are carrying on a mediaeval religious disputation without knowing it. Psychiatrists tend to be uncertain about concepts such as culpability and equally uncertain about human behaviour in general. Psychiatric theory whether it acknowledges it or not is considerably influenced by psychoanalytic theory and assigns prime importance to conflict, unconscious motivation, early experience and so on. The psychiatrist is likely to look for sickness as a model of antisocial behaviour, whereas the jurist may see a criminal act as a deliberate antisocial act or as part of a career of criminality. On the other hand it should be realised that the concept of free will raises man above the level of being a mere decision-making machine, programmed by his environment, incapable of exercising free choice, and entirely governed by whims and fortuitous events.

The legal position regarding responsibility for actions is summed up in the quotation 'actus non facit reum nisi mens sit rea', *i.e.* there cannot be a guilty act unless there is a guilty mind.

The question of responsibility for actions is taken for granted in daily life where people are assumed to be responsible people who contribute to their own and their family welfare, to the common good, and that they have a general though unstated awareness of their obligations and relationships to their fellows, so that responsibility for one's own actions is called to question usually when a person behaves in an unexpected and unpredicted way, the most extreme example of this in our society being murder, where the deliberate killing of a person is intolerable. When capital punishment for murder existed the problem of responsibility was questioned, *i.e.* 'to act like that a man must be sick (*i.e.* mad)'—thus he is less than responsible for his actions. Now in English law murder is distinguished from manslaughter entirely on the basis of intent, *i.e.* the person intended the death of the victim. The question of responsibility for murder has caused considerable legal disagreement. Murder is a crime that has for centuries been intolerable to any society that tries to preserve its safety and as societies became more organised, murder became less acceptable through corporate murder in the name of society is given spurious dignity in the name of war.

There has to be some way of deciding whether someone is less than responsible for an act such as murder and one way is to say that the killer is sick; that he did not intend the victim's death because his judgement, moral sense and self-control were diminished by being ill. Responsibility for murder was questioned long before capital punishment was abolished since it was obvious that murder was often committed by people who did not know what they were doing—in the eyes of the law such a person could be held to be so abnormal as to be incapable of forming intent. Culpability was for many years subject to the McNaghten rules which were a legal attempt to define criminal responsibility. They arose out of the trial of Daniel McNaghten, a paranoid schizophrenic who in 1843 killed Sir Robert Peel's secretary, under the impression that he was Sir Robert Peel whom he believed to be persecuting him. This prompted Queen Victoria to comment that she could not see how anyone could be judged to be insane who tried to murder a Conservative Prime Minister. McNaghten was acquitted on the grounds of insanity, and subsequently 15 judges in the House of Lords formulated a series of answers to questions—and the answers came to be known as the McNaghten rules and were applied as a test of criminal responsibility.

The basic statement of the rules was that every man is presumed to be sane and to possess 'a sufficient degree of reason to be responsible for his crimes unless proved to the contrary and that to establish a defence on grounds of insanity it must be clearly proved that at the time of the committing of the act, the party accused was labouring under such a defect of reason from disease of the mind, as not to know the nature and quality of the act he was doing: or if he did know it, that he did not know he was doing what was wrong'. The other statement made by the rules was in effect that delusion could only be used as a defence in cases where if the delusions were true that it could justify the offence.

The McNaghten rules were never really satisfactory since they, on the one hand, referred to 'disease of the mind' as a mitigating factor but at the same time restricted the use of such a defence by virtually limiting it to certain types of mental illness. For instance a depressive psychotic may kill a close relative believing that this will save them from eternal damnation but be judged sane by the McNaghten rules and executed, and this in fact used to happen.

In Scotland in the mid 19th Century the law had already recognised diminished responsibility in murder when in 1867 a Judge advised a jury in a murder case that 'It was not beyond their province to find a verdict of culpable homicide' in the case being tried since the accused 'had his mind weakened by successive attacks of disease'—which might be thought of as 'an extenuating circumstance'. But the McNaghten rules remained the test of criminal responsibility for murder in England until the Homicide Act 1957 in which section 2 (1) provides that 'Where a person kills or is a party to the killing of another, he shall not be convicted of murder if he was suffering from such abnormality of mind (whether arising from a condition of arrested or retarded development of mind or any inherent causes or induced by disease or injury) as substantially impaired his mental responsibility for his acts and omissions in doing or being a party to the killing'. In practice this means that in cases of alleged murder where the accused can be clearly shown to be psychotic, mentally subnormal or psychopathic, then this will be accepted as diminished responsibility and the offence if proved will be manslaughter.

The concept of diminished responsibility has come in for some criticism since some feel that it calls into question the notion of any sort of responsibility for one's acts at all, while others seem to think it yet another sign of the deteriorating standards of an age in which people are dangerously self-indulgent and permissive, ignoring free will and making men into dehumanised machines etc.

This is a topic which psychiatrists must think about. It is not quite good enough to have a vague assumption that all offenders are sick people, the victims of bad upbringing, in need of treatment etc. This does not fit the facts. In cases of murder the incidence of psychosis and psychopathy is high, but in England murder is rare—the bulk of criminality is thieving and here the role of frank mental disorder is minor.

The psychiatrist and crime

A crime is said to occur 'when a society with recognised ways of behaving or when a part of society which has power and authority to do so categorises certain varieties of extreme or damaging behaviour as being liable to punishment'. In considering the incidence of crime in any country one relies on the criminal statistics provided by official agencies. In England offences are divided broadly into two groups, those which are indictable and those which are not. Non-indictable offences are common and include such behaviour as drunkenness, the taking and driving away of motor vehicles, dangerous driving and certain sexual offences. Yet public attention is constantly directed towards the increase in delinquent behaviour amongst the young much of which is relatively trivial. Delinquent behaviour has to be seen against the general social background of the UK. This is mainly a single culture nation with a more or less stratified society. There is little organised crime and the historical and economic climate is one of gradual social development influenced by moderate radicalism. The welfare state has produced a new range of opportunity for self-betterment and on the whole a modestly acceptable degree of equality of educational opportunity.

There has been a steady increase in juvenile offences in the last 10 years. There was a sharp rise after the war up until 1951, little change between the years 1951 and 1957, and then a renewed increase. The main recent rise in juvenile delinquency occurred in the 16 to 20 age group, but, as pointed out by West (1967), the peak age of conviction is 14. Of the people found guilty of indictable offences 50% lie between the ages of 10 and 21, but by the age of 25 the number convicted is half that of people aged 14. As in most developed countries, the main problems of delinquent behaviour concern young boys. The factors contributing to delinquent behaviour are numerous and the evidence for their importance is profuse and, at times, conflicting. For instance between the years 1935–6 and the years 1941–2 the sharp rise in conviction rates amongst the young produced the idea of a 'delinquent generation', an idea now disregarded.

It is wise, to be cautious about accepting figures provided by official agencies. For instance recorded increases may be affected by a number of factors. There may be changes in reporting patterns used by the police, or the public may be more ready to report certain offences, particularly those involving violence. Also victims of assault tend nowadays to report the offence more readily than formerly.

Another fact is that there is a clear sex difference in delinquent behaviour. In general the ratio of male to female offenders is in the order of six to one, but this ratio decreases with age. Many investigations have been carried out which suggest that girls and women in general have more conformist views on ethical and moral behaviour, and of course there are many offences which lie beyond their physical capabilities. In England, at any rate, the main offences involving women are shoplifting, prostitution, abortion, and assaults against other women and children. Also certain crimes committed by women occur within the context of a special relationship, and so never get reported at all: for instance, the prostitute's client who has his money stolen would normally be reluctant to report her.

In general the main offences committed by the juvenile male offender in the UK are minor larcenies, taking and driving away cars, damage to property and absconding. Juvenile offences are common in large cities. and many social workers have put together a broad picture of the typical young juvenile offender. Great stress has been laid on the frequency with which these youngsters come from 'broken homes'. In this context it appears that divorce or separation of the parents is of greater significance than the loss of one parent by death. There is no apparent correlation between delinquency rates and intelligence as such, but the youngsters studied usually show evidence of low educational attainment. This may be because they tend to come from a background where expectations are low and where little interest is taken in their future. The one factor that emerges clearly is that juvenile delinquency is disproportionately high in slum areas, and that there is a real correlation between delinquency and both poverty in the material sense and poverty of expectation in a more subtle sense.

In the USA investigation of the juvenile offender has concentrated on ethnic factors. It has been found, for instance that disproportionate numbers of offenders are Negro slum dwellers. However, the delinquency rates amongst blacks and whites tend to level out when black populations move into areas where they enjoy better conditions of living. An overall consideration of the juvenile offender in slum areas in the USA shows that these youngsters usually live in physical environments which are extremely bad. They are brought up in an expectation of failure in a climate of extreme disorganisation of family life. Loss of one parent through separation or divorce is common, and discipline in the home often shows itself as an inconsistent mixture of permissiveness and harshness. Rejection by one or other parent is extremely common. There seems to be a failure of identification of the son with the father in the process of growing-up.

In the UK extreme degrees of poverty and social disorganisation are rare, so that the picture of the ghetto-dwelling delinquent youngster, drawn from American studies, has little relevance here. On the other hand two important factors do stand out: these are the clear relevance of age and sex. Boys are in general more delinquent than girls, and the young are more delinquent than the old.

If the official crime statistics are anything to go by, it could well be argued that delinquent behaviour is self-limiting since the number of offences falls off with age. The economic background to crime in this country probably relates to periods of financial hardship rather than to conditions of permanent poverty. For example, someone would be more likely to commit a crime when unemployed than when in work. A further point which has emerged from a large number of studies undertaken both in the UK and in the USA is that the delinquent youngster usually comes from a large family. Belonging to a large family means that a youngster drifts into delinquency through lack of adequate supervision. Even if the father is earning a reasonably good wage, supporting a large family is bound to strain his financial resources. The control and training of many children is also harder for the mother, particularly if she is in poor health. The lack of general supervision in large families can be reflected by such indications as the rates of truancy.

It is important to realise that there is apparently no single cause for criminal behaviour. Many studies have been devoted to the social backgrounds, personal characteristics, psychological attributes etc. of young people involved in criminal acts, and certain general observations have emerged. However, it must be conceded that, with the exception of the age and sex factors mentioned earlier, no single factor can be cited to predict criminal behaviour. As West (1967) has commented 'although no single type of hardship has a monopoly in relation to delinquency, it could be that delinquents experience an accumulation of adverse pressures which build up to the point where restraints are overcome and crimes occur'. It is this sort of balanced statement that is badly needed when considering the juvenile offender.

The Mental Health Act

By any standards the Mental Health Act 1959 is a good piece of law. It is liberal and it encourages informal admission in preference to compulsion and custodialism. Previously the laws were cumbersome and mainly concerned with the regulation of mental hospitals, compulsory treatment and the protection of the patient's rights. These were admirable aims which arose following the squalid disclosures of the 18th Century in which the mentally ill were usually treated in a dreadful way. They were bullied, assaulted, neglected and exploited in ways that cause horror to 20th Century man who has learnt to accept genocide as part of history. The abuse of mental patients became a public spectacle—fashionable people went to mock the lunatics in Bedlam in the same way that they attended public executions.

Legal attempts to control this were the beginnings of custodialism—now a dirty word, but originally an honest attempt to house, feed and clothe defenceless psychotics, that is to provide them with asylum. In the early part of the 19th Century there emerged the 'moral treatment of the insane', *i.e.* treating mental patients as responsible human beings and encouraging them to be self-reliant individuals. Hospitals such as the Retreat in York and physicians such as Connolly were leaders in this movement. The sad thing is that many of these early lessons were overlooked and forgotten in the late 19th Century emphasis on a scientific and medical model of psychiatry.

The Lunacy Act 1890 was a comprehensive law which protected patient's rights, guarded his property and protected against unlawful detention. This was done by covering admission procedures by the presence of a Justice of the Peace who could act as a person unbiased by medical influence or mistaken diagnosis. The description of the mental state had to be set out in such a way as to make sense to a layman and convince him of the need to deprive a citizen of his liberty on the grounds of mental illness. Mental hospitals were supervised and inspected by the Board of Control who ferreted out abuse and neglect. But the Act was rigid and prevented people from getting hospital treatment without compulsion so that mental hospitals tended to become more established in a rigid custodial role and were unable to take advantage of such therapeutic advances as came along, *e.g.* as late as the late 1930s when insulin coma treatment for schizophrenia came in at least one County Council forbade its use no doubt in a spirit of benign paternalism and wooden bureaucratic ignorance. The stigma of mental hospital admission got worse since everyone knew that only the worst cases were in such places. The Mental Treatment Act of 1930 helped to improve matters but the Mental Health Act made the whole situation more rational.

The main provisions of the Act are as follows:

1 The control and supervision of psychiatric hospitals becomes the responsibility of the National Health Service through the Department of Health and Social Security and Area Health Authorities. However direct supervision of special hospitals such as Broadmoor and Rampton is retained by the Department of Health

2 Informal admission is proclaimed as the ideal whilst compulsory admission is reserved for emergencies, observation and special cases needing compulsory treatment or other cases needing treatment related to criminality. In practice this has resulted in the fact that over 90% of mental hospital patients are informal patients having the same rights and status as any patient in any general hospital.

3 The procedures surrounding compulsory admission for observation or treatment are made clinical in tone rather than formal and intimidating.

4 The local authority is empowered and encouraged to provide after care and rehabilitation services.

On the first three counts the Mental Health Act has been an unqualified success, on the last it has failed mainly because Local Authorities have lacked sufficient funds to provide appropriate services. The Act is divided into nine parts.

Part 1 repeals previous legislation, defines and classifies mental disorder and proclaims informal admission   (Sec. 1–5)

Part 2 deals with the role of the local authority   (Sec. 6–13)

Part 3 deals with nursing homes etc.   (Sec. 14–24)

Part 4 deals with compulsory admission to hospital   (Sec. 25–59)

Part 5 deals with criminal patients   (Sec. 60–80)

Part 6 deals with transfer of patients (Sec. 81–96)

Part 7 deals with special hospitals (for dangerous and violent patients) (Sec. 97–99)

Part 8 deals with management of property and affairs of patients (Sec. 100–121)

Part 9 Miscellaneous (Sec. 122–154)

The Act defines mental disorder, psychopathic disorder and mental subnormality. Mental disorder is rather vaguely defined as mental illness, arrested or incomplete development of mind, psychopathic disorder and any other disorder or disability of mind. This is a definition that leaves the impression that 'mental disorder' is a term in general rather than particular.

Psychopathic disorder is a persistent disorder or disability of mind (whether or not including subnormality of intelligence) which results in abnormally aggressive or seriously irresponsible conduct on the part of the patient, and requires or is susceptible to medical treatment.

Subnormality is a state of arrested or incomplete development of mind (not amounting to severe subnormality) which include subnormality of intelligence and is of a nature and degree which requires or is susceptible to medical treatment or other special care or training of the patient.

Severe subnormality is a state of arrested or incomplete development of mind which includes subnormality of intelligence and is of such a nature or degree that the patient is incapable of living an independent life or of guarding himself against serious exploitation, or will be so incapable when of an age to do so.

Psychiatrists should be familiar with the Mental Health Act particularly those sections relating to compulsory admission. In every case of compulsory admission the intention of the Act is to make this as short a period as possible and to this end it employs two principles: firstly an application for admission, preferably made by the nearest relative, or if unavailable a Mental Welfare Officer and secondly a medical recommendation usually made by two doctors at least one of whom must be a doctor recognised as having special psychiatric experience under Section 28 of the Act. The requirements of medical recommendation vary. Opposite are summarised the essential requirements of the relevant sections.

Section	Object	Application made by	Medical recommendation	Comment
25	Admission for observation	Nearest relative or MWO	Two doctors; one recognised as having special experience	Duration is 28 days. This is the preferred method of compulsory short term admission
26	Admission for compulsory *treatment*	Nearest relative or MWO	Two doctors; one recognised as having special experience	This lasts for 1 year. It should only be used where informal admissions have clearly failed. The patient and family may appeal to a Mental Health Review Tribunal after 3 months
29	Emergency admission for observation	Nearest relative or MWO	Any doctor	Lasts for 3 days; should only be used in *genuine* emergencies *e.g.* acutely suicidal or homicidal behaviour and *not* as a convenient way to get rid of noisy or elderly patients
30	To retain a patient in *any* hospital if after admission he is disturbed enough to warrant it		Hospital doctor, usually consultant	
60	To provide compulsory treatment for offenders		Two doctors; usually a Prison Medical Officer and a visiting consultant	The hospital order (60) is made by a judge on the grounds of mental illness, mental subnormality or psychopathic disorder. The hospital consultant has the right to discharge the patient unless the Judge makes a recommendation restricting discharge under Section 65

Section	Object	Application made by	Medical recommendation	Comment
136	To provide a facility for the examination of patients found by the Police and thought to be of unsound mind in public			The Police may take such a person to a 'place of safety' to be examined by a doctor and a mental welfare officer

In practice Section 29 and Section 25 are the most commonly used sections of the Act. The spirit of the Act favours Section 25 where admission for observation is recommended by *two doctors* but there is a general impression that Section 29 has been used too frequently usually to transfer noisy and unacceptable patients to psychiatric hospitals. This tendency should be resisted, it is a very serious matter to deprive a person of his liberty for however short a period; and any doctor who abuses this duty behaves irresponsibly.

The admission for compulsory treatment (Section 26) is also an important question. It may be used for mental illness, subnormality and psychopathic disorder (under the age of 21) but properly it should only be used if (a) there are *really* adequate clinical indications which can be set out in the medical recommendation and (b) if informal treatment has failed and compulsory treatment offers some hope of recovery. This latter is an important point, there really is little humanity in imposing compulsory treatment on a patient if the treatment offers no hope of improvement, to do so seems a euphemism for imprisonment. Also it is debatable whether one should use compulsory treatment 'because the patient will not improve without it'. The efficacy of psychiatric treatment is not so good as to be backed up by such a vague claim.

Danger to others is a very important criterion; society must be protected from violent people whether mentally ill or not but the risk of suicide is another matter. It may be used as grounds for short term admission but it is hardly admissible as grounds for long term compulsory admission. In the case of patients admitted under Section 60 the psychiatrist has a special responsibility since he has the right to discharge an offender who may present a real danger to society in terms of violence or homicide.

Here the psychiatrist must accept the proposition that society's needs may take precedence of the needs of the patient's apparent clinical recovery and the discharge is something that should be treated cautiously using periods of leave of absence as 'parole' during which the patient may be carefully tested out. In these cases the psychiatrist must recognise his dual responsibility to society and patient.

All doctors should try to combine respect for the patient with responsibility for his case. This is, on the whole, not a difficult thing to do providing the doctor remembers always that the patient is a real person whose individuality must ever be respected—and that is what good medicine and good psychiatry is all about.

REFERENCES

Contents

Affective disorders—biochemistry
Affective disorders—genetic studies
Alcoholism and addiction
Anorexia nervosa
Antidepressants
Anxiety
Aphasia
Behaviour therapy
Bereavement
Biochemistry
Cerebral tumour
Delinquency
Depersonalisation
Depression
Epidemiology
Epilepsy—psychiatric aspects
Family influences in psychiatric disorders
Lithium
Monoamine oxidase inhibitors
Morbid jealousy
Munchausen syndrome
Myxoedema
Neuroleptics

Neurosis
Nosology—diagnosis
Obsessional disorder
Old age
Old age—late onset schizophrenia
Organic syndromes
Phobias
Puerperal disorders
Psychiatry—transcultural aspects
Psychological theory
Psychopathic disorder
Psychosurgery
Psychopharmacology
Psychosomatic disorders
Schizophrenia
Schizophrenia—epidemiology
Schizophrenia—genetics
Senile dementia
Sexual disorders
Sleep
Sociology and psychiatry
Suicide and attempted suicide
Other topics

Affective disorders—biochemistry

CADE J.F.L. (1964) A significant elevation of plasma magnesium levels in schizophrenia and depressive states *Med. J. Australia,* **1,** 195

COPPEN A., SHAW D.M. & MANGORIC A. (1962) Total exchangeable sodium in depressive illness *Brit. Med. J.,* **ii,** 295

COPPEN A., SHAW D.M., MALLESON A. & COSTAIN R. (1966) Mineral metabolism in mania *Brit. Med. J.,* **1,** 71

CRAMMER J.L. (1959) Water and sodium in two psychotics *Lancet,* **1,** 1122

FLACH F.F. (1964) Calcium metabolism in states of depression *Brit. J. Psychiat.,* **110,** 588

GIBBONS J.L. (1968) Biochemistry of the affective illnesses *Brit. J. Hosp. Med.,* 1164

KLEIN R. (1950) Clinical and biochemical investigations in a manic-depressive with short cycles *J. Ment. Sci.,* **96,** 293

KLEIN R. & NUNN R.F. (1945) Clinical and biochemical analysis of a case of manic depressive psychosis showing regular weekly cycles *J. Ment. Sci.,* **91,** 79

Affective disorders—genetic studies

HOPKINSON G. (1964) A genetic study of affective illness in patients over 50 *Brit. J. Psychiat.,* **110,** 244

HOPKINSON G. & LEY P. (1969) A genetic study of affective disorder *Brit. J. Psychiat.,* **115,** 917

PERRIS C. (1966) *Acta Psychiat. Scand.,* **42** Suppl. 194

PRICE J.S. (1967) The dominance hierachy and evolution of mental illness *Lancet,* **ii,** 243

PRICE J.S. (1968) Genetics of the affective illnesses *Brit. J. Hosp. Med.,* 1172

RODGER T.F. (1961) *Acta psychiat. Scand.,* **37** Suppl. 162

SLATER E.T.O. (1953) Psychotic and neurotic illness in twins, Special Report Series, MRC, London No. 278

STENSTEDT A. (1959) *Acta Psychiat. neurol. Scand.,* Suppl. 127

WILSON D.C. (1951) *Dis. Nerv. Syst.,* **12,** 362

WINOKUR G. & CLAYTON P. (1967) *Recent Advances in Biological Psychiatry,* **9,** 35

WINOKUR G. & PITTS F.N. (1964) *J. Nerv. Ment. Dis.,* **138,** 541

Alcoholism and addiction

ADVISORY COMMITTEE ON DRUG DEPENDENCE (1968) *Cannabis* HMSO, London

ADVISORY COMMITTEE ON DRUG DEPENDENCE (1970) *Amphetamines and L.S.D.* HMSO, London

ANDREASSON R. (1962) *Alcohol and Road Traffic: an international survey of the discussion.* Proceedings of the Third International Conference on Alcohol and Road Traffic, London

BAILEY M.B., HABERMAN P.W. & ALSKNE H.J. (1965) *Quart. J. Stud. Alcohol,* 26, 19

BALES R.R. (1946) Cultural differences in rates of alcoholism *Quart. J. Stud. Alcohol,* **6,** 480

BATCHELOR I.R.C. (1954) Alcoholism and attempted suicide *J. Ment. Sci.,* **100,** 451

BEWLEY T.H. (1966) Recent changes in patterns in drug dependence in the UK *Bull. Narcot.,* **28,** 1

BEWLEY T.H., BEN ARIE O. & JAMES I.P. (1968) Morbidity and mortality from heroin dependence *Brit. Med. J.,* 1, 725

BEWLEY T.H. (1970) An introduction to drug dependence *Brit. J. Hosp. Med.,* **4,** 150

CHEIN I., GERARD D.L., LEE R.S. & ROSENFELD E. (1964) *Narcotics, Delinquency and Social Policy—the road to H* Tavistock, London

CLOWARD R.A. & OHLIN L.E. (1960) *Delinquency and Opportunity: a Theory of Delinquent Gangs* Free Press of Glencoe, New York

COCKETT R. (1971) *Drug Abuse and Personality in Young Offenders* Butterworth, London

CONNELL P.H. (1958) *Amphetamine Psychosis* Maudsley Monographs. Chapman and Hall, London

D'ALARCON R. (1969) *Bull. Narcot.,* **21,** 17

D'ALARCON R. & RATIIOD N.H. (1967) Prevalance and early detection of heroin use. *Brit. Med. J.,* **62,** 549

GERARD D.L. & KORNETSKY C. (1955) Adolescent opiate addiction: Study of control and addict subjects *Psychiat. Quart.,* **29,** 457

GILLESPIE D., GLATT M.M., HILLS D.R. & PITTMAN D.J. (1967) Drug dependence and abuse in England *Brit. J. Addict.* **62,** 155

GLATT M.M., PITTMAN D.J., GILLESPIE D.G. & HILLS D.R. (1967) *The Drug Scene in Great Britain* Edward Arnold, London

GLATT M.M. (1970) Alcoholism and drug dependence amongst Jews *Brit. J. Addict.,* **64,** 297

KESSEL N. & GROSSMAN G. (1961) Suicide in alcoholics. *Brit. Med. J.,* **ii,** 1671

KESSEL N. (1965) Self poisoning *Brit. Med. J.,* **2,** 1265

KOSVINER A., MITCHESON M.C., MYERS K., OGBORNE A., STIMSON G.V., ZACUNE J., & EDWARDS G. (1968) Heroin use in a provincial town *Lancet,* **1,** 1189

HORTON D. (1943) Function of alcohol in primitive societies *Quart. J. Stud. Alcohol,* **4,** 199

INDIAN HEMP DRUGS COMMISSION (1894) Report Simla

JAMES I.P. (1967) Suicide and mortality amongst heroin addicts in Britain *Brit. J. Addict.,* **62,** 277

JAMES I.P. (1969) Delinquency and heroin addiction in Britain *Brit. J. Criminol.,* **9,** 108

JELLINEK E.M. (1960) *The Disease Concept of Alcoholism* Hillhouse Press, New Haven Conn.

MITCHESON M., DAVIDSON J., HAWKS D.V., HITCHENS L. & MALONE S. (1970) Sedative abuse by heroin addicts *Lancet,* **1,** 606

MOSS M.C. & BERESFORD DAVIES E. (1967) *A Survey of Alcoholism in an English County* St. Ann's Press, London

MOWRER H.R. & MOWRER E.R. (1945) Ecological and familial factors associated with inebriety *Quart. J. Stud. Alcohol,* **6,** 36

MULFORD H.A. & MILLER D.E. (1960) Drinking in Iowa, II. The extent of drinking and selected socio-cultural categories *Quart. J. Stud. Alcohol,* **21,** 26

PLYMAR W. (1955) The relation of alcohol to highway accidents alcohol and road traffic. Proceedings of the Second International Conference of Alcohol and Road Traffic

PREBLE E. & CASEY J.J. (1969) Taking care of business—the heroin user's life on the street *Int. J. Addict.,* **4,** 1

RINGEL E. & ROTTER H. (1957) The problem of attempted suicide during intoxication Wien Z. Nervenheilk, **13,** 406

SAARENHEMO E. (1952) Sociological studies on suicides *Alkoholik Ysynys.,* **20,** 5

SCHUR E.M. (1963) *Narcotic Addiction in Britain and America* London, Tavistock

SNYDER C.R. (1958) Alcohol and the Jews: A cultural study of Drinking and Sobriety. Rutgers Center of Alcohol Studies. Monograph No. 1. New Brunswick, N.J. Rutgers Center of Alcohol Studies Publication Division

SPEAR H.B. (1969) The growth of heroin addiction in the United Kingdom *Brit. J. Addict.,* **64,** 245

WILLIS J.H. (1969) The natural history of drug dependence: some comparative observations on United Kingdom and United States subjects in *Scientific Basis of Drug Dependence.* Ed. Steinberg. Churchill London

WILLIS J.H. (1969) Drug dependence: some demographic and psychiatric aspects in UK and US subjects *Brit. J. Addict.,* **64,** 135

ZACUNE J., MITCHESON M. & MALONE S. (1969) Heroin use in a provincial town—one year later *Int. J. Addict.,* **4,** 557

Anorexia nervosa

BHANJI S. & THOMPSON J. (1974) Operant conditioning in the treatment of anorexia nervosa. A review and retrospective study of 11 cases *Brit. J. Psychiat.,* **124,** 166

BIANCO F. (1971) *Behaviour therapy in anorexia nervosa* Report of Vth World Congress of Psychiatry, Mexico

DALLY P. & SARGANT W. (1966) Treatment and outcome of anorexia nervosa *Brit. Med. J.,* **ii,** 793

WRIGHT W.J., MANWELL M.K.C. & MERRITT J.K. (1969) Anorexia nervosa: a discriminant function analysis. *Brit. J. Psychiat.,* **115,** 827

Antidepressants

BURROWS G.D. & DAVIES B. (1971) Antidepressants and barbiturates *Brit. Med. J.,* **iv,** 113

CARLSSON A., CAERODI H., FUXE K. & HÖKFELD T. (1969) *European J. Pharmacol.,* **5,** 357

DAVIS J.M. & JALOWSKY D.S. (1974) Recent advances in the treatment of depression *Brit. J. Hosp. Med.,* **219**

KAY D.W., FAHY T. & GARSIDE (1970) A trial of amitryptiline and diazepam in ECT treated depressed patients *Brit. J. Psychiat.,* **117,** 667

KLEIN D.F. (1966) *Can. Psychiat. Assoc. J.,* **11,** 146

MINDHAM R.H.G., HOWLAND C. & SHEPHERD M. (1972) *Lancet,* **ii,** 561

PAYKEL E.S., PRICE J.S., GILLAN R.V., PALMAI G. & CHESSER E.S. (1968) In Proc of 4th World Congress of Psychiatry Sept. 1966 Pt III I.C.S. No. 150 Excerpta Medica 2090

PEREL J.M. & GLASSMAN A. (1973) The clinical pharmacology of imipramine *Arch. Gen. Psychiat.,* **28,** 659

RASKIN A., SCHUTTERBRANDT J.G., REATIG N. & MCKEAN J.J. (1970) Differential reponse to chloropromazine, imipramine and placebo *Arch. Gen. Psychiat.,* **23,** 164

Anxiety

ADLER A. (1951) *The Theory and Practice of Individual Psychology* Humanities Press, New York

FREUD S. (1936) *The Problem of Anxiety* W.W. Norton, New York

FROMM E. (1941) *Escape from Freedom* Farrar and Rinehart, New York

HORNEY K. (1950) *Neurosis and Human Growth* W.W. Norton, New York

LADER M.H. (1969) Psychophysiological aspects of anxiety in studies of anxiety *Brit. J. Psychiat.* (Special publication), **3,** 53

LADER M.H. & Marks I.M. (1971) *Clinical Anxiety* Heinemann Medical, London

LADER M.H. & MATTHEWS A.M. (1970) Physiological changes during spontaneous panic attacks *Journal of Psychosomatic Research,* **14,** 377

LEVITT E.E. (1968) *The Psychology of Anxiety* Staples Press, London

LEWIS A.J. (1967) Problems prescribed by the ambiguous word 'anxiety' as used in psychopathology *Israel. Ann Psychiat. rel. Discip.,* **5,** 105

MAY R. (1950) *The Meaning of Anxiety* Ronald Press, New York

RANK O. (1952) *The Trauma of Birth* Robert Bremner, New York

Aphasia

BENSON D.F. (1973) Psychiatric aspects of aphasia *Brit. J. Psychiat.,* **123,** 555

BENSON D.F. & GESCHWIND N. (1971) *Aphasia and Related Disturbances in Clinical Neurology* ed Baker A.B. & Baker L.H. Harper and Row, New York

GOODGLASS H. & KAPLAN E. (1963) Disturbance of gesture and pantomime in aphasia. *Brain,* **86,** 703

Behaviour therapy

BARRETT C.L. (1969) Systematic desensitisation versus implosive therapy *J. Abnormal. Psychol.,* **74,** 587

DE MOOR W. (1970) Systematic desensitisation versus prolonged high intensity stimulation (flooding) *Journal of Behaviour Therapy and Experimental Psychiatry,* **1,** 45

EYSENCK H.J. (1960) *Behaviour Therapy and the Neuroses* Pergamon Press, Oxford

GELDER M.G., BANCROFT J.H.J., GATH D.H., JOHNSTON D.W., MATTHEWS A.M. & SHAW D.M. (1973) Specific and non specific factors in behaviour therapy *Brit. J. Psychiat.,* **123,** 445

GELDER M.G., MARKS I.M. & WOLFF H.H. (1967) Desensitisation and psychotherapy in the treatment of phobic states: A controlled enquiry *Brit. J. Psychiat.*, **113,** 53

GELDER M.G. & MARKS I.M. (1968) Desensitisation and phobias: a cross-over study *Brit. J. Psychiat.*, **114,** 323

GELDER M.G. & MARKS I.M. (1966) Severe agoraphobia: a controlled prospective study of behaviour therapy *Brit. J. Psychiat.*, **112,** 309

MARKS I.M., BOULOUGOURIS J. & MAKSET P. (1971) Flooding vs desensitisation in the treatment of phobic disorders: a cross-over study *Brit. J. Psychiat.*, **119,** 353

RACHMAN S. (1959) The treatment of anxiety and phobic reactions by systematic desensitisation in psychotherapy *J. Abn. Soc. Psychol.*, **58,** 259

WOLPE J. (1958) *Psychotherapy by Reciprocal Inhibition* Stanford University Press, California

Bereavement

ANDERSON C. (1949) Aspects of pathological grief and mourning *Int. J. Psychoanal* **30,** 48

BOWLBY J. (1951) Maternal Care and Mental Health W.H.O. Monograph no. 2 Geneva

BOWLBY J. (1960) Grief and mourning in infancy *Psychoanalytic study of the child*, **15,** 9

BOWLBY J. (1961) Childhood mourning and its implications for psychiatry *Amer. J. Psychiat.*, **118,** 481

CLAYTON P.J., HALILXAS J.A. & MAURICE W.L. (1972) The depression of widowhood *Brit. J. Psychiat.*, **120,** 71

ENGEL G.L. (1961) Is grief a disease? *Psychosom. Med.*, **23,** 18

LINDEMANN E. (1944) Symptomatology and management of acute grief *Amer. J. Psychiat.*, **101,** 141

MARIS P. (1958) *Widows and their families* Routledge & Kegan Paul, London

PARKES C.M. (1964) Recent bereavement as a cause of mental illness *Brit. J. Psychiat.*, **110,** 198

PARKES C.M. (1964) The effects of bereavement on physical and mental health—a study of the medical records of widows *Brit. Med. J.*, **ii,** 274

PARKES C.M. (1965) Bereavement and mental illness *Brit. J. Med. Psychol.*, **38,** 1; **38,** 13

ROTH M. (1959) The phobic-anxiety depersonalisation syndrome *Proc. Roy. Soc. Med.*, **52,** 587

STERN K., WILLIAMS G.M. & PRADOS M. (1951) Grief reactions in later life *Amer. J. Psychiat.*, **108,** 289

Biochemistry

BANNISTER D. (1968) The myth of physiological psychology *Bull. Brit. Psychol. Soc.*, **21,** 229

FRIEDHOFF A.J. & VAN WINKLE E. (1962) Isolation and characterisation of a compound from the urine of schizophrenics *Nature*, **194,** 897

GREINER A.C. & NICHOLSON G.A. (1965) Hypothesis schizophrenia—melanosis *Lancet*, **ii,** 1165

HEATH R.G., NESSELHOF W. & TIMMONS E. (1966) D.L. Methionine–dl–sulphoxi-mine effects in schizophrenic patients *Arch. Gen. Psychiat.,* **14,** 213

KETY S.S. (1969) Biochemical hypotheses and studies in *The Schizophrenic Syndrome* Ed. Bellak L., Loeb L. Grune & Stratton, New York

MEDNICK S.A. & McNEIL T.F. (1968) Current methodology in research on the aetiology of schizophrenia. Serious difficulties which suggest the use of the high-risk group method *Psychological Bulletin,* **70,** 681

McISAAC W.M. (1961) A biochemical concept of mental disease *Postgrad. Med.,* **20,** 111

SHATTOCK F.M. (1950) The somatic manifestations of schizophrenia. A clinical study of their significance *J. Ment. Sci.,* **96,** 32

SMYTHIES J.R. (1967) Biochemical abnormalities associated with schizophrenia *Brit. J. Hosp. Med.,* **573**

Cerebral tumour

BLEULER M. (1951) Psychiatry of cerebral diseases *Brit. Med. J.,* **ii,** 1233

CRITCHLEY M. (1953) *The Parietal Lobes* Edward Arnold, London

CUSHING H. (1932) Intra cranial Tumours: Notes upon a series of 2,000 verified cases with surgical-mortality percentages pertaining thereto. C.C. Thomas, Springfield, Illinois

DAVIDOFF L.M. (1930) *New York State. J. Med.,* **30,** 1205

DAVIDOFF L.M. & FERRARO A. (1929) Intra cranial tumours among mental hospital patients *Amer. J. Psychiat.,* **855,** 599

KESCHNER M., BENDER M. & Strauss I. (1938) Mental symptoms associated with brain tumour. A study of 530 verified cases *J. Amer. Med. Ass.,* **110,** 714

RUBERT S.L. & REMINGTON F.B. (1962) Why patients with brain tumours come to a psychiatric hospital: A 30 year survey *Amer. J. Psychiat.,* **119,** 256

WAGGONER R.W. & BAGCHI B.K. (1954) Initial masking of organic brain changes by psychic symptoms *Amer. J. Psychiat.,* **110,** 904

WAGGONER R.W. (1967) in *Comprehensive Psychiatry* **20,** 789 Ed. Freeman A.M. & Kaplan H.I. Williams and Wilkins, Baltimore

WALTHER B.H. (1951) *Psychiatry of Cerebral Tumours and the problem of Focal Syndromes and of Psychological Localisation* Vienna

Delinquency

GLUECK S. & GLUECK E.T. (1950) *Unravelling Juvenile Delinquency* Commonwealth Fund, New York

GLUECK S. & GLUECK E.T. (1959) *Predicting delinquency and Crime* Harvard University Press, Cambridge, Mass.

McCORD W. & McCORD J. (1959) *Origins of Crime* Columbia University Press, New York

ROBINS L.N. (1966) *Deviant children grown up: A Sociological and psychiatric study of scoiopathic personality* Williams & Wilkins, Baltimore

WEST D.J. & FARRINGTON D.P. (1973) *Who becomes deliquent?* Heinemann, London

P

Depersonalisation

ACKNER B. (1954) Depersonalisation *J. Ment. Sci.,* **100,** 838

DAVIDSON K. (1964) Episodic depersonalisation *Brit. J. Psychiat.,* **110,** 505

DIXON J.C. (1963) Depersonalisation phenomena in a sample of college students *Brit. J. Psychiat.,* **109,** 371

KENNA J.C. & SEDMAN G. (1965) Depersonalisation in temporal lobe epilepsy and organic psychoses *Brit. J. Psychiat.,* **111,** 293

ROTH M. (1960) The phobic anxiety depersonalisation syndrome and some general aetiological problems in psychiatry *J. Neuropsychiat.,* **1,** 293

SEDMAN G. & KENNA J.C. (1963) Depersonalisation and mood changes in schizophrenia *Brit. J. Psychiat.,* **109,** 699

SEDMAN G. & REED G.F. (1963) Depersonalisation phenomena in obsessional personalities *Brit. J. Psychiat.,* **109,** 376

SHORVON H.J. & HILL J.D.N. (1946) Depersonalisation syndrome *Proc. Roy. Soc. Med.,* **39,** 779

Depression

BLACKWELL B. (1963) Hypertensive crises due to monoamine-oxidase inhibitors *Lancet,* **ii,** 849

BROWN F.W. (1942) Heredity in the psychoneuroses *Proc. Roy. Soc. Med.,* **35,** 785

CARNEY M.W.P., ROTH M. & GARSIDE R.F. (1965) The diagnosis of depressive syndromes and the prediction of E.C.T. response *Brit. J. Psychiat.,* **111,** 659

CURRAN D. (1937) The differentiation of neuroses and manic-depressive psychosis *J. Ment. Sci.,* **83,** 156

CURRAN D. & MALLINSON W.P. (1941) Depressive states in war *Brit. Med. J.,* **i,** 305

EYSENCK H.J. (1970) The classification of depression *Brit. J. Psychiat.,* **117,** 538, 241

GURNEY C., ROTH M., KERR T.A. & SCHAPIRA K. (1970) The bearing of treatment on the classification of the affective disorders *Brit. J. Psychiat.,* **117,** 538, 251

GURNEY C., ROTH M., GARSIDE R.F., KERR T.A. & SCHAPIRA K. (1972) Studies in the classification of affective disorder. The relationship between anxiety states and depressive illness *Brit. J. Psychiat.,* **121,** 561; 162

HAMILTON M. & WHITE J.M. (1959) Clinical syndromes in depressive states *J. Ment. Sci.,* **105,** 895

HOPKINSON G. & LEY P. (1969) A genetic study of affective disorder *Brit. J. Psychiat.,* **115,** 525; 917

KAY D.W.K., GARSIDE R.F., ROY J.R. & BEAMISH P. (1969) Endogenous and neurotic syndromes of depression: A 5 to 7 year follow up of 104 cases *Brit. J. Psychiat.,* **115,** 521; 389

KAY D.W.K., GARSIDE R.F., BEAMISH P. & ROY J.R. (1969) Endogenous and neurotic syndromes of depression: A factor analytic study of 104 cases *Brit. J. Psychiat.,* **115,** 521; 377

KILOH L.G. & GARSIDE R.F. (1963) The independence of neurotic and endogenous depression *Brit. J. Psychiat.,* **109,** 451

KILOH L.G., ANDREWS G., NEILSON G. & BIANCHI G.N. (1972) The relationship of the syndromes called endogenous and neurotic depression *Brit. J. Psychiat.*, **121,** 561; 183

LEWIS A.J. (1934) Melancholia: a clinical survey of depressive states *J. Ment. Sci.*, **80,** 277; 378

LEWIS A.J. (1936) Melancholia: a prognostic study and case material *J. Ment. Sci.*, **82,** 488

LEWIS A.J. (1938) States of depression: their clinical and aetiological differentiation *Brit. Med. J.*, **ii,** 875

POLLITT J.D. (1965) Depression: suggestions for a physiological classification *Brit. J. Psychiat.*, **111,** 489

ROTH M., GURNEY C., GARSIDE R.F. & KERR T.A. (1972) Studies in the classification of affective disorder: The relationship between anxiety states and depressive illness *Brit. J. Psychiat.*, **121,** 561; 147

SCHAPIRA K., ROTH M., KERR T.A. & GURNEY C. (1972) The prognosis of affective disorders: The differentiation of anxiety states from depressive illnesses *Brit. J. Psychiat.*, **121,** 561; 175

SLATER E. (1936) The inheritance of manic depressive insanity *Proc. Roy. Soc. Med.*, **29,** 981

STENSTEDT A. (1952) A study in manic depressive psychosis. Clinical, social and genetic investigations *Acta. Psychiat. Scand.* (KBH) Suppl. 79

STOREY P.B. (1968) Pathogenetic and other aspects of depression *Brit. J. Hosp. Med.*, 1157

Epidemiology

ADLER A. (1943) Neuro psychiatric complications in victims of Boston's Coconut Grove disaster *J. Amer. Med. Assoc.*, **123,** 1098

BRILL H. & PATTON R.E. (1962) Clinical-statistical analysis of population changes in New York mental hospitals since introduction of psychotropic drugs *Amer. J. Psychiat.*, **119,** 20

BREMNER J. (1951) Social psychiatric investigation of a small community in Northern Norway *Acta. Psychiat. Neurol. Scand.* Suppl. 62

BROWN G.W. & BIRLEY J.L. (1968) Social change and the onset of schizophrenia *J. Hlth. Soc. Behav.*, **9,** 203

CHEYNE G. (1973) The English Malady: or a treatise of nervous disorders of all kinds, as spleen, vapours, lowering of spirits, hypochondriacal and hysterical distempers etc. AMS Press, New York

CHRISTOPHERSON E. (1946) Results of the Norwegian Scientific expedition to Tristan da Cunha 1937–1938 Norske Videnskaps Akademi, Oslo

COOPER B. & SHEPHERD M. (1970) Life change, stress and mental disorder the ecological approach in *Modern Trends in Psychological Medicine* Ed. Price J.H., **5,** 102 Butterworth, London

GOLDHAMMER & MARSHALL (1953) *Psychosis and Civilization: Two Studies in the Frequency of Mental Disease* Free Press, Glencoe Illinois

HARE E.H. (1952) The ecology of mental disease *J. Ment. Sci.*, **98,** 579

HARE E.H. (1955) Mental illness and social class in Bristol *Brit. J. Prev. Soc. Med.,* **9,** 191

HARE E.H. (1956) Family setting and the urban distribution of schizophrenia *J. Ment. Sci.,* **102,** 753

HARE E.H. (1967) The epidemiology of schizophrenia in *Recent Developments in Schizophrenia* Ed. Coppen A. Walk A. Roy. Medico. Psych. Assoc., London

HOLLINGSHEAD A.B. & REDLICH F.C. (1958) *Social Class and Mental Illness: a Community Study* Wiley, New York

JONES M. (1953) *The Therapeutic Community* Basic Books, New York

KESSEL N. & SHEPHERD M. (1962) Neurosis in hospital and general practice *J. Ment. Sci.,* 108

LIN T-Y. & Standley C.C. (1962) The scope of epidemiology in psychiatry Public Health Papers No. 16 W.H.O. Geneva

MEZEY A.G. (1960) Personal background, emigration and mental disorder in Hungarian refugees *J. Ment. Sci.,* **106,** 618

Millbank Memorial Fund (1950) *Epidemiology of Mental Disorder* New York

MISCHLER L. & SCOTCH P. (1960) Epidemiology of schizophrenia *Int. J. Psychiat.,* **1,** 2; 261

MORRIS J.N. (1957) *Uses of Epidemiology* Livingstone, Edinburgh

Ødegaard Ø. (1932) Emigration and insanity *Acta Psychia. Neurol. Scand.,* Suppl. 4.

RAWNSLEY K. & LONDON S.B. (1964) Epidemiology of mental disorder in a closed community *Brit. J. Psychiat.,* **110,** 830

REID D.D. (1960) Epidemiological methods in the study of mental disorders. Public Health Papers. No. 2. W.H.O. Geneva

SHEPHERD M. (1957) *A Study of the Major Psychoses in an English County* Maudsley Monogr. Chapman & Hall, London

SHEPHERD M. & COOPER B. (1964) Epidemiology of mental disorder: a review *J. Neurol. Neuro surg. Psychiat.,* **27,** 277

SHEPHERD M., COOPER B., BROWN A.C. & KALTAR G.W. (1966) *Psychiatric Illness in General Practice* Oxford University Press, Oxford

SROLE L., LANGNER T.S., MICHAEL S.T., OPLER M.K. & RENNIE T.A.C. (1962) *Mental Health in a Metropolis: The Mid town Manhattan Study* McGraw-Hill, New York

STATE OF MASSACHUSSETTS (1855) Report of a commission to examine statistics of lunacy and conditions of asylums in the State of Massachussetts 1855

WING J.K. (1970) in *Psychiatric Epidemiology: an International Symposium* Ed. Hare E.H. & Wing J.K. Oxford University Press, London

WING J.K. (1972) Epidemiology of schizophrenia *Brit. J. Hosp. Med.,* **4,** 364

Epilepsy—psychiatric aspects

BARTLETT J.E.A. (1957) Chronic psychosis following epilepsy *Amer. J. Psychiat.,* **114** 338

FALRET J. (1860) De l'etat mental des epileptiques *Archs. Gen. Med.,* **16** 666; **17,** 461; **18,** 423

GRUHLE H.W. (1936) Uber den Wahn bei epilepsie *Zeitschr. ges. Nem. Psychiat.,* **154,** 395

HILL D. (1953) Psychiatric disorders of epilepsy *Med. Press,* **20,** 473

POND D.A. (1957) Psychiatric aspects of epilepsy *J. Indian Med. Prof.,* **3,** 1441

POND D. (1963) Maturation, epilepsy and psychiatry *Proc. Roy. Soc. Med.,* **56,** 710

SLATER E. & BEARD A.W. (1963) The schizophrenia like psychoses of epilepsy *Brit. J. Psychiat.,* **109,** 95

TAYLOR D.C. (1967) Factors related to mental state in patients with temporal lobe epilepsy treated by temporal lobectomy M.D. Thesis Univ. of London

TOMKIN O. (1971) *The Falling Sickness* The John Hopkin Press, Baltimore

WALKER A. (1961) Murder or Epilepsy *J. Nerv. Ment. Dis.,* **133,** 430

Family influences in psychiatric disorders

BATESON G. (1960) Minimal requirements for a theory of schizophrenia *Arch. Gen. Psychiat.,* **2,** 477

BIRLEY J.L.T. & BROWN G.W. (1970) Crisis and life changes preceding the onset or relapse of acute schizophrenia: clinical aspects *Brit. J. Psychiat.,* **116,** 327

BROWN G.W. & BIRLEY J.L.T. (1968) Crisis and life changes and the onset of schizophrenia *J. Health and Social Behaviour,* **9,** 203

BROWN, G.W., BIRLEY J.L.T. & WING J.K. (1900) Influence of family life on the course of schizophrenic disorders: a replication *Brit. J. Psychiat,* **121,** 241

HALEY J. (1959) The family of the schizophrenic: a model system. *Journal Nerv Ment. Dis.,* **129,** 372

HIRSCH S.R. & LEFF J.P. (1971) Parental abnormalities of verbal communication in the transmission of schizophrenia *Psychol. Med.,* **1,** 118

JACKSON D.D. (1960) *The Etiology of Schizophrenia* Basic Books, New York

LAING R. (1960) *The Divided Self* Tavistock Publications, London

LIDZ T. (1963) *The Family and Human Adaptation,* 53 New York University Press, New York

LIDZ T., FLECK S. & CORNELISON A.R. (1966) *Schizophrenia and the Family* International Universities Press, New York

MEYER A. (1907) An attempt at analysis of the neurotic constitution *Amer. J. Psychiat.,* **14,** 90

MEYER A. (1909) After care and prophylaxis *State Hosp. Bull.,* **1,** 631

MEYER A. (1911) Case work in social service. Proc. Nat. Conf. Charities and Correction 275

SPIEGEL J.P. & BELL N.W. (1959) The family of the psychiatric patient in *American Handbook of Psychiatry* Ed. Arieti S. 5, 114. Basic Books, New York

VENABLES P.H. (1968) Experimental psychological studies of chronic schizophrenia, in *Studies in Psychiatry* Ed. Shepherd M. & Davies D.L. Oxford University Press, London

WARING M. & RICKS D. (1965) Family patterns of children who become schizophrenics *J. Nerv. Ment. Dis.,* **140,** 351

WYNNE L.C. & SINGER M.T. (1963) Thought disorder and family relations of schizophrenics *Arch. Gen. Psychiat.* **9,** 191

Lithium

CADE J.F.J. (1949) *Med. J. Aust.,* **36,** 349

CHRISTODOULOU G.N. (1968) The use of lithium in psychiatry *Brit. J. Hosp. Med.,* 1181

MAGGS R. (1963) Treatment of manic illness with lithium carbonate. *Brit. J. Psychiat.,* **109,** 56

SCHOU M., JUEL NIELSEN N., STRONGREN E. & VOLDBY H. (1954) *J. Neurol. Neurosurg. Psychiat.,* **17,** 250

SCHOU M. (1959) Psychopharmacologia (Berl.) 1. 65

Monoamine oxidase inhibitors

COLLINS G.G.S., SANDLER M., WILLIAMS E. & Youdrin M.B.H. (1970) *Nature,* **225,** 817

HOLLISTER L.E. (1969) *Clin. Pharmacol. Ther.,* **10,** 170

JARVIK M.E. (1970) in *Pharmacological Basis of Therapeutics* 4th edn. Ed. Goodman L.S. & Gilman A. MacMillan, London

PARE M., REES W.L. & SAINSBURY M.J. (1962) *Lancet,* **ii,** 1340

SARGANT W. (1966) Psychiatric treatment in general teaching hospitals: a plea for a mechanistic approach *Brit. Med. J.,* **ii,** 257

SLATER E. & ROTH M. (1969) *Clinical Psychiatry* 3rd edn. Ballière Tindall & Cassell, London

TYRER P. (1973) Current status of monoamine oxidase inhibitors in psychiatry *Brit. J. Hosp. Med.,* **9,** 6 795

YOUDRIN M.B.H. & SANDLER M. (1967) *Biochem. J.,* **105,** 43

Morbid jealousy

BRIERLEY H.C. (1932) *Homicide in the United States* Chapel Hill

EY H. (1950) 'Jalousie Morbide' in *Etudes Psychiatriques* Tome II Paris. Desclée de Brower et cie

EAST W.N. (1936) *Medical Aspects of Crime* Churchill, London

HOPWOOD J.S. & MILNER K. (1940) Alcoholism and criminal insanity *Brit. J. Ineb.,* **38,** 51

MOONEY H.B. (1965) Pathologic jealousy and pharmacotherapy *Brit. J. Psychiat.,* **111,** 1023

SHEPHERD M. (1961) Morbid jealousy *J. Ment. Sci.,* **167,** 687

Munchausen syndrome

ASHER R. (1951) *Lancet,* **i,** 339

BARKER J.C. (1962) The syndrome of the hospital addiction (Munchausen syndrome) *J. Ment. Sci.,* **108,** 167

BLACKWELL B. (1965) Munchausen at Guy's *Guy's Hospital Reports,* **114,** 3, 257

FRANKEL E. (1951) *Lancet,* **i,** 911

Myxoedema

ASHER R. (1949) Myxoedematous madness *Brit. Med. J.,* **ii,** 555

BROWNING T.B., ATKINS R.W. & WEINER M.D. (1954) Cerebral metabolic disturbances in hypothyroidism *A.M.A. Arch. Intern. Med.,* **93,** 938

GULL W.W. (1873) On a cretinoid state supervening in adult life in women *Trans. Clin. Soc. Lond.,* **7,** 180

ORD W.M. (1878) On myxoedema, a term proposed to be applied to an essential condition in the cretinoid affection occasionally observed in middle-aged women *Med. Clin. Trans.,* **61,** 57

SAVAGE G.H. (1880) Myxoedema and its nervous symptoms *J. Ment. Sci.,* **25,** 517

TONKS C.M. (1964) Mental illness in hypothyroid patients *Brit. J. Psychiat.,* **110,** 706

Neuroleptics

BAN T.A. & LEHMANN H.E. (1970) Nicotinic acid in the treatment of schizophrenics. Progress Report 1. Canadian Mental Health Assoc., Toronto

HIRSCH S., GAIND R. ROHDE B., STEVENS B. & WING J. (1973) Outpatient maintenance of chronic schizophrenic patients with long acting fluphenazine: Double blind placebo trial *Brit. Med. J.,* **i,** 627

HOLLISTER L.E., OVERALL J.E., KATZ G., HIGGINBOTHAM W.E. & KIMBELL I. (1972) Oxypertine and thiothixene in newly admitted schizophrenic patients: A further search for specific indication of antipsychotic drugs *Clinical Pharmacology and Therapeutics* **12,** 3, 531

MCGRATH S.S., O'BRIEN D.T., POWER P.J. & SHEA J.R. (1972) Nicotinamide treatment of schizophrenia *Schizophrenia Bulletin,* **5,** 74

PAULING L. (1967) Orthomolecular psychiatry *Science,* 160, 265

RAMSEY R.A., BAN T.A., LEHMANN H.E., SAXENA B.M. & BENNETT J. (1970) Nicotinic acid as adjuvant therapy in newly admitted schizophrenic patients *Can. Med. Assoc. J.,* **102,** 939

STEVENS B.C. (1973) Role of fluphenazine decanoate in lessening of the burden of chronic schizophrenics in the community *Psych. Med.,* **3,** 2, 141

Neurosis

ERIKSON E.H. (1959) Identity and the life cycle. *Psychol. Issues,* **1,** 1, 751

GOLDBERG D.P. & BLACKWELL B. (1970) Psychiatric illness in general practice a detailed study using a new method of case identification *Brit. Med. J.,* **ii,** 439

HORNEY K. (1942) *Self Analysis* W.W Norton, New York

HORNEY K. (1945) *Our Inner Conflicts* W.W. Norton, New York

HORNEY K. (1937) *The Neurotic Personality of our Time* W.W. Norton, New York

KESSEL W.N. (1960) Psychiatric morbidity in a London general practice *Brit. J. Prevent. Soc. Med.,* **14,** 16

LOGAN W.P.D. & CUSHION A.A. (1958) *Morbidity Studies in General Practice General Register Office: Studies in Medical and Population Subjects* HMSO, London

MEYER A. (1921) The contribution of psychiatry to the understanding of life problems. Address at 100th anniversary of Bloomingdale Hospital

ROGERS C. (1951) *Client Centred Therapy* Houghton Mifflin, Boston

Nosology—diagnosis

BANNISTER D., SALMON P. & LEIBERMANN D. (1964) Diagnosis: treatment relationships in psychiatry—a statistical analysis *Brit. J. Psychiat.,* **110,** 776

BECK A.T. (1962) Reliability of psychiatric diagnoses; a critique of systematic studies *American Journal of Psychiatry,* **119,** 210

CAMERON N. (1944) *The Functional Psychoses—in Personality and the Behaviour Disorders* Ed. Hunt J.V. Ronald Press, New York

COOPER J.E., KENDELL R.E., GURLAND B.J., SHARPE L., COPELAND J.R.M. & SIMON R. (1972) *Psychiatric diagnosis in New York and London* Maudsley Monograph. No. 20. Oxford University Press, London

COPELAND J.R.M., COOPER J.E., KENDELL R.E. & GOURLAY A.J. (1971) Differences in usage of diagnostic labels amongst psychiatrists in the British Isles *British Journal of Psychiatry,* **118,** 629

DEGAN J.W. (1952) Dimensions of functional psychosis *Psychometr. Monograph.* 6.

EYSENCK H.J. (1957) *The Dynamics of Anxiety and Hysteria* Routledge & Kegan Paul, London

EYSENCK H.J. (1961) *Handbook of Abnormal Psychology* 1, 3 Basic Books New York

GAURON E.F. & DICKINSON J.K. (1966a) Diagnostic decision making in psychiatry: information usage *Archives of General Psychiatry,* **14,** 225

GAURON E.F. & DICKINSON J.K. (1966b) Diagnostic decision making in psychiatry: diagnostic styles *Archives of General Psychiatry,* **14,** 233

KENDELL R.E., EVERITT B., COOPER J.E., SARTORIUS N. & DAVID M.E. (1968) The reliability of the 'Present State Examination' *Social Psychiatry,* **3,** 123

KENDELL R.E. (1973) Psychiatric diagnoses: A study of how they are made *Brit. J. Psychiat.,* **122,** 437

KENDELL R.E. (1973) The influence of the 1968 glossary on the diagnoses of English psychiatrists *Brit. J. Psychiat.,* **123,** 527

KRAUPL TAYLOR (1967) The role of phenomenology in psychiatry *Brit. J. Psychiat.,* **113,** 500, 765

KREITMAN N., SAINSBURY P., MORRISSEY J., TOWERS J. & SCRIVENER J. (1961) The reliability of psychiatric assessment: an analysis *Journal of Mental Science,* **107,** 887

LEWIS A.J. (1970) Paranoia and paranoid: a historical perspective *Psychological Medicine,* **1,** 2

LIDZ R.W. & LIDZ T. (1950) An interpretation of the perspectives of American psychiatry *Nervenarzt.,* **21,** 490 2

MARZOLF S. (1945) Symptom and syndrome statistically interpreted *Psychol. Bull.,* **42,** 162

SULLIVAN H.S. (1953) *The Interpersonal Theory of Psychiatry* 750 Norton, New York

SZASZ T. (1957) The problem of psychiatric nosology. A contribution to a situational analysis of psychiatric operations *Amer. J. Psychiat.,* **114,** 405

SZASZ T. (1960) The myth of mental illness *American Psychologist,* **15,** 113

TROUTON D.S. & MAXWELL A.E. (1956) The relation between neurosis and psychosis *J. Ment. Sci.,* **102,** 1

Obsessional disorder

GRIMSHAW L. (1965) The outcome of obsessional disorder: a follow up study of 100 cases *Brit. J. Psychiat.,* **111,** 1051
KRINGLEN E. (1965) Obsessional neurotics—a long term follow up *Brit. J. Psychiat.,* **111,** 709
LEWIS A.J. (1935) Problems of obsessional illness *Proc. Roy. Soc. Med.,* **29,** 325
POLLITT J. (1960) Natural history studies in mental illness *J. Ment. Sci.,* **106,** 442
POLLITT J. (1969) Obsessional states *Brit. J. Hosp. Med.,* 1146

Old age

BERGMANN K. (1969) Epidemiology of senile dementia *Brit. J. Hosp. Med.,* 727
COMFORT A. (1961) The position of fundamental age studies *Amer. Heart J.,* **62,** 293
CORSELLIS J.A.N. (1962) *Mental Illness and the Ageing Brain* Maudsley Monograph No. 9. Oxford University Press, London
CUMMING E. & HENRY W.E. (1961) *Growing Old* Basic Books, New York
ESQUIROL J.E.D. (1838) *Traité des Maladies Mentales* Trans. Hunt E.K. 1845
GELLERSTEDT N. (1932) Upsala Läk *FörenForh,* **38,** 193
GRIESINGER W. (1845) *Pathologie und Therapie de Psychiatrischen Krankheiten* Trans. Robertson C.L. New Sydenham Society Publications No. 33 (1862), London
KALLMANN F.J. (1956) in *Mental disorders in Later Life* 2nd edn. Ed. Kaplan O. Stanford University Press, California
KAY D.W.K., BEAMISH P. & ROTH M. (1964a) (1964b) Old age mental disorders in Newcastle upon Tyne *Brit. J. Psychiat.,* 110, 146, 668
KAY D.W.K., BERGMANN K. & GARSIDE R.F. (1966) In Proc. of IVth World Congress of Psychiatry Abstr 610 in Excerpta Medica Int. Congress Series. Excerpta Medica Foundation
LARSSON T. (1964) *Age with a Future* Munksgaard, Copenhagen
LARSSON T., SJOGREN T. & JACOBSON G. (1963) *Acta Psychiat. Scand.,* Suppl. 167
LECHLER H. (1950) Die Psychosen der Alten *Arch. Psychiat. Nervenkr.,* **185,** 465
LODGE PATCH I.C., POST F. & SLATER P. (1965) Constitution and the psychiatry of old age *Brit. J. Psychiat.,* **111,** 405
LORGE S. & TUCKMAN J. (1958) Retirement and the industrial worker Columbia University Press, New York
McDONALD C. (1969) Clinical heterogeneity in senile dementia *Brit. J. Psychiat.,* **115,** 267
MACMILLAN D. (1960) Preventitive geriatrics *Lancet,* **ii,** 439
MEDAWAR P.B. (1957) *The Uniqueness of the Individual* Methuen, London
MUELLER C. (1959) *Uber das Senium des Schizophrenen* Kargel, Basel
POST F. (1965) *The Clinical Psychiatry of Late Life* Pergamon Press, Oxford
POST F. (1944) Some problems arising from a study of mental patients over the age of 60 *J. Ment. Sci.,* **90,** 554

Post F. (1962) *The Significance of Affective Symptoms in Old Age* Maudsley Monograph No. 10. Oxford University Press, London

Roth M., Tomlinson B.E. & Blessed G. (1966) Correlation between scores for dementia and counts of senile plaques in cerebral grey matter of elderly subjects. *Nature,* **209,** 109

Roth M. (1963) Neurosis, psychosis and the concept of disease in psychiatry *Acta. psychiat. Scand.,* **39** (i), 128

Rothschild D. (1937) *Amer. J. Psychiat.,* **93,** 957

Sheps J. (1958) Paranoid mechanisms in the aged *Psychiatry,* **25,** 399

Townsend P. (1962) *The Last Refuge. A Survey of Residential Institutions for the Aged in England and Wales* Routledge & Kegan Paul, London

Klein Ashley (1972) *Population Trends in the Elderly* New Society

Old age—late onset schizophrenia

Bleuler M. (1943) *Fortsch. Neur. Psychiat.,* **15,** 29

Bleuler M. (1963) *Proc. Roy. Soc. Med.,* **59,** 945

Bleuler M. (1965) *Int. J. Psychiat.,* **1,** 501

Fish F. (1960) Senile schizophrenia *J. Ment. Sci.,* **106,** 938

Funding T. (1961) *Acta Psychiat. Scand.,* **37,** 267

Kay D.W.K. & Roth M. (1961) Factors in schizophrenia of old age *J. Ment. Sci.,* **107,** 649

Kay D.W.K. & Roth M. (1963) *Acta Psychiat. Scand.,* **39,** 159

Lechler H. (1950) *Arch. Psychiat. Nerven K.R.,* **185,** 456

Post F. (1967) Schizophrenic reaction type in late life *Proc. Roy. Soc. Med.,* **60,** 249

Post F. (1966) *Persistent Persecutory States of the Elderly* Oxford University Press, London

Organic syndromes

Bastrem A. (1930) *General Paralysis; Bumke's Handbook of Mental Diseases* Vol. 8. Berlin

Bleuler M. (1951) Psychiatry of cerebral diseases *Brit. Med. J.,* **ii,** 1233, 393

Brain R. & Henson R.A. (1958) Neurological syndromes associated with carcinoma *Lancet,* **2,** 971

Davenport C.D. (1916) *Huntington's Chorea in Relation to Heredity and Eugenics* Cold Spring Harbor, Long Island

Denny Brown D. (1945) Disability arising from closed head injury *J. Amer. Med. Assoc.,* **127,** 429

Dewhurst K. (1909) The neurosyphilitic psychoses today. *Brit. J. Psychiat.,* **115,** 31

Edwin E., Holten K., Norman K.R., Schumpf A. & Skang O.E. (1965) Vitamin B_{12} hypovitaminosis in mental disease *Acta Med. Scand.,* **177,** 689

Engel G.L. & Romano J. (1944) Delirium II. Reversibility of the E.E.G. with experimental procedures *Arch. Neurol. Psychiat.,* **51,** 378

Engel G.L. & Romano J. (1959) Delirium, a syndrome of cerebral insufficiency *J. Chronic Dis.,* **9,** 260

GOLDSTEIN K. (1939) *The Organism: A Holistic Approach to Biology derived from Pathological data on Man* American Book Co., New York

GOLDSTEIN K. (1939) The significance of special mental tests for diagnosis and prognosis in schizophrenia *Amer. J. Psychiat.*, **96**, 575

HARE E.H. (1959) The origin and spread of dementia paralytica *J. Ment. Sci.*, **105**, 594

HERBERT V. (1959) *The Megaloblastic Anaemias* Grune & Stratton, New York

HORDERN A. (1968) in *Psychopharmacology—dimensions and perspectives* Ed. Joyce C.R.B. 95, 102. Tavistock, London

HUNTER R. & MACALPINE I. (1963) *Three Hundred years of Psychiatry, 1575–1860* Oxford University Press, London

HUNTER R. & MATTHEWS D.M. (1965) Mental symptoms in vitamin B_{12} deficiency *Lancet*, **ii**, 738

JACOBOWSKY B. (1965) General paresis and civilisation *Acta Psychiat. Scand.*, **41**, 267

LEVIN M. (1959) *Toxic Psychoses in American Handbook of Psychiatry* 2, 1222, Basic Books, New York

LEVY R. (1969) The neurophysiology of dementia *Brit. J. Hosp. Med.*, 688

MAYER GROSS W. & GUTTMANN E. (1937) Schema for the examination of organic cases *J. Ment. Sci.*, **83**, 440, 45

MAYER GROSS W., SLATER E. & ROTH M. (1969) *Clinical Psychiatry* 3rd edn. Ballière Tindall, London

MCGOVERN G.P., MILLER D.H. & ROBERTSON (1959) A mental syndrome associated with lung carcinoma *Arch. Neurol. Psychiat.*, **81**, 341

MINSKI L. & GUTTMAN E. (1938) Huntington's chorea: A study of thirty four families *J. Ment. Sci.*, **84**, 21

POWER T.D. (1930) The aetiology of general paralysis of the insane *J. Ment. Sci.*, **76**, 524

SHULMAN R. (1967) Vitamin B_{12} deficiency and psychiatric illness *Brit. J. Psychiat.*, **113**, 252

SHULMAN R. (1967) A survey of vitamin B_{12} deficiency in an elderly psychiatric population *Brit. J. Psychiat.*, **113**, 241

ROMANO J. & ENGEL G.L. (1944) Delirium I E.E.G. Data *Arch. Neurol. Psychiat.*, **51**, 356

ROTH M. & MYERS D.M. (1969) The diagnosis of dementia *Brit. J. Hosp. Med.*, **705**

RUSSELL W.R. (1959) *Brain—memory, learning* Oxford University Press, London

STRACHAN R.M. & HENDERSON J.Y. (1967) Dementia and folate deficiency *Quart. J. Med.*, **36**, 189

VESSIE P.R. (1932) On transmission of Huntington's chorea for 300 years Bures family group *J. Nerv. Ment. Dis.*, **76**, 553

WOOLF H.G. & CURRAN D. (1935) Nature of delirium and allied states *Arch. Neurol. Psychiat.*, **33**, 1175

Phobias

MARKS I.M. (1969) *Fears and Phobias* Heinemann, London

MARKS I.M. & GELDER M. (1966) Different onset ages in varieties of phobia *Amer. J. Psychiat.*, **123**, 218

MARKS I.M. & GELDER M. (1965) A controlled retrospective study of behaviour therapy in phobic patients *Brit. J. Psychiat.*, **111**, 571

Puerperal disorders

ENGELHARA J.L.B. (1912) On puerperal psychoses and the influence of the gestation period on psychiatric and neurological disease already in existence. *Z. Geburtsh. Gynäk.*, **70**, 727

MARTIN M.E. (1958) Puerperal mental illness—a follow up study of 75 cases *Brit. Med. J.*, **ii**, 737

PROTHEROE C. (1969) Puerperal psychoses: A long term study 1927–1961 *Brit. J. Psychiat.*, **115**, 58, 9

SEAGER C.P. (1960) A controlled study of post partum mental illness. *J. Ment. Sci.*, **106** 214

Psychiatry—transcultural aspects

ARENSBERG C.M. & KIMBALL S.T. (1940) *Family and Community in Ireland* Cambridge, Massachusetts

BHATTACHARJYA B. (1949) On the wartime incidence of mental diseases in the Indian Army *Ind. J. Neurol. Psychiat.*, **1**, 51

CROCETTI G.M. *et al.* (1964) Selected aspects of the epidemiology of schizophrenia in Croatia (Yugoslavia) *Milbank Mem. Fund Q.*, **42**, 9

KADRI Z.N. (1963) Schizophrenia in the university students *Singapore Med. J.*, **4**, 113

MALZBERG, B. (1940) *Social and Biological Aspects of Mental Disease* Utica

MURPHY, H.B.M. (1959) Cultural factors in the mental health of Malayan students, in Funkenstein D.H. *The Student and Mental Health: An International View, World Federation for Mental Health,* pp. 164–222

MURPHY H.B.M. (1965) The epidemiological approach to transcultural psychiatric research, in *Transcultural Psychiatry, A Ciba Foundation Symposium,* Eds. de Reuck & Porter, pp. 303–27 London

MURPHY H.B.M., WITTKOWER E.D., FRIED J. & ELLENBERGER H.A. (1963) Cross cultural survey of schizophrenic symptomatology *Int. J. Soc. Psychiat.*, **9**, 237

POLLOCK H.M. (1913) A statistical study of the foreign-born insane in New York state hospitals *State Hospitals Bull.* 10–27 of special number.

POLLOCK H.M. (1928) Frequency of schizophrenia in relation to sex, age, environment, nativity and race *Schizophrenia (Assn. Res. Nerv. Ment. Dis., 5),* New York

SINGH K. (1946) Psychiatric practice among Indian troops *Ind. Med. Gazette,* **81**, 394

SPITZKA, E.C. (1880) Race and insanity *J. Nerv. Ment. Dis.*, **7**, 342

SWIFT H.M. (1913) Insanity and race *Am. J. Insanity,* **70**, 143

WILLIAMS A.H. (1950) A psychiatric study of Indian soldiers in the Arakan *Brit. J. Med. Psychol.*, **23**, 131

Psychological theory

ADLER A. (1930) Individual psychology in *Psychologies of 1930* 749. Clark University Press, Worcester, Mass.

BANNISTER D. (1970) *Perspectives in Personal Construct Theory* Academic Press, London
BECKER W.C. (1960) Cortical inhibition and extraversion-introversion *J. Abnorm. Soc. Psychol.*, 61, 52
CHAMPION R.A. (1961) Some comments on Eysenck's treatment of modern learning theory *Brit. J. Psychol.*, **52**, 167
CHRISTIE R. (1956) Eysenck's treatment of the personality of communists *Psychol. Bull.*, **53**, 411
EYSENCK H.J. (1961) *Handbook of Abnormal Psychology* Basic Books, New York
EYSENCK H.J. (1952) *Scientific Study of Personality* Routledge & Kegan Paul, London
EYSENCK H.J. (1959) *Structure of Human Personality* Methuen, London
FOULDS G.A. (1961) The logical impossibility of using hysterics and dysthymics as criterion groups in the study of introversion and extraversion *Brit. J. Psychol.*, **52**, 385
HAMILTON V. (1959) Eysenck's theories of anxiety and hysteria—a methodological critique *Brit. J. Psychol.*, **50**, 48
LYKKEN D.J. (1959) Review of Eysenck's 'The Dynamics of Anxiety and Hysteria' *Contemp. Psychol.*, **4**, 377
STORMS L.H. & SIGAL J.J. (1958) Eysenck's personality theory with special reference to the dynamics of anxiety and hysteria *Brit. J. Med. Psychol.*, **228**

Psychopathic disorder

ALLPORT G.W. (1937) *Personality* Holt, New York
BOWLBY J.M. (1951) *Maternal Care and Mental Health* W.H.O., Geneva
BRANDON S. (1960) *An Epidemiological Study of Maladjustment in Children* M.D. Thesis. Univ. Durham
BRIDGE E.M. (1949) *Epilepsy and Convulsive Disorders in Children* McGraw, Hill, New York
CLECKLEY H. (1964) *The Mask of Sanity* C.V. Mosby, St. Louis
CRAFT M. (1965) *Ten Studies into Psychopathic Personality* John Wright, Bristol
CURRAN D. & MALLINSON P. (1944) Psychopathic personality *J. Ment. Sci.*, **90**, 266
EHRLICH S.K. & KEOUGH R.P. (1956) The psychopath in a mental institution *Arch Neurol. Psychiat.*, **76**, 286
ESSEN-MOLLER E. (1956) Individual traits and morbidity in a Swedish rural population *Acta Psychiat. Scand.*, Suppl. 100
FERGUSON T. (1952) The young delinquent in his social setting. Oxford University Press, London
GESELL A. (1941) *Wolf Child and Human Child* Methuen, London
GIBBENS T.C.N. & WALKER A. (1956) *Cruel Parents* Inst. Study. Delinq., London
GIBBENS T.C.N. (1957) The sexual behaviour of young criminals *J. Ment. Sci.*, **103**, 527
GIBBENS T.C.N., POND D.A. & STAFFORD-CLARK D. (1959) A follow up study of criminal psychopaths *J. Ment. Sci.*, **105**, 108
GLUECK S.S. & GLUECK E.T. (1943) *Criminal Careers in Retrospect* Commonwealth Fund, New York

GLUECK S.S. & GLUECK E.R. (1950) *Unravelling Juvenile Delinquency* Harvard University Press, Cambridge, Mass.

GLUECK S.S. & GLUECK E.T. (1956) *Physique and Delinquency* Harper, London, New York

GOLDFARB W. (1945) Effects of psychological deprivation in infancy and subsequent stimulation *Amer. J. Psychiat.,* **102,** 18

GRUNBERG F. & POND D.A. (1957) Conduct disorder in young children *J. Neurol. Psychiat.,* **20,** 65

GUZE S.B. (1964) A study of recidivism based upon a follow up of 217 consecutive criminals *J. Nerv. Ment. Dis.,* **138,** 575

HARRINGTON J.A. & LETEMENDIA F.J.J. (1958) Persistent psychiatric disorders after head injuries in children *J. Ment. Sci.,* **104,** 1295

HENDERSON D.K. (1939) *Psychopathic States* W.W. Norton, New York

KAHN E. (1931) *Psychopathic Personalities* Yale University Press, New Haven, Conn.

KOCH J.L.A. (1889) *Leit faden der Psychiatrie* 2nd ed. Dorn, Ravensburg

KRAEPELIN E. (1909) *Psychiatrie,* J.A. Banth, Leipzig

KARPMAN B. (1951) Psychopathic behaviour in infants and children. A critical survey of the existing concepts *Amer. J. Orthopsychiat.,* **21,** 223

LANGE J. (1931) *Crime and Destiny* George Allen, London

LEWIS H.N. (1954) *Deprived Children* Oxford University Press, London

LOWRY L.G. (1940) Personality distortion and early institutional care *Amer. J. Orthopsychiat.,* **10,** 576

MANNHEIM H. & WILKINS L.J. (1955) *Prediction methods in relation to Borstal training* HMSO, London

MACFARLANE J.W., ALLEN L. & HENZIK M.P. (1954) A development study of the behaviour problems of normal children between 21 months and 14 years Univ. Calif. Publ. Child develpms.

McCORD W. & McCORD J. (1956) *Psychopathy and Delinquency* Grune & Stratton, New York

PRICHARD J.C. (1835) *A Treatise on Insanity and other Disorders Affecting the Mind* Sherwood, Gilbert & Piper, London

PRINGLE K. (1961) The incidence of some supposedly adverse family conditions and of left-handedness in schools for maladjusted children *Brit. J. Ed. Psychol.,* **31,** 183

PUNTIGAM F. (1950) Verursacht die encephalitis Post Cassinationem Bei Jugendlichen Kriminogene Personlichkeits Verander-ungen. Ost. 2 Kinderheilk 4, 142

ROBINS L.N. (1966) *Deviant children group up: a sociological and psychiatric study of Sociopathic Personality* Williams & Wilkins, Baltimore

ROWE A.W. (1931) A possible endocrine factor in the behaviour problems of the young *Amer. J. Orthopsychiat.,* **1,** 451

ROSANOFF A.J., HANDY L.M. & ROSANOFF L.A. (1934) Criminality and delinquency in twins *J. Crimin. Law and Criminol.,* **24,** 923

ROSANOFF A.J., HANDY L.M. & PLESSETT I.R. (1941) Aetiology of child behaviour *Psychiatr. Monogr.,* 1

RUSH B. (1812) Medical inquiries and observations upon the diseases of the Mind Philadelphia

SCHNEIDER K. (1958) *Psychopathic Personalities* Cassell, London

SCOTT P.D. (1962) Psychopathic personalities *Curr. Med. Drugs,* **2,** 19

SLATER E.T. (1948) Psychopathic personality as a genetical concept *J. Ment. Sci.,* **94,** 277

SLATER E.T. (1943) The neurotic constitution *J. Neurol. Neurosurg. Psychiat.,* **6,** 1

THOMPSON G.N. (1945) Psychiatric factors influencing learning *J. Nerv. Ment. Dis.,* **101,** 347

WILLIS B.E. (1959) A case of extreme isolation in a young child *Bull. Brit. Psychol. Soc.* **38,** 68

ZUCKERMANN M., BARNETT B.H. & BRAGIEL R.M. (1960) Parental attitudes of parents of child guidance cases *Child Development,* **31,** 401

Psychosurgery

FALCONER M. & SCHURR P. (1958) in *Recent Progress in Psychiatry III* Ed. Fleming G.W. & Walk A. Churchill, London

FREEMAN W. & WATTS J.W. (1942) *Psychosurgery* Thomas, Springfield, Illinois

KNIGHT G.C. (1964) *Brit. J. Surg.,* **51,** 114

LEWIN W.S. (1961) Observations on selective leucotomy *Journal of Neurology, Neurosurgery and Psychiatry,* **24,** 37

MacLEAN P.D. (1958) *Journal of Nervous and Mental Disease,* **127,** 1

MONIZ E. (1936) *Tentatives operatoires dans le traitement de certaines psychoses* Massn., Paris

PAPEZ J.W. (1937) *Archives of Neurology and Psychiatry,* **38,** 725

SCOVILLE W.B. (1949) *Journal of Neurosurgery,* **6,** 65

SCHURR P. (1973) Psychosurgery *Brit. J. Hosp. Med.,* **53,** 60

Psychopharmacology

DELAY J. & DENIKER P. (1952) *Annales Medico-psychologiques,* **110,** 564

HOFFMAN (1955) *Sandoz Excerpta,* **1,** 1, 435. Hanover, New Jersey

HORDERN A. (1968) Psychopharmacology: some historical considerations in *Psychopharmacology: Dimensions and Perspectives* Ed. Joyce C.R.B. 4. 95 Tavistock, London

JOYCE C.R.B. (1968) *Psychopharmacology: Dimensions and Perspectives* Tavistock, London

KLINE N.S. (1954) *Annals of New York Academy of Sciences,* **59,** 107

KOHN R. (1957) *Schweizerische Medizinische Wochenschrift,* **87,** 1135

LOOMER H.P., SANDERS J.C. & KLINE N.S. (1957) *Psychiatric Research Reports of the American Psychiatric Research Association,* **8,** 129

REES W.L. (1966) Drugs used in the treatment of psychiatric disorders *Abst. World Medicine,* **39,** 3, 129

REES W.L. (1972) New horizons in psychopharmacology *Proc. Roy. Soc. Med.,* **65,** 813

RODDIS L.H. (1951) *James Lind, Founder of Nautical Medicine* Heinemann, London

SHEPHERD M., LADER M. & RODNIGHT R. (1968) *Clinical Psychopharmacology* English Universities Press, London

Psychosomatic disorders

ANSTEE B.H. (1972) The pattern of psychiatric referrals in a general hospital *Brit. J. Psychiat.*, **120**, 631

CRISP A.H. (1968) The role of the psychiatrist in the general hospital *Post. Grad. Med. J.*, **44**, 267

CROWN S. (1973) Psychiatry and the Medical Service *Medicine*, **10**, 2, 661

ROSE G.A. & BLACKBURN H. (1968) *Cardiovascular Survey Methods* (W.H.O. Monograph series 66.) W.H.O. Geneva

Schizophrenia

BANNISTER D. (1960) Conceptual structure in thought disordered schizophrenics *J. Ment. Sci.*, **106**, 1230

BANNISTER D. & FRANSELLA F. (1966) A Grid Test of schizophrenic thought disorder *Brit. J. Clin. Psychol.*, **5**, 95

BROWN G.W., MONCK E.M., CARSTAIRS G.N. & WING J.K. (1962) Influence of family life on the course of schizophrenic illness *Brit. J. Prev. Soc. Med.*, **12**, 55

BLEULER E. (1911) *Dementia Praecox or the Group of Schizophrenias* International Universities Press, New York

CAMERON N. (1938) Reasoning, regression and communication in schizophrenics *Psychol. Monogr.*. **50**, 1

CAMERON N. (1939) Deterioration and regression in schizophrenic thinking *J. Abnorm. Social Psychol.*, **34**, 265

CHAPMAN J. (1966) Schizophrenia: early symptoms *Brit. J. Psychiat.*, **112**, 255

FEIGHNER J.P., ROBINS E., GUZE S.B., WOODRUFF R.A., WINOKUR & MUNOZ R. (1972) *Arch. Gen. Psychiat.*, **26**, 57

GOLDSTEIN K. (1943) The significance of psychological research in schizophrenia *J. Nerv. Ment. Dis.*, **97**, 201

HERRON W.G. (1962) The process reactive classifications of schizophrenia *Psychol. Bulletin*, **59**, 329

HESTON L.H. (1966) Psychiatric disorders in foster home reared children of schizophrenic mothers *Brit. J. Psychiat.*, **112**, 819

HOCH P.H. & POLATIN P. (1949) Pseudoneurotic forms of schizophrenia *Psychiat. Quart.*, **23**, 248

JACKSON D. (1965) Family rules *Arch. Gen. Psychiat.*, **12**, 589

KENDELL R.E. (1972) Schizophrenia, the remedy for diagnostic confusion *Brit. J. Hosp. Med.*, **8**, 4, 383

KIND H. (1966) Psychogenesis of schizophrenia *Brit. J. Psychiat.*, **112**, 337

LANGFELDT G. (1939) *The Schizophreniform Psychoses* Munksgaard, Copenhagen

LIDZ T., WILD C., SCHAFER S., ROSMAN B. & FLECK S. (1963) Thought disorder in the parents of schizophrenic patients: a study utilising the object sorting test. *J. Psychiatric Res.*, **1**, 193

MAYER GROSS W. (1924) *Self Descriptions from Confusional States—The Oneroid Experience* 206 Berlin

MEDUNA L.J. & McCULLOCH W.S. (1945) The modern concept of schizophrenia *Med. Clin. N. Amer.*, **29**, 147, 262

MISCHLEV E.G. & WAXLER N.E. (1969) Family interaction processes and schizophrenia. A review of current Theories *Int. J. Psychiat.*, 375

MURPHY H.B.M. (1967) *Cultural Factors in the Genesis of Schizophrenia* Pergamon, London

SINGER W.T. & WYNNE L.C. (1963) Differentiation characteristics of parents of childhood schizophrenics, childhood neurotics and young adult schizophrenics *Amer. J. Psychiat.*, **120**, 234

SINGER W.T. & WYNNE L.C. (1963) Thought disorder and family relations of schizophrenics I *Arch. Gen. Psychiat.*, **9**, 191

SINGER W.T. & WYNNE L.C. (1963) Thought disorder and family relations of schizophrenics II. A classification of forms of thinking *Arch Gen. Psychiat.*, **9**, 199

SINGER W.T. & WYNNE L.C. (1965) Thought disorder and family relations of schizophrenics III. Methodology using projective techniques *Arch. Gen. Psychiat.*, **12**, 187

SMYTHIES J.R., COPPEN A. & KREITMAN N. (1968) *Biological Psychiatry* Heinemann, London

VON DOMARUS (1944) The specific laws of logic in schizophrenia in *Language and Thought in Schizophrenia* Ed. Kasanin J.S. 104. University of California Press, Berkeley

WARING M. & RICKS D. (1965) Family patterns of children who become adult schizophrenics *J. Nerv. Ment. Dis.*, **140**, 351

WILLIS J.H. & BANNISTER D. (1965) The diagnosis and treatment of schizophrenic: a questionnaire study of psychiatric opinion *Brit. J. Psychiat.*, **111**, 1165

Schizophrenia—epidemiology

BÖÖK J.A. (1953) *Acta Genet* (Basel), **4**, 1.

BÖÖK J.A. (1961) in *Causes of Mental Disorders: A Review of Epidemiological Knowledge* Ed. Gruenberg, E.M. & Huxley M. Milbank Memorial Fund, New York

COHEN B. & FAIRBANK R. (1938) *Amer. J. Psychiat.*, **94**, 1153

CROCETTI G.M., KULCAR Z., KESIC B. & LEMKAU P.V. (1964) Selected aspects of the epidemiology of schizophrenia in Croatia. *Millbank Mem. Fund. Quart.*, **42**, 2, 9

FARIS, R.E.L. & DUNHAM H.W. (1939) *Mental Disorders in Urban Areas* Hafner, Chicago

HARE E.H. (1967) in *Recent Developments in Schizophrenia* Ed. Coppen A. & Walk A. Royal Medico-Psychological Association, London

KRAMER M. (1969) *Amer. J. Psychiat.*, suppl. 125, 1

LEMKAU P.V. & CROCETTI G.M. (1958) Vital statistics of schizophrenia in *Schizophrenia: a review of the syndrome* Ed. Bellak L. Logos Press, New York

MEZEY A.G. (1960) *J. Ment. Sci.*, **106**, 618

MURPHY H.B.M. (1965) in *Mobility and Mental Health* Ed. Kantor M. C.C. Thomas, Springfield, Illinois

ØDEGAARD Ø. (1932) Emigration and insanity *Acta. psychiat. neurol. scand.*, Suppl. 4.

ØDEGAARD Ø. (1946) *J. Ment. Sci.,* **92,** 35
ØDEGAARD Ø. (1952) *Psychiat. Quart.,* **26,** 212
STEVENS B. (1969) *Marriage and Fertility of Women Suffering from Schizophrenia or Affective Disorders* Oxford University Press, London
WING J.K. (1970) in *Psychiatric Epidemiology: An International Symposium* Ed. Hare E.H. & Wing J.K. Oxford University Press, London
WING J.K. & BROWN G.W. (1970) *Institutionalism and Schizophrenia* Cambridge University Press, London
WING J.K. (1972) Epidemiology of schizophrenia *Brit. J. Hosp. Med.,* 364

Schizophrenia—genetics

FRASER ROBERTS J.A. (1970) *An Introduction to Medical Genetics* Oxford University Press, London
HUMAN GENETICS (1972) A memorandum prepared by D.H.S.S.
GOTTESMAN I.I. & SHIELDS J. (1966) Schizophrenia in twins. 16 years consecutive admissions to a psychiatric clinic *Brit. J. Psychiat.,* **112,** 809
KALLMAN F.J. (1946) The genetic theory of schizophrenia: an analysis of 691 schizophrenic twin index families *Amer. J. Psychiat.,* **103,** 309
KRINGLEN E. (1964) Schizophrenia in male monozygotic twins *Acta. Psychiat. Scand. Suppl.* 178
ØDEGAARD Ø. (1963) The psychiatric disease entities in the light of a genetic investigation *Acta. Psychiat. Scand.,* **39,** 5, 169
PENROSE L.S. (1971) Critical survey of schizophrenia genetics *Modern Perspectives in World Psychiatry,* **2,** 3
ROSENTHAL D. (1961) Problems of sampling and diagnosis in the major twin studies of schizophrenia *J. Psychiat. Res.,* **1,** 116
SHIELDS J. (1965) A review of Tienari P. (1963) *Brit. J. Psychiat.,* **111,** 777
SLATER E. (1953) *Psychotic and Neurotic Illness in Twins* Med. Res. Council Spec. Rept. Series 278 HMSO, London
SLATER E. & COWIE V. (1971) *The Genetics of Mental Disorders* Oxford University Press, London
TIENARI P. (1963) Psychiatric illness in identical twins *Acta Psychiat. Scand.,* **39,** S 171, 9

Senile dementia

ALZHEIMER A. (1907) On a peculiar disease of the cerebral cortex *Allg. Z. Psychiat.,* **64,** 146
BERGMANN K. (1972) Psychogeriatrics *Medicine,* **9,** 643. Medical Educ. Int., London
BERGMANN K. (1969) The epidemiology of senile dementia *Brit. J. Hosp. Med.,* **727**
CORSELLIS J.A.N. (1962) *Mental Illness and the Ageing Brain* Maudsley Monograph No. 9 Oxford University Press, London
GOLDFARB A.I. (1961) Current trends in management in *Psychopathology of Ageing*
KALLMAN F.J. (1968) in *Mental Disorders in Later Life* 2nd ed. Ed. Kaplan D. Stanford University Press, California
KAY D.W.K. (1962) *Acta psychiat. Scand.,* **38,** 249
KAY D.W.K., BEAMISH P. & ROTH M. (1964) *Brit. J. Psychiat.,* **110,** 146

KAY D.W.K., BEAMISH P. & ROTH M. (1964) *Brit. J. Psychiat.*, **110**, 668
LARRSON T. (1964) *Age with a Future* Munksgaard; Copenhagen
LARRSON T., SJOGREN & JACOBSON G. (1963) *Acta Psychiat. Scand.*, suppl. 167
MALZBERG B. (1963) *Acta Psychiat. Scand.*, **39**, 19
ROTH M. (1955) *J. Ment. Sci.*, **101**, 281
SAINSBURY P., COSTAIN W.R. & GRAD J. (1965) in *Psychiatric Disorders in the Aged* Proceedings World Psychiatric Association Symposium, London 23
SJOGREN H., SJOGREN T. & LINDGREN (1952) Morbus Alzheimer and Morbus Pick *Acta. Psychiat. Kbh.*, Suppl. 82

Sexual disorders

KINSEY A.C., POMEROY W.B. & MARTIN C.E. (1948) *Sexual Behaviour in the Human Male* Saunders, Philadelphia
KINSEY A.C. & GEBHARD P.H. (1953) *Sexual Behaviour in the Human Female* Saunders, Philadelphia
MASTERS W.H. & JOHNSON V.E. (1966) *Human Sexual Response* Little, Brown, Boston
MASTERS W.H. & JOHNSON V.E. (1970) *Human Sexual Inadequacy* Little, Brown, Boston
STEKEL W. (1929) *Sadism and Masochism* Liveright, New York
STEKEL W. (1930) *Sexual Aberrations: The Phenomenon of Fetishism in Relation to Sex* Liveright, New York
STORR A. (1964) *Sexual Deviation* Penguin, Middlesex, England
WOLPE J. (1958) *Psychotherapy by Reciprocal Inhibition* Stanford University Press, Stanford, California

Sleep

CRISP A.H. & STONEHILL E. (1973) Aspects of the relationship between sleep and nutrition: a study of 375 psychiatric outpatients. *Brit. J Psychiat*, **122**, 379
BERGER R.J. & OSWALD I. (1962) Effects of sleep deprivation *J. Ment. Sci.*, **108**, 457
DEMENT W.C. & KLEITMAN N. (1957) *J. Exp. Psychol.*, **53**, 339
DEMENT W.C. & KLEITMAN (1957) Cyclic variations in E.E.G. during sleep and their relation to eye movements, bodily motility and dreaming *Electroenceph. clin. neurophysiol.*, **9**, 673
DEMENT W.C. (1960) The effect of dream deprivation *Science*, **131**, 1705
DEMENT W.C. (1965) Recent studies on the biological role of rapid eye movement sleep *Amer. J. Psychiat.*, **122**, 401
EVANS J.I. & OSWALD I. (1966) Some experiments in the chemistry of narcoleptic sleep *Brit. J. Psychiat.*, **112**, 401
HINTON J. (1963) Patterns of insomnia in depressive states *J. Neurol. Neurosurg. Psychiat.*, **26**, 184
KLEITMAN N. (1963) *Sleep and Wakefulness* University of Chicago Press, Chicago
McGHIE A. (1966) The subjective assessment of sleep patterns in psychiatric illness *Brit. J. Med. Psychol.*, **39**, 221
OSWALD I. & THACORE K.R. (1963) *Brit. Med. J.*, **ii**, 427
OSWALD I. (1970) Sleep, dreams and drugs in *Modern Trends in Psychological Medicine* Ed. Price J.H. 3, 53. Butterworth, London

OSWALD I. (1962) *Sleeping and Waking* Elsevier Press, Amsterdam
OSWALD I., BERGER R.J., JARAMILLO R.A., KEDDIE K.M.G., OLLEY P.C. & PLUNKETT G.B. 1963 Melancholia and barbiturates: a controlled EEG, body and eye movement study of sleep *Brit. J. Psychiat.*, **109,** 66
OSWALD I. & PRIEST R. (1965) Five weeks to escape the sleeping pill habit *Brit. Med. J.,* **ii,** 1093
RATNA L. (1973) *Brit. J. Hosp. Med.,* 203

Sociology and psychiatry

DURKHEIM E. (1951) *Suicide: a Study in Sociology* Illinois Free Press, Glencoe
DURHAM H.W. (1965) Social class and schizophrenia *Amer. J. Orthopsychiatry,* **34,** 634
GOLDHAMMER H. & MARSHALL A. (1953) *Psychosis and Civilisation* Illinois Free Press, Glencoe
GOFFMAN E. (1968) *Asylums—Essays on the Social Situations of Mental Patients and Other Inmates* Penguin Books, London
GOFFMAN E. (1961) On the characteristics of total institutions in *The Prison* Ed. Cressey, D.R. Holt Reinhart and Winston
LAING R.D. (1967) *The Politics of Experience* Pelican, London
OLDHAM A.J. (1969) Community psychiatry in London. A three year analysis *Brit. J. Psychiat.,* **115,** 521, 465
RUESCH J. (1961) Research and training in social psychiatry in the United States *Int. J. Soc. Psychiat.,* **7,** 2, 87
SIEGLER M. & OSMOND H. (1966) Models of madness *Brit. J. Psychiat.,* **112,** 1193
SIEGLER M., OSMOND H. & MANN H. (1969) Laing's models of madness *Brit. J. Psychiat.,* **115,** 947
SMYTHIES J.R., JOHNSTON V.S. & BRADLEY R.J. (1969) Behavioral models of psychosis *Brit. J. Psychiat.,* **115,** 518, 55
STANTON A.H. & SCHWARTZ, M.S. (1954) *The Mental Hospital* Basic Books, New York
WEINBERG K. (1967) *The Sociology of Mental Disorders* Aldine, Chicago

Suicide and attempted suicide

DOUGLAS J.D. (1967) *The Social Meaning of Suicide* Princeton
DUBLIN L. (1963) *Suicide: A Sociological and Statistical Study* The Ronald Press Company, New York
KENNEDY P. & KREITMAN N. (1973) An epidemiological survey of parasuicide (attempted suicide) in general practice *Brit. J. Psychiat.,* **123,** 23
KESSEL N. (1965) Self poisoning *Brit. Med. J.,* **ii,** 1265; **ii,** 1336
KREITMAN N. & CHOWDHURY N. (1973) Distress behaviour: A study of selected samaritan clients and parasuicides (attempted suicide) patients 1. General aspects *Brit. J. Psychiat.,* **123,** 1; 2. Attitudes and choice of action *Brit. J. Psychiat.,* **123,** 9
MINTZ R.S. (1964) A pilot study of the prevalence of persons in the City of Los Angeles who have attempted suicide. Paper presented at the 120th Meeting of the American Psychiatric Association, Los Angeles, California, May 1964

MYERS J.K., LINDENTHAL J.J. & PEPPER M.P. (1971) Life events and psychiatric impairment *Journal of Nervous and Mental Disease,* **152,** 149

MYERS J.K., LINDENTHAL J.J., PEPPER M.P. & OSTRANDER D.R. (1972) Life events and mental status: a longitudinal study *Journal of Health and Social Behaviour,* **13,** 398

OVENSTONE I.M.K. (1973) A psychiatric approach to the diagnosis of suicide and its effect upon the Edinburgh statistics *Brit. J. Psychiat.,* **123,** 15

PARKIN D. & STENGEL E. (1965) Incidence of suicide attempts in an urban community *British Medical Journal,* **2,** 133

PAYKEL E.S., MYERS J.K., LINDENTHAL J.J. & TANNER J. (1974) Suicidal feelings in the general population: A prevalence study *Brit. J. Psychiat.,* **124,** 460

POKORNY A.D. (1964) Suicide rates in various psychiatric disorders *Journal of Nervous and Mental Disease,* **139,** 499

SAINSBURY P. (1955) *Suicide in London: An Ecological Study* Maudsley Monograph No. 1. Chapman and Hall, London

SAINSBURY P. (1973) Suicide: opinions and facts *Proc. Roy. Soc. Med.,* **66,** 579

SAINSBURY P. & BARRACLOUGH B. (1968) *Nature,* **220,** 1252

SCHNEIDMAN E.S. & FARBEROW N.L. (1961) Statistical comparisons between attempted and committed suicides in *The Cry for Help* Eds. Farberow N.L. & Schneidman E.S. McGraw Hill Book Company, New York

STENGEL E. & COOK N.G. (1958) *Attempted Suicide.* Oxford University Press, London

STENGEL E. (1959) *Suicide* Pelican, London

Other topics

BASTIAN H.C. (1893) *Various forms of hysterical functional paralysis* 1, Lewis, London

BASTIAN H.C. (1886) *Paralyses: Cerebral Bulhar and Spinal* 600, Lewis, London

BIRCH H.G., RICHARDSON S.A., BAIRD D., HOROBIN G. & ILLSLEY R. (1970) *Mental Subnormality in the Community: A Clinical and Epidemiologic Study* Williams & Wilkins, Baltimore

CHAUDHURI A.K.R. (1972) Electroconvulsive therapy *Antiseptic,* **69,** 735

FLEMINGER J.F., HORNE D.J. & NORTH P.N. (1970) Unilateral ECT and cerebral dominance: Effect of R & L sided electrode placement in verbal memory *J. Neurol. Neurosurg. Psychiat.,* **33,** 408

FLEMINGER J.F. (1973) Personal communication

HOWELL J. (1965) *Modern Perspectives in Child Psychiatry* Oliver & Boyd, Edinburgh and London

HOWELL J. (1971) *Modern Perspectives in Adolescent Psychiatry* Oliver & Boyd, Edinburgh and London

KIRMAN B. (1972) The clinical assessment of mental handicap *Brit. J. Hosp. Med.,* 128

KRAEPELIN E. (1920) Symptoms of mental disease *Z. ges Neurol. Psychiat.,* **62,** 1. 252

LEONHARD K. (1959) *Anfteilung der Endogen Psychosen* 2nd Ed. Springer Verlag, Berlin

LEVY R. (1968) The clinical evaluation of unilateral ECT. *Brit. J. Psychiat.,* **114,** 559

NIELSEN J. (1968) Chromosomes in senile dementia *Brit. J. Psychiat.,* **114,** 303

NIELSEN J. (1963) *Acta psychiat. Scand.,* **38,** 307

OSMOND H. & SMYTHIES J.R. (1952) Schizophrenia: a new approach *J. Ment. Sci.,* **98,** 309

RUTTER M. (1971) in *Mental Retardation: an Annual Review III* Ed. Wortis J. Grune & Stratton, New York

RUTTER M. (1972) Psychiatric disorder and intellectual impairment in childhood *Brit. J. Hosp. Med.,* 137

SHAPIRO M.B., POST F., LOFRING B. & INGLIS J. (1956) Memory function in psychiatric patients over sixty; some methodological and diagnostic implications. *Journal Ment. Sci.,* **102,** 233, 246

SCOTT D. (1967) Alcoholic hallucinosis *Brit. J. Psychiat.,* **62,** 113, 125

SLATER E. (1965) Diagnosis of hysteria *Brit. Med. J.,* **1,** 1395

STAFFORD-CLARK D. (1970) Personal communication

WITHERS E. & HINTON J. (1971) The usefulness of the clinical tests of the sensorium *Brit. J. Psychiat.,* **119,** 9

WITHERS E. & HINTON J. (1971) Three forms of the clinical tests of the sensorium and their reliability *Brit. J. Psychiat.,* **119,** 1

Index

Abnormality, as used in psychiatry   4
Abreaction   216
Acalculia   137
Accedie   8
Acromegaly   148
Acting out   83
Addiction, drug   285–305
  aetiology   298
  amphetamine type   294
  barbiturate/alcohol type   294
  cannabis   297, 298
  classification   293ff.
  cocaine   294
  definitions   288
  epidemiology   285–8
  hallucinogenic type   295–7
  historical aspects   290–3
  legal aspects   301–5
  morphine type   293–4
  patterns of   293–8
  treatment   299–301
Addison's disease   148
Adler, A.   85
Adolescence, see Childhood and
    adolescence   327–34
Aetiology of psychiatric disorders   77–
    109
Affect, definition   30, 31

Affective disorders   161–88
  aetiology   163ff.
  symptomatology   161ff.
  see also Depression, Mania and Hypo-
    mania
Agoraphobia   200–3
Agraphia   137
Alcoholism   305–12
  aetiology   307–8
  criminality and   310
  definitions   305, 307
  diagnosis   307
  epidemiology   308, 309
  psychiatric syndromes associated with
      310, 311
    alcoholic hallucinosis   310
    Alcoholics Anonymous (AA)
        312
    delirium tremens   310
    Korsakov's syndrome   147, 148,
        310
    paranoid states   310
    pellagra and   145
    road accidents and   310
    suicide and   310
    treatment   311, 312
    Wernicke's encephalopathy   146,
        147, 310

463

Aliphatic phenothiazines, *see* Phenothiazines
Alzheimer's disease 144
Amaurotic family idiocy 153
Amitriptyline 385
Amnesia 47–9
see also Memory
Amok 419
Amphetamine, abuse 294
psychosis 294
Anaemia, pernicious 145
Angina 339
Anorexia nervosa 342–4
Anosognosia 137
Antidepressant drugs 385–92
monoamine oxidase inhibitors 390–
391
isocarboxazid 391
phenelzine 391
tranylcyplomamine 391
tricyclic antidepressants 385–
390
amitriptyline 385
clomipramine 385
dothiepin 385
doxepin 385
imipramine 385
iprindole 385
nortriptyline 385
protriptyline 385
trimipramine 385
Antisocial personality disorder 279–
281
see also Psychopathy
Anxiety 28, 32, 195–205
diagnosis 197–8
dynamic concepts 193
phobic 199
symptomatology 197ff.
Aphasia 352–4
Apraxia 137
Aquinas, Thomas 8
Archetype 86
Aristotle 23
Arousal 198–9
Autism 331, 332

Barbiturates 155
see also Addiction
Behaviour therapy 397–9
conditioned avoidance 397, 398
desensitisation 398
flooding 398
reciprocal inhibition 398
Bender-Gestalt Test 74
Benzodiazepines 384, 385
Bereavement 170–4
Bernheim 14
Biochemistry and psychiatry 89–92
Bleuler, E. 224, 225
Brain and behaviour 87–9
Brain damage, *see* Organic cerebral
syndromes
Breuer 15
Bromides 154
Burton 10
Butyrophenones 377, 378

Camberwell Case Register 97, 101–5
Cannabis 90, 297, 298
Carbohydrate metabolism 149
Carbon monoxide 156
Carcinoma, psychiatric aspects of
156
Cardiovascular disease 337–9
Catastrophic reaction 119
Catatonic schizophrenia 249
Cerebral dysrhythmia, *see* Epilepsy
Cerebral trauma 138–42
acute 138, 140
coma 138
concussion 139
post-traumatic amnesia 140
post-traumatic delirium 139–41
Cerebral tumour 131–8
frontal lobe 135
parietal lobe 136–8
symptoms 131–5
temporal lobe 135, 136
Ceruloplasmin 151
Charcot 14, 15
Cheyne 96

Child psychiatry, childhood and
    adolescence 327–34
  adolescence 331–4
  aggression in 334
  autism in 331, 332
  crisis of identity, adolescent 333
  eating disorders 328, 329
  excretion disorders 329, 331
  general comments 327, 328
  school refusal and truancy 334
Chlordiazepoxide 384
  see also Benzodiazepines
Chlorpromazine 377
  see also Phenothiazines
Chorea, Huntington's 152–3
Chromosomal abnormalities, in mental
    subnormality 319–21
Chronic brain syndromes, *see* Organic
    cerebral syndromes and
    Dementia
Cicero 7
Citrullinuria 318
Classification of psychiatric disorders
    23–6
Cocaine 294
Cognitive function
  concentration 66
  examination 66–8
  information 66
  memory 66
  orientation 66
Colitis, ulcerative 340, 341
Coma 138
Compensation 83
Complexes 86, 87
Compulsions, *see* Obsessional disorder
Concussion 138–9
Conditioned avoidance 397, 398
Confabulation 147, 148, 310
Confusional states 111, 114
Connolly, J. 12
Consciousness 87–9
Conversion hysteria, *see* Hysteria
Cornell Medical Index 105, 106
Corpus Juri Civilis 7
Cotard's syndrome 420

Cowan 96
Crime and psychiatric disorders 422–
    428
Cushing's syndrome 148
Cyclothymic personality 31

Darwin 13
Defence mechanisms, *see* Mental mech-
    anisms 82–4
Déjà vu 159, 160
Delinquency, aetiology 272, 273
Delirium 28, 111–14
Delirium tremens 310
Delusion 28, 33–7
  erotic 36
  grandiose 36
  jealousy 36
  litigious 37
  persecutory 36
  reference 37
Delusional awareness 34
Delusional ideas 28
Delusional perception 34
Delusional reference 34
Dementia 28, 111, 112, 116–18
  clinical features 116
  diagnosis 120, 124, 125
  investigation 121–3
Dementia praecox, *see* Schizophrenia
Denial 83
Dependence, drug, *see* Addiction
Depersonalisation 28, 37–9
Depression 28, 161ff.
  aetiology 163ff.
  bereavement and 170–4
  biochemistry 164–6
  classification 174–7
  diagnosis 181–4
  endogenous and reactive 161, 162
  life events and 168
  personality and 168, 169
  prognosis in 184
  social class 167
  suicide and 180–1
  treatment 184, 185

Depression (*cont.*)
  see also Management of psychiatric
    disorders
Derealisation 28, 37–9
Desensitisation 398
Diagnosis of psychiatric disorders 22,
  23
  in general practice 97, 105–9
Diazepam 384
Dickens 12
Diphenyl-butyl-piperidines 379
Disorientation 44, 113ff.
  see also Organic cerebral syndromes
Displacement 83
Distractibility 185
Disulfiram 312
DMPE 91
Double-bind 238
Dreaming 93–5
Drugs, *see* Psychopharmacology, Anti-
  depressant drugs, Neuroleptic
  drugs, Psychotropic drugs,
  Tranquillosedative drugs
Duodenal ulcer 340
Dysmnesic syndrome 111, 116

Echolalia 260
Echopraxia 260
Ecstasy 31
Ego 80
  defence system 82, 83
Elation 31
Electroconvulsive therapy (ECT) 399–
  401
  contraindications 400
  indications for 400, 401
  mode of action, theories 401
  uses 399, 400
Electroencephalography 92, 93
Emotions, disturbances
  in affective disorders 127, 161, 162
  in organic syndromes 113ff.
  in schizophrenia 262, 263
Endocrine disorders and psychiatry
  148–53

Enuresis 329–31
Epidemiology
  alcoholism 308–9
  Camberwell Case Register Study 97,
    101–5
  drug dependence 285–8
  Midtown Manhattan Study 97, 99–
    101
  psychiatric illness in general practice
    97, 105–9
  psychiatry and 95–109
  social class and mental illness 97–9
  Tristan da Cunha 96–7
Epilepsy 156–60
  altered mental states and 156, 157
  psychosis and 158, 159
  temporal lobe epilepsy 159, 160
  violence and 157, 158
Euphoria 31

Family, interaction studies in schizo-
    phrenia 231–41
Fetishism 372
Flight of ideas 28
Flooding 398
Fluphenazine
  decanoate 377
  enanthate 377
Folie à deux 418
Free association 79
Freud, Sigmund 15, 54, 55, 77–82
  ego defence system and 82–5
  theory of mind 79
  theory of personality development
    81, 82
  see also Psychoanalysis and related
    theories
Fugue 49, 160

Galactosaemia 318
Ganser syndrome 418
Gastrointestinal disorders 339–41
Gaucher's disease 319

General hospital, the psychiatrist and 335–54
  anorexia nervosa 342–4
  cardiovascular disease 337–9
  gastrointestinal disorders 339–41
  general comments 335–6
  Munchausen syndrome 341–2
  myocardial infarction 339
  peptic ulcer 340
  psychosomatic disorders 336–49
  puerperal psychosis 344–7
  suicide and attempted suicide 347–352
  ulcerative colitis 340, 341
Goldstein 118, 119
Goldstein Scheerer Test 74
Grandeur, delusions of 36
Griesinger 232
Group therapy, *see* Psychotherapy

Haliperidol 378
Hallucinations 29, 39–41
  auditory 40
  olfactory 41
  tactile 41
Hartnup disease 318
Hashish 90
  see also Cannabis
Head injury 138–42
Hebephrenic schizophrenia 246, 247
Heraclitus 6
Heroin, *see* Addiction
Hippocrates 7
Histidinuria 318
Homosexuality 371, 372
Hospitalisation, effects 406–8
Hughlings Jackson 14
Huntington's Chorea 152–3
Hurler's disease 319
Hypochondriasis 29, 205
Hypomania 184, 185
Hypomanic personality 185–7
Hysteria 208–17
  amnesia 49

Id 80
Ideas of reference 29
Identity, crisis in adolescence 331–4
Illusions 29, 41–2
Iminodibenzyl derivatives 385
Imipramine 385
Impotence 369–71
Inadequate personality 283
Incoherence of thought 258, 259
Industrial toxins 155–6
  carbon monoxide 156
  lead 155
  manganese 155
  mercury 155
Insight 50–1, 67
Intellectualisation 83
Intelligence 71, 314–16
Intoxication 153–6
  see also Addiction and Alcoholism
Iprindole 385
Islam, influence in psychiatry 9
Isocarboxazid 391

Jakob-Creutzfeldt disease 144, 145
Jamais vu 159, 160
Janet, Pierre 14
Jaspers 14, 34ff.
Jung 85, 86

Kayser-Fleischer ring 151
Klinefelter's syndrome 320
Koro 419
Korsakov's syndrome 147, 148, 310
Kraepelin 13, 23, 26, 232, 275

Language, of psychiatry 27–51
Latah 419
Law and psychiatry 421–33
  criminal responsibility 422–5
  crime, the psychiatrist and 425–6
  general comments 421, 422
  McNaghten Rules 423, 424
  Mental Health Act 1959 428–33
Legal responsibility 422–5

Leucotomy, see Psychosurgery
Libido 86
Life style 85
Limbic system 88, 89
Lipoidoses 317ff.
Lithium 382–4
  dosage 382
  side effects 383
LSD 295
  see also Addiction

Malleus Maleficarum 8
Malingering 208–17
  see also Hysteria
Malnutrition, see Vitamin deficiency
Management of psychiatric disorders
  373ff.
Mania 185, 186
Manic depressive syndromes, see
  Affective disorder, Mania and
  Hypomania
Mannerisms 247
Maple Syrup disease 318
Marihuana, see Cannabis
Masochism 372
'Medical model', of psychiatry 1
Memory 45–50
Mental mechanisms 82–4
  see also Neurosis
Mental state, examination 53–70
  attention 68
  delusions 65
  emotional state 64, 68
  hypochondriacal ideas 65
  obsessional/compulsive pheno-
    mena 65
  perception 65
  talk 63, 64
  thought content 64
Mental subnormality 313–25
  aetiology 317–22
  associated handicap 316–17
  chromosomal defects and 319–21
  definitions 313, 314, 315
  family and 322

Mental subnormality (cont.)
  intelligence and 314
  I.Q. 314–16
    measurement 314ff.
  management 322–5
    children, special needs 322, 323
    educational 323, 325
    general 323–5
    metabolic defects and 317ff.
Mescaline 296
Meyer, A. 55
Middle Ages 8–9
Minnesota Multiphasic Personality In-
  ventory 76
Models of psychiatric illness 19–26
  family/social 20, 21
  medical/analytic 20
  political/conspiratorial 21, 22
Mood, disturbances, see Affective dis-
  order
Morbid jealousy 415–18
Moreau de Tours 90
Munchausen syndrome 341–2
Myocardial infarction 339
Myxoedema 150

Neoplasm, see Cerebral tumour
Neuroleptic drugs 1, 375–82
  butyrophenones 377, 378
    haliperidol 378
    trifluoperidol 378
  diphenyl-butyl-piperidenes 379
    prinozide 379
  phenothiazines 376–82
    aliphatic
      chlorpromazine 377
      promazine 377
      fluopromazine 377
      methotrimeprazine 377
    piperazine
      fluphenazine 377
      long acting, fluphenazine enan-
        thate 377
      long acting, fluphenazine
        decanoate 377

Neuroleptic drugs (*cont.*)
  piperazine (*cont.*)
    prochlorperazine   377
    perphenazine   377
    thiopropazate   377
    trifluoperazine   377
  piperidine
    thioridazine   377
    pericyazine   377
  rauwolfia and allied drugs   378
  side effects   380–2
  thioxarthines   378
Neurosis   29, 82–5, 189–229
Neurosyphilis   125, 126–30
Nightingale, Florence   95
Noradrenaline   89–92
Nortriptyline   385

Obesity, in childhood   329
Obsessional disorder   29, 217–22
Obsessions   42
Old age
  admission to hospital   365
  affective disorders   364
  ageing process   356, 357
  delirious states, acute and subacute   363
  dementia, senile   363
  depressive reactions   364
  general comments   355, 356
  history taking and examination, importance   361, 362
  mania and hypomania   364
  organic cerebral disorders   363
  paranoid syndromes   364
  personality disorders   364
  psychiatric disorders
    classification   358, 361
    diagnosis   361–4
    epidemiology   359, 360
    management   364, 365
Organic cerebral syndromes   111–60
  cerebral arteriosclerosis and   142, 143
  cerebral impairment, tests   73, 74
  classification   111

Organic (*cont.*)
  clouded states   111, 114
  deficiency disorders and   145–8
    B_{12} deficiency   145
    Korsakov's syndrome   147, 148, 310
    pellagra   145
    Wernicke's encephalopathy   146, 147
  dementia   111, 112, 116–18, 120–3
  dysmnesic syndrome   111, 116
  endocrine and metabolic disorders   148–53
    acromegaly   148
    Addison's disease   148
    Cushing's syndrome   148
    hepatolenticular degeneration   151
    hypoglycaemia   149
    myxoedema   150
    porphyria   150, 151
    thyrotoxicosis   149, 150
  genetic causes   152–3
  'organicity'   118–20
  presenile dementia   143–5
  symptomatology of   112, 113
  toxins and   153–6
  trauma and   138–42
  tumours, cerebral   131–8
  types   125, 126

Paranoid   29
Paranoid delusions   35
Paranoid personality   282–3
Paraphrenia, late   358, 359
Passivity, feelings   30
Pavlov
Pellagra   145
Peptic ulcer   340
Perception   88, 89, 255, 261
Persecutory delusions   35
Perseveration   112–13
Persona   86
Personality   269
  normal and abnormal   269–72
  tests   74–6

Personality disorders, *see* Psychopathy
Phenothiazines 376–82
  aliphatic 377
  piperazine 377
  piperidine 377
Phenylketonuria 317, 318
Phobic states 199
Physiology anxiety and 198, 199
Pick's disease 144
Pimozide 379
Pinel 232
Plato 6
Pleasure principle 80
Post-traumatic amnesia 48, 49
  see also Memory
Preconscious 79
Presenile dementia 143–5
Prichard 294
Projection 83
Promazine 377
Psilocybin 296
Psychiatric examination, and history
    taking 53–70
  of patients with suspected organic
    disease 67–70
  of stuporose patients 70
Psychiatry
  concepts 1–4, 19–26
  definition 6
  history 5–17
Psychoanalysis and related theories
    77–87
Psychology 71, 72, 314–16
Psychometry 71, 314–16
Psychoneurosis, *see* Neurosis
Psychopathology 27–51
Psychopathy and personality disorder
    269–83
  aetiology 276–9
  childhood and 277–9
  definition problems 274–6
  genetic factors and 276, 277
  typology of 279–83
Psychopharmacology 373–92
  historical aspects 373
  see also Antidepressant drugs, Neuro-

leptic drugs, Psychotropic drugs,
    and Tranquillosedative drugs
Psychosexual disorders 367–72
  bestiality 372
  deviant sexual behaviour 372
  fetishism 372
  frigidity 371
  general comments 367–9
  homosexuality 371–2
  impotence 369–71
  necrophilia 372
  pedophilia 372
  sado-masochism 372
Psychosis, definition 191–2
Psychosomatic disorders 336, 344
Psychosurgery 401–2
Psychotherapy 392ff.
  definitions 392
  existential 396
  influence of psychoanalysis on 393,
    395
  relationship to concept of Thera-
    peutic Community 394
  supportive 396
  see also Psychoanalysis
Psychotropic drugs 373ff.
  classification 374
  clinical trials 373ff.
  use 379
Puerperal psychosis 344–7

Rare and unclassifiable syndromes,
    415–20
Rationalisation 83
Rauwolfia 378
Reaction formation 83
Reality principle 80
Recall 47
  see also Memory
Reference, ideas of 29
Registration 47
  see also Memory
Regression 83
Retention 47
  see also Memory

REM sleep 93, 94
Renaissance 9
Repression 82
Reserpine 378
Retardation 178, 181
Reticular activating system 88, 89
Retrograde amnesia 48
  see also Memory
Rorschach 74
Rush, Benjamin 274

Schizoid personality 281, 282
Schizophrenia 223–68
  aetiology 228–46
  biochemistry and 245, 246
  catatonic 249
  clinical types 246–53
  community care and 266, 267
  delusions in 254, 255
  diagnosis 225–8
  differential diagnosis 263–5
  emotional symptoms in 262, 263
  epidemiology 229, 230
  family interation studies in 231–41
  genetics and 241–4
  hebephrenia 246, 247
  historical aspects 223–4
  latent 251
  late onset 251–3
  life changes and 231
  management of 265–8
  motor and behavioural symptoms 260, 261
  oneirophrenia 251–2
  paranoid 247–9
  perceptual disorder in 261, 262
  personality and 230, 231
  physical illness and 231
  prognosis and outcome 265–8
  pseudoneurotic 252
  psychological factors 231ff.
  residual 251
  schizoaffective disorder 252
  simple 249, 250
  symptomatology 253–63

Schizophrenia (*cont.*)
  thought and language disorder in 250–60
  treatment of 265–8
Senile dementia 363
Sexual disorders 367–72
Shaman 5
Shell shock 194
Sleep 93–5
Snow, John 95
Social psychiatry 402–13
  general 402–6
  industrial therapy 412, 413
  institutions, effects 406–8
  occupational therapy 412
  patient role 408, 409
  rehabilitation 411–13
  social work and psychiatry 410, 411
  therapeutic community 394, 409, 410
  token economy 413
  see also Epidemiology
Sociopathic disorders, *see* Psychopathic personality
Soranus 7
Speech disorders 352–4
Sprenger and Kramer 8
St Augustine 8
Stereotypy 261
Subacute delirium 111–14
Sublimation 83
Suicide and attempted suicide 347–52
  epidemiology 347, 348
  psychiatric aspects 350–2
  suicidal ideas, in the general population 349
  see also Affective disorder, Personality disorder, Schizophrenia
Superego 80
Sydenham 10
Syphilis 125, 126–30

Taboparesis 129
Tay Sach's disease 153
Thematic Apperception Test (TAT) 74
Thioridazine 377

Thioxanthenes   378
Thought and talk   43–4
  circumstantiality   43
  control of thought   44
  incoherent talk   43
  interruption in flow   43
  in schizophrenia   250–60
Time sense   44
Tranquillosedative drugs   384–5
  benzodiazepines   384
  chlordiazepoxide   384
  diazepam   384
  medazepam   384
  nitrazepam   384
  oxazepam   384
  side effects   384–5
Trauma, cerebral   134–42
Treatment, psychiatric   373–413
  psychopharmacology   373–92
  psychotherapy   392–6

Trifluoperidol   378
Trifluoperazine   377
Trisomy   21, 320
Tuke   11, 13
Tumours, cerebral   131–8
Turner's syndrome   321

Ulcerative colitis   340, 341

Vitamin deficiency, and psychiatric
  syndromes   145–8

Wechsler Adult Intelligence Scale
  (WAIS)   73, 74
Wernicke's encephalopathy   146, 147
Withdrawal syndromes   293–8, 310–11